PRINCIPLES AND PRACTICE OF CHEMOTHERAPY

Principles and Practice of Chemotherapy

Major Mirza Qaiser Baig MOBC MD
Assistant Professor and Head
Radiation Oncology Division
Department of Radiotherapy
BRD Medical College
Gorakhpur, UP, India

JAYPEE BROTHERS MEDICAL PUBLISHERS (P) LTD
New Delhi • Panama City • London

Jaypee Brothers Medical Publishers (P) Ltd.

Headquarter

Jaypee Brothers Medical Publishers (P) Ltd
4838/24, Ansari Road, Daryaganj
New Delhi 110 002, India
Phone: +91-11-43574357
Fax: +91-11-43574314
Email: jaypee@jaypeebrothers.com

Overseas Offices

J.P. Medical Ltd.,
83 Victoria Street London
SW1H 0HW (UK)
Phone: +44-2031708910
Fax: +02-03-0086180
Email: info@jpmedpub.com

Jaypee-Highlights Medical Publishers Inc.
City of Knowledge, Bld. 237, Clayton
Panama City, Panama
Phone: 507-317-0160
Fax: +50-73-010499
Email: cservice@jphmedical.com

Website: www.jaypeebrothers.com
Website: www.jaypeedigital.com

Inquiries for bulk sales may be solicited at: jaypee@jaypeebrothers.com

Principles and Practice of Chemotherapy
First Edition: **2012**

ISBN: 978-93-80704-79-1

Printed at Rajkamal Electric Press, Plot No. 2, Phase-IV, Kundli, Haryana.

Dedicated to

My son Amaan and Indian Army Soldiers who did their supreme sacrifices during Kargil Military Operation, because I am *per se* a witness of Kargil War, and thus, decided to provide free consultation services to Indian Army Soldiers and their family throughout life.

And needless to say, to my patients whom I learn a lot on day-to-day basis.

Preface

Principles and Practice of Chemotherapy is one of the most useful books on oncology presently available in the market. It presents all aspects of cancer management including recent advances. It throws light on biologic and pharmacologic aspects as well as basics of chemotherapy, including clinically relevant new understanding of cellular mechanisms that direct cancer cell growth and its potential control with molecular targeted therapy.

The book focuses on primary indication, usual dosage, schedule and side effects of new drugs, and targeted agents that oncologists have begun to use in the last five years as well as also on new data regarding information for many of the older agents.

The book contains wealth of information for surgical, medical and radiation oncologists, as well as non-oncology physicians, oncology nurses, pharmacists and medical students. It can be read and understood by many patients and their attendants who want information about their cancer and what chemotherapy they have been prescribed by their oncologists.

Chemotherapy has been long-time aspiration for many of the people engaged in cancer research and treatment. The book is a new ray of hope for those people. Current traits which are exploring never targeted therapy alone and in combination with chemotherapy continue to offer a realistic control of cancer in the decade ahead.

I am thankful to Dr Rahat Hadi for his full support as well as contributing a chapter in this book.

Major Mirza Qaiser Baig

Contents

Section-A: Medical Oncology

Section-B: General Management in Oncology

Section-C: Common Cancer and its Management

Section-D: Radiation Oncology

Plate 1

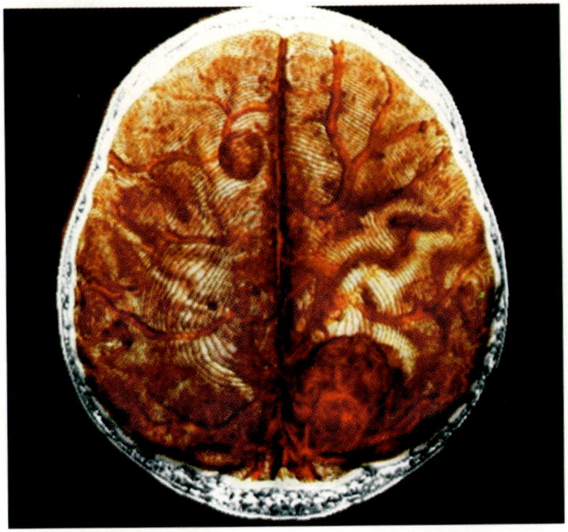

Fig. 21.3: Brain metastasis in lung cancer

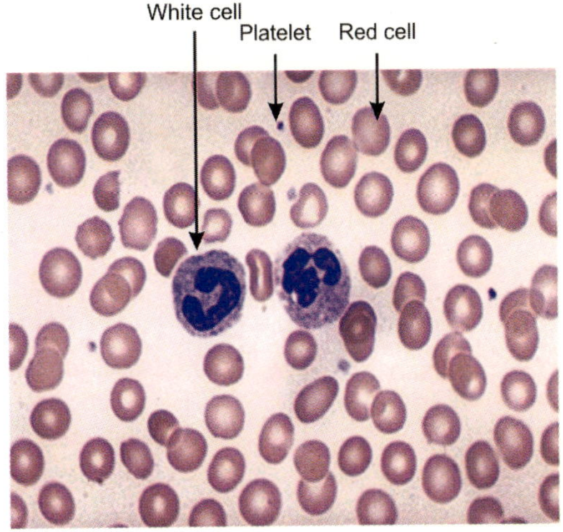

Fig. 25.2: Normal human blood

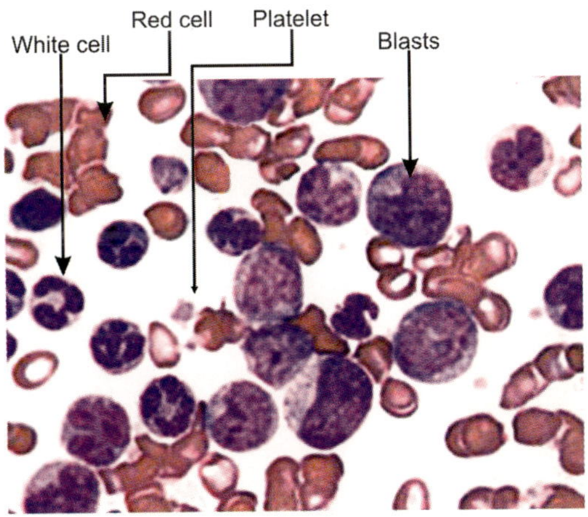

Fig. 25.3: Blood with leukemia

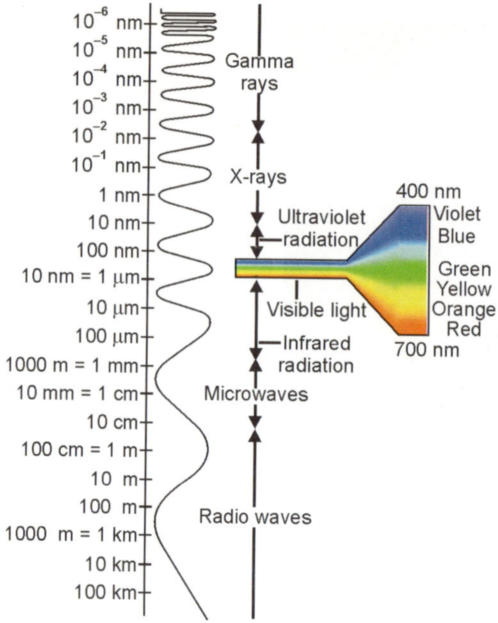

Fig. 27.2: Type of electromagnetic waves

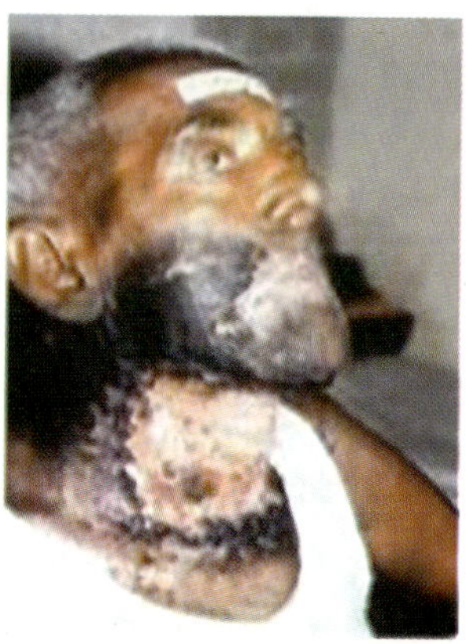

Fig. 31.1: Severe skin reaction

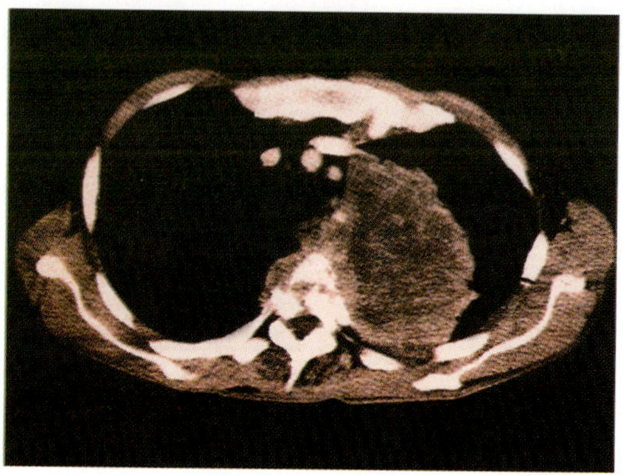

Fig. 33.1: CECT thorax showing left lung mass

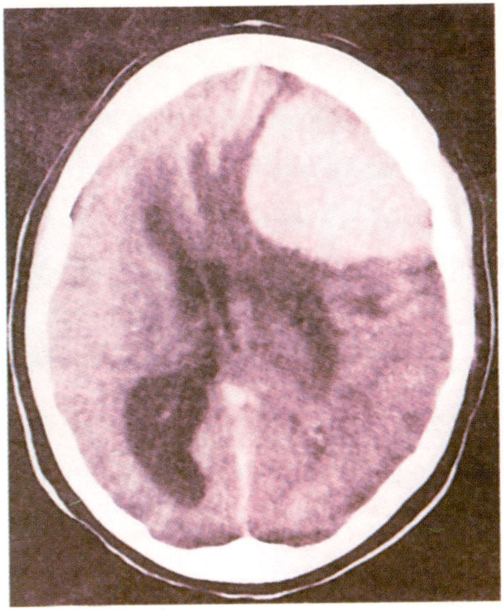

Fig. 33.2: CECT head, meningioma left frontal

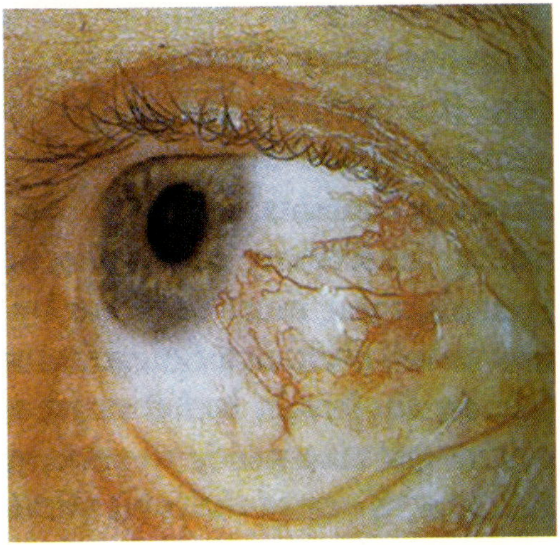

Fig. 34.1: Pterygium

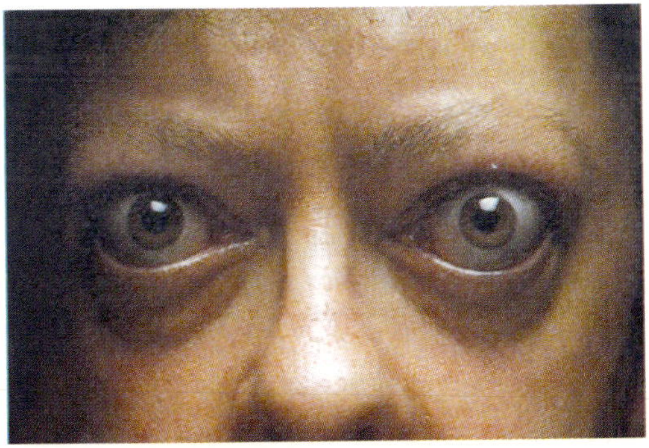

Fig. 34.2: Grave's ophthalmopathy

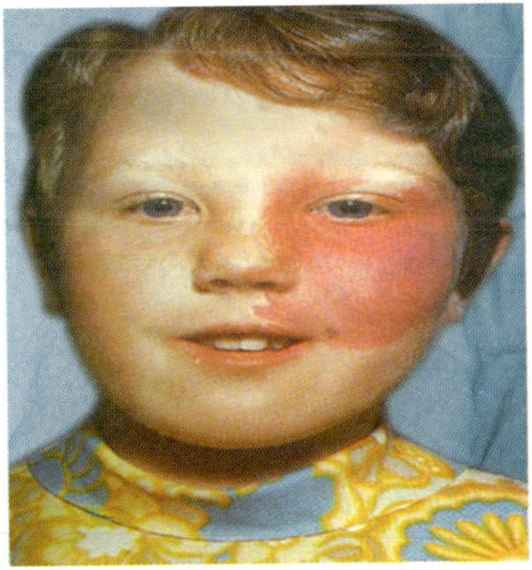

Fig. 34.3: Hemangioma

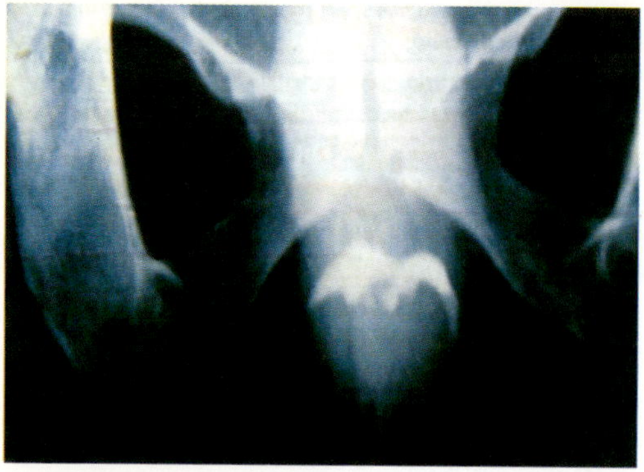

Fig. 34.4: Peyronie's disease of penis

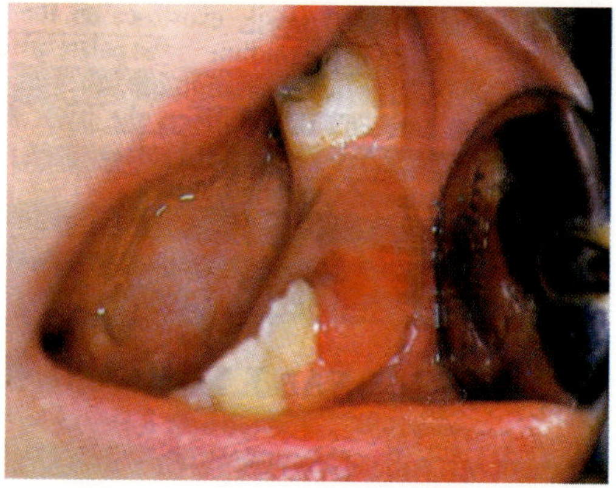

Fig. 34.5: Ameloblastoma of jaw

Section-A

Medical Oncology

Chapter 1 Concepts of Cancer Chemotherapy

FIRST PERSON DR PAUL EHRLICH (20TH CENTURY) USED TERM CHEMOTHERAPY (FIG. 1.1)

The use of drugs to treat disseminated cancer has developed into a specialized discipline. The first successful effort to control cancer with the help of drugs is attributed to Li *et al.* (1956) who demonstrated permanent remission in metastatic trophoblastic disease.

Tumor cell kinetics: A fundamental characteristic of malignant tumors is the rapid proliferation of malignant cells. These rapidly proliferating cells keep repeating a cycle of biochemical events continuously which culminate in cell division.

Since each proliferative cell gives rise to two daughter cells that continue the proliferative process, the cell population increases geometrically (Fig. 1.2).

A tumor is described as consisting of four types of cells.

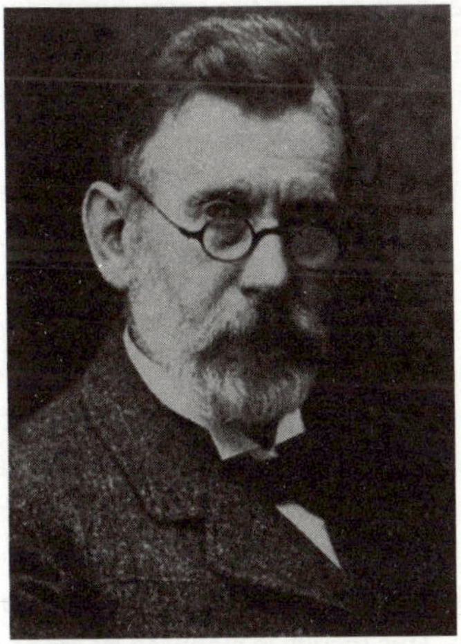

Fig. 1.1: Dr Paul Ehrlich

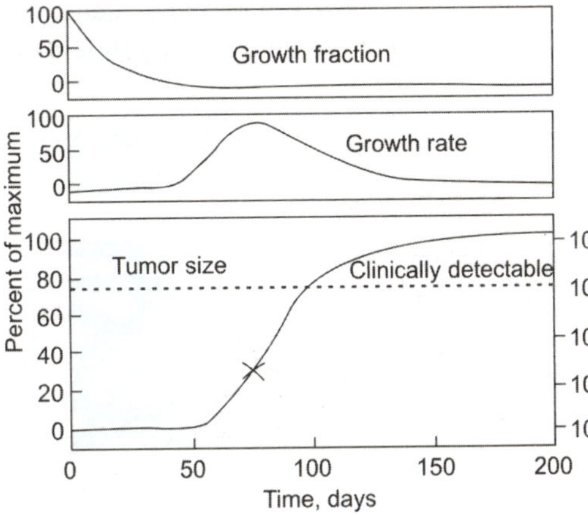

Fig. 1.2: Tumor growth pattern, tumor cell grows as Gompertzian curve

How Tumor Spread via Vascular System (Fig. 1.3)?

1. *Dividing tumor cells:* This is the only compartment that adds to the cell population.
   Cells postsynthetic gapG2
   DNA synthetic periods
   Mitosis
   Presynthetic gapG1.
2. *Resting cells:* These are nondividing cells resting temporarily (cells in G0 phase). They are refractory to chemotherapeutic agents. During this phase, the cells are not part of the active replication cycle (Fig. 1.4).
3. *Differentiated cells:* These cells have lost their dividing potential, and are awaiting natural death. Since they do not have malignant potential, they are of little concern to the chemotherapist.
4. *Dying cells:* These are terminal cells. The protocol of cytotoxic drug therapy should aim at achieving maximum tumor cell kill with minimal side effects. Small rapidly growing tumors have many more rapidly dividing and growing cells, hence the doubling time is short. However, these are the same tumors which have a high number of cells sensitive to cell-cycle specific cytotoxic drugs. As the tumor mass enlarges, the growth rate progressively slows down, doubling time becomes longer, the cell input may equal loss, hence a stationary size may be reached, and the sensitivity to cell-specific drugs diminishes. Another factor to be considered during cancer chemotherapy is the tumor load present at the commencement of therapy. Reduction in the burden of tumor cell load will bring an apparent remission. But during the interval between successive courses of cancer chemotherapy, the tumor growth recurs. This results in stepwise decrease in tumor

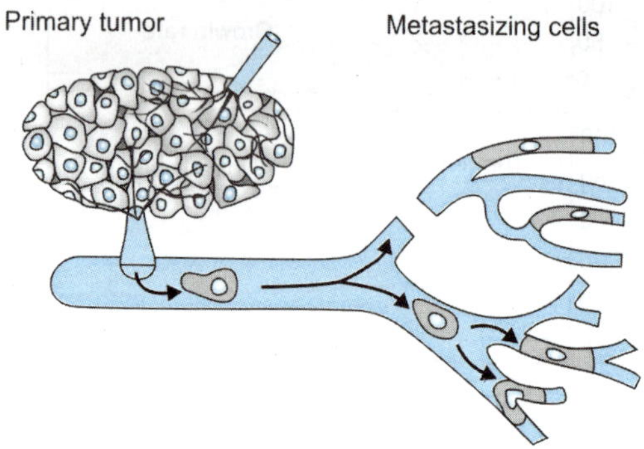

Fig. 1.3: Metastasis process via vascular channel

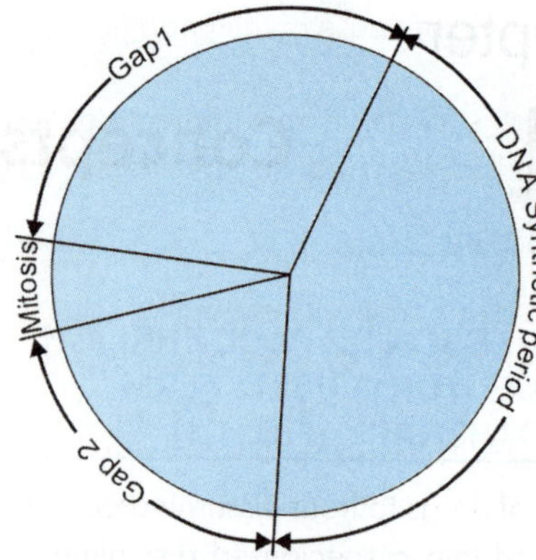

Fig. 1.4: Cell cycle

cell mass, because of the changing number of cells.

In order to attain maximum tumor cell kill, certain principles must be considered and these are:

1. The chemotherapist must be well aware of the "total tumor cell kill concept".
2. Tumor cell kill by cytotoxic drugs follow the pattern demonstrated by Skipper and Perry (1970), that the killing of tumor cells by cytotoxic agents occurs in an exponential fashion, so that a given dose kills a constant fraction of the population, irrespective of its initial size.
3. There is a clear dose response relationship.
4. Prolonged treatment may be necessary to reduce the malignant cell population to a low number which will then to be dealt with by the host immune mechanism.
5. Chemotherapy is most effective, when it is started early because the number of tumor cell population is low and the rapidly growing and dividing cells are sensitive to cancer chemothereapy (Figs 1.5A and B).
6. Chemotherapy must aim at different cell kill. The dose must be so adjusted that maximum destruction of tumor cell is achieved with minimal damage to normal cells.
7. Many cytotoxic drugs in present use show some degree of tissue selectivity.
8. Combination drug regimes and/or sequential drug regimes achieve superior tumor cell control with lowered side effects.

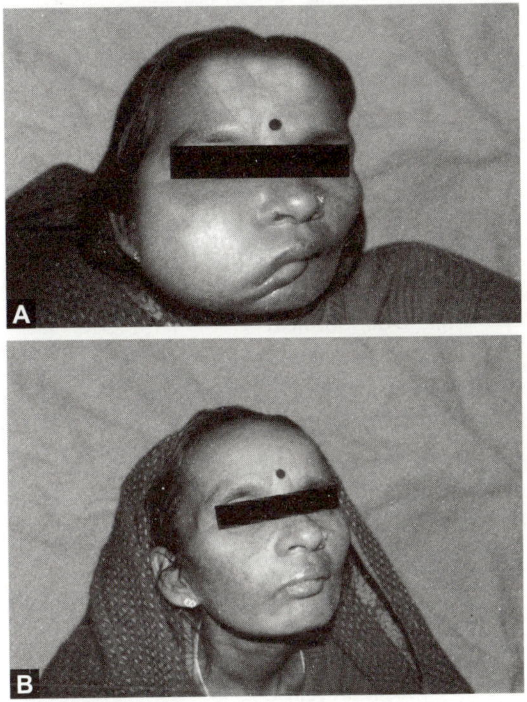

Figs 1.5A and B: (A) Prechemotherapy of NHL patient; (B) Postchemotherapy of same patient

9. The problem of drug resistance must be constantly borne in mind. Classification of cancer chemotherapeutic agents.

Classification of these drugs-based on their mechanism of action:

A. Drugs interfering with the biosynthesis of DNA, RNA and tissue proteins:
   1. Antimetabolites

   i. Folic acid
   ii. Ethylene amines (triethylene melamine (TEM), hexamethyl melamine, triethylene thiophosphoramide – thio TEPA)
   iii. Sulfonic esters (piperazine derivatives, Mitomycin-C)
2. Drugs interfering with transcription
   i. Actinomycin-D
   ii. Mithramycin
   iii. Daunorubicin
   iv. Quinacrine
3. Drugs interfering with translation
   i. Puromycin

B. Agents with radiomimetic effects
   i. Ethylene amines (triethylene melamine (TEM), hexamethyl melamine, triethylene thiophosphoramide – thio TEPA)

C. Sulfonic esters (piperazine derivatives, Mitomycin-C)
   i. Drugs interfering with transcription
      - Actinomycin-D
      - Mithramycin
      - Daunorubicin
      - Quinacrine
   ii. Drugs interfering with translation
      - Puromycin

D. Agents with radiomimetic effects
   i. Bleomycin
   ii. Streptonigrin

E. Agents interfering with mitotic spindle
   i. Colchicine
   ii. Vincristine
   iii. Vinblastine

F. Inhibitors of protein synthesis
   i. L-Asparaginase
   ii. Azaserine

G. Other drugs
   i. DTIC
   ii. Triolone
   iii. Chalones
   iv. Vitamin A

H. New drugs
   i. Cisplatin
   ii. Carboplatin
   iii. Etoposide, Taxol singly or in combination.

Clinical Considerations during Chemotherapy

1. Administration of cytotoxic agents. Drug therapy may be administered in one of the following ways:
   a. Single drug therapy
   b. Sequential drug therapy
   c. Combination therapy

   Combination chemotherapy is the treatment of choice today because:

– It is possible to achieve greater therapeutic response with less toxicity.
– The chance of developing drug resistance is diminished or delayed.
– It achieves a higher rate of complete remission with longer disease free intervals.

However, the disadvantages are:

– Hospitalization is required.
– Careful and well-supervised monitoring is mandatory.
– The cost of treatment is high.

Work-up and Supervision of the Patient that Involves

1. Pathological diagnosis and extent of the disease must precede initiation of therapy.
2. Evaluation of the general condition of the patient to determine fitness to withstand therapy. The performance status and response to therapy is periodically reviewed.
3. Evaluation of essential organ functions, e.g. bone marrow, liver, kidney and under special circumstances, heart and lungs.
4. Levels of tumor markers before and after therapy.

Essential Investigations during Chemotherapy

1. Hemogram and platelet count.
2. Blood urea, uric acid, creatinine and creatinine clearance (when nephrotoxic drugs like methotrexate or cisplatin are used).
3. Baseline ECG and serial left ventricular ejection fraction before and after using cardiotoxic drug like adriamycin.
4. Baseline and periodic pulmonary function tests for patients receiving a pulmonary toxic drug like bleomycin.
5. Liver function tests and periodic enzyme studies because many drugs are detoxicated in the liver.
6. Serum electrolytes as required.

Special Precautions during Chemotherapy

1. Nausea and vomiting require an antiemetic (metoclopramide diphenhydramine, or rarely chlorpromazine) half an hour prior to drug therapy.
2. When administering a renal/bladder toxic agent, e.g. cytoxan, the patient must be hydrated well before and after treatment, and encouraged to void frequently.
3. If a vesicant drug is administered (adriamycin, actinomycin-D, vincristine), a short silastic catheter (angiocath) should be used for intravenous access, and care is taken that the drug does not extravasate.
4. Inspect oral, axillary and perineal areas, as an immunosuppressed patient may develop candidal infections
5. If granulocyte count falls below 1000 mm stop chemotherapy temporarily and give blood transfusion.
6. If platelets fall below 40000 mm, stop chemotherapy and give blood transfusion. Observe for hemorrhages, especially IV sites, old injection sites mucus membranes and joints.

Chapter

2 Chemotherapeutic Drugs

Cancer drug therapy is a recent addition in the cancer care. Nitrogen mustard (mustine) was the first chemotherapeutic agent introduced in 1941 in the cancer treatment. The field of medical oncology has come a long-way since then, and an array of agents are available today. In curable cases, chemotherapy is used as an adjuvant or primary measure to enhance the long-term survival, while in case of incurable cancers, chemotherapy primarily has a palliative role to play steps of cancer drug development are shown in (Fig. 2.1). The chemotherapy regimens in the treatment of lymphomas, leukemias, germ cell tumors, and Wilms' tumor provide the best examples of success in medical oncology. The immediate responses of chemotherapy are objectively assessed as complete, partial or no response.

INDUCTION CHEMOTHERAPY

Initiated as a first line therapy prior to the main modality of treatment is known as induction, anterior or neoadjuvant chemotherapy. Induction chemotherapy theoretically ensures better drug delivery and, aims at reduction of the tumor bulk. With the help of this type of treatment, tumors can be down staged and the organs can be preserved such as in esophagus, bladder and breast cancer. The neoadjuvant chemotherapy by

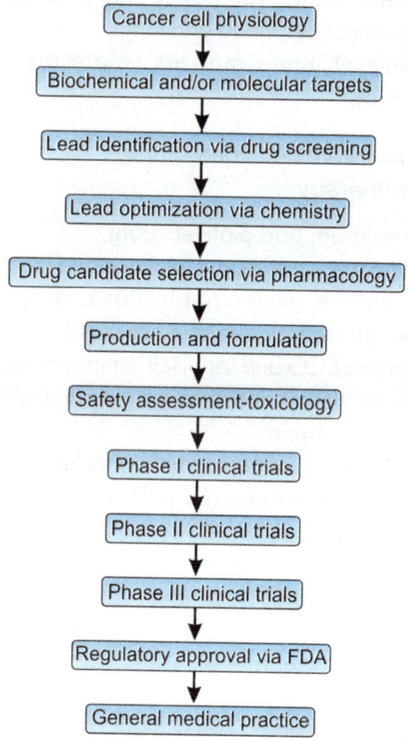

Fig. 2.1: Steps of cancer drug development

producing tumor shrinkage could theoretically allow reoxygenation and reduction of the hypoxic component, and thereby renders the tumor more vulnerable to radiation cell kill. Disadvantage of induction chemotherapy is that, it delays the local treatment either by surgery or radiotherapy.

ADJUVANT CHEMOTHERAPY

Adjuvant chemotherapy when the disease is localized and has been controlled primarily by another therapeutic modality (surgery or radiation therapy). For a vast majority of solid tumor where surgery and radiotherapy remain the local treatment modality, the patient may have the risk of local recurrence, lymph node or distant metastasis. The locoregional relapse rate can be reduced in these patients by the adjuvant chemotherapy. The benefits of adjuvant systemic treatment in a particular neoplasm is critically linked to the properly selected chemotherapy regimen. Suitable and specific, regimens have been evolved over the years in certain tumors, e.g. Wilms' tumor, osteogenic sarcoma, breast cancer and colorectal malignancies.

PRIMARY CHEMOTHERAPY

In chemoresponsive tumors, chemotherapy is administered as the treatment of choice such as in leukemias, lymphomas, choriocarcinoma and nonseminomatous germ cell tumors. Currently, chemotherapy usually consisting of a combination of several *combination chemotherapy*. Drugs that have shown antitumor activity against the disease are delivered in specific dose and schedules.

Principles for the Combination Chemotherapy

1. Only those agents of proven effectiveness should be used.
2. Each agent used should have a different mechanism of action.
3. Each drug should have a different spectrum of toxicity.
4. Each drug should be used at maximum.
5. Drug combination should be administered in shortest interval between therapy cycles to allow for the recovery of normal tissues.

The dose modification is needed when the patient has myelotoxicity (low blood counts), renal or hepatic dysfunction or poor tolerance to the given regimen. The response to the chemotherapy is periodically evaluated after every 2 to 3 cycles.

CONCOMITANT CHEMORADIOTHERAPY

Rationale for this strategy is utilization of direct interaction of radiotherapy and chemotherapy. Drug delieved to have radiation enhancing properties are utilized in this approach. The drugs known to have this property are hydroxyurea, 5-FU and cisplation. However, there are certain drugs which can cause dramatic increase in cutaneous and mucosal reactions and prove deleterious at times. Simultaneous chemoradiotherapy is given to improve the local control as well as to decrease the incidence of distant metastasis. Radiation combined with hydroxyurea proved more effective than radiation alone in a randomized trial in advanced cervical cancer. The chemoirradiation has also been tried as an alternative to the traditional surgery and radiotherapy combination in advanced laryngeal cancer.

SALVAGE CHEMOTHERAPY

Whenever, the first line of therapy, i.e. surgery, radiotherapy, chemotherapy or combinations fail, the patient is considered for salvage therapy . The salvage chemotherapy is generally attempted when the patient has a good performance status, there is reasonable expectancy of life, and the neoplasm is potentially chemosensitive. Radiotherapy and chemotherapy alone can control about 20 to 30 percent of cancers. The multimodal holistic approach in cancers, has resulted in some completely curable cancers, namely, childhood. ALL, Wilms' tumor, Ewing's sarcoma, testicular tumor and medulloblastoma.

ALDESLEUKIN

Other names: Interleukin-2 (IL-2), Proleukin.

Mechanism of Action

Enhançes mitogenesis of T cells, natural killer cells, and lymphokine-activated killer cells; augments cytotoxicity of natural killer and lymphokine-activated killer cells; induces interferon gamma sign.

Primary Indications

1. Renal cell carcinoma
2. Melanoma.

Usual Dosage and Schedule

A wide range of doses and routes (IV or SC) have been used. In any of the schedules, therapy may be stopped prematurely for severe constitutional symptoms indicative of cardiovascular, renal, hepatic, neurologic, pulmonary, or hematologic toxicity.

1. 6000,000 IU/kg (22 $\times$ 10^6 IU/m^2) as a.15 min IV infusion

   Immunosuppressants, Gene Therapy 9

   Every 8 hours for up to 14 doses on days 1 to 5. Repeat on days 15 to 19. Repeat cycle in 6 to 12 weeks if stable or responding disease.
2. 18 $\times 10^6$ IU/m^2/24 hours as a continuous IV infusion daily for up to 5 days. Repeat in 2 weeks. Repeat cycle in 6 to 12 weeks if stable or responding disease.
3. 22 $\times 10^6$ IU/m^2 SC or as a 15 min IV infusion for 5 consecutive days for 2 successive weeks. Repeat every 3 to 6 weeks as tolerated. In some regimens, it is preceded by 3 days with a single dose of low-dose cyclophosphamide 350 mg/m^2 IV push.
4. 9 $\times$ 10^6 IU/m^2 daily by continuous IV infusion on days 1 to 4 (96 hours), together with chemotherapy (cisplatin, vinblastine, dacarbazine) and interferon in melanoma.

Schedules 1, 2 and 4 require hospitalization. Schedule 3 can be given in an outpatient setting but may require several hours of observation after treatment.

Special Precautions

Patients must be carefully monitored after treatment using any of the dosing regimens.

Outpatient regimens require that patients have cardiovascular status observed for up to 5 liter, particularly after the first several doses. With higher doses, capillary leak syndrome resulting in hypotension, pulmonary edema, myocardial infarction, arrhythmias, azotemia, and alterations in mental status may occur. Intensive care, controlled volume replacement, and intubation may be required lower doses can be given in an outpatient setting (Table 2.1).

Table 2.1: Safety of high-dose intravenous bolus recombinant interleukin-2 therapy: The national cancer institute experience

Adverse event	*1985 Incidence (%)*	*1997 Incidence (%)*
Hypotension	81	31
Diarrhea	92	12
Neuropsychiatric toxicity	19	8
Line sepsis	18	4
Pulmonary complications	12	3

Toxicity

1. All are dose dependent
2. Safety of high-dose intravenous bolus recombinant
3. Interleukin-2 therapy. The national cancer institute experience
4. Adverse event hypotension 81:31
5. Diarrhea 92:12
6. Neuropsychiatric toxicity 19:8
7. Line sepsis 18:4
8. Pulmonary complications 12:3.

Note: With patient selection and experience in managing side effects, high-dose recombinant interleukin-2 is safe. No treatment-related deaths in 809 consecutive patients. Incidence of grade 3 to 4 adverse events has been greatly reduced a 720,000 IU/kg every 8 hours.

1. *Myelosuppression and other hematologic effects:* Uncommon at lower doses and common but rarely serious at higher doses. Anemia requiring transfusion is common at higher doses. Thrombocytopenia is common at higher doses.
2. *Nausea, vomiting and other gastrointestinal effects:*
   a. Anorexia, nausea, vomiting and diarrhea are common.
   b. Transient liver function abnormalities including hyperbilirubinemia, hypoalbuminemia, and elevation of the prothrombin time and partial thromboplastin time are common.
   c. Colonic perforations are rare.
3. *Mucocutaneous effects:* Mucositis is occasional to common. Alopecia is uncommon. Pruritic erythematous rash is common.
4. *Cardiovascular effects:*
   a. Arrhythmias are common and dose-related.
   b. Hypotension is dose-related but is occasionally seen at the lower-dose schedules.

c. Myocardial injury is seen primarily at the higher-dose schedules.
d. Pulmonary edema from capillary leak syndrome is common with intensive-dose regimens.

e. Weight gain is common from edema, particularly in more intensive-dose regimens.

5. *Neuropsychiatric effects:*
   a. Mental status changes are common, with dose-related severity.
   b. Dizziness or light-headedness is common.
   c. Blurry vision and other visual disturbances are occasional.
   d. Seizures are uncommon to rare at lower-dose regimens.
6. *Renal function impairment:* Common but reversible. More frequent laboratory abnormalities include creatinine elevation, hypomagnesemia, acidosis, hypocalcemia, hypophosphatemia, hypokalemia, hypouricemia and hypoalbuminemia.
7. *Fever:* With or without chills, universal and may be severe.
8. *Bacterial infection:* Occasional probably related to chemotactic defect induced in granulocytes.
9. *Myalgias and arthralgias:* Occasional to common.
10. *Malaise and fatigue:* Common and dose-related.

Prophylaxis of Acute Toxicity

1. Acetaminophen 650 to 1,000 mg PO 1 hour before therapy and every 3 hours for two doses.
2. Cimetidine 800 mg PO or other histamine H_2-receptor antagonist before therapy and daily for duration of treatment.
3. Antiemetics such as granisetron, ondansetron or other 5-HT3 antagonist, metoclopramide, and prochlorperazine may be used. Do not use dexamethasone.
4. Meperidine 25 to 50 mg IV, when chills start after first dose. For subsequent doses, meperidine 150 mg PO 1.5 hour before chills are predicted to start, based on the first treatment.
5. Diphenhydramine 50 mg PO every 3 hours for three doses may be substituted for meperidine in patients who tolerate the latter drug poorly.
6. Diphenoxylate with atropine (Lomotil) 1 tablet up to eight times daily for diarrhea.
7. Hydroxyzine 25 to 50 mg PO every 4 to 6 hours for itching.

AMIFOSTINE

Other name: Ethyol.

Mechanism of Action

The prodrug, amifostine, is dephosphorylated to an active free thiol metabolite that can reduce the toxic effects of cisplatin. The differential activity between normal and cancer tissue is thought to be related to higher capillary alkaline phosphatase activity and better vascularity of normal tissue. Pretreatment reduces cumulative renal toxicity from cisplatin.

Primary Indications

1. For reduction of cumulative renal toxicity associated with repeated administration of cisplatin in patients with advanced cancer.
2. For reduction of moderate to severe xerostomia from radiation of the head and neck where the radiation port includes a substantial portion of the parotid glands.

Usual Dosage and Schedule

1. *Reduction of cumulative renal toxicity with chemotherapy:* 910 mg/m^2 IV over 15 min once daily, starting 30 min before cisplatin chemotherapy.
2. *Reduction of xerostomia from radiation to the head and neck:* 200 mg/m^2 administered once daily as a 3 min IV infusion, starting 15 to 30 min prior to standard fraction radiation. **Immunosuppressants, Gene therapy 13** therapy (1.8–2.0 Gy).

Special Precaution

To minimize hypotension during the infusion, patients should be adequately hydrated prior to the amifostine infusion and kept in a supine position during the infusion. Blood pressure should be monitored every 5 min during the infusion and thereafter as clinically indicated. Interrupt the infusion if the decrease in systolic pressure is more than 20 to 25 percent of the baseline systolic pressure.

Toxicity

1. *Myelosuppression and other hematologic effects:* Not increased by amifostine.
2. *Nausea, vomiting and other gastrointestinal effects:* Nausea and vomiting are common and may be severe.
3. *Mucocutaneous effects:* Skin rash is rare.
4. Miscellaneous effects:
   a. Transient hypotension during the infusion is common. Loss of consciousness may occur, but is usually easily reversed.
   b. Flushing and feeling of warmth are occasional.
   c. Chilling and feeling of coldness are occasional.
   d. Dizziness, somnolence, hiccups and sneezing are occasional.
   e. Allergic reactions are rare but have included anaphylactic reactions.
   f. Hypocalcemia is rare.
   g. Seizures are rare.

AMINOGLUTETHIMIDE

Other name: Cytadren.

Mechanism of Action

Inhibits aromatization and cytochrome P-450 hydroxylating enzymes, thereby blocking the conversion of androgens to estrogens and the biosynthesis of all steroid hormones. This drug causes, in effect, a reversible chemical adrenalectomy.

Primary Indications

1. Adrenocortical carcinoma
2. Ectopic Cushing's syndrome
3. Previously used in breast cancer, but uncommonly now, because of more specific aromatase inhibitors.

Usual Dosage and Schedule

1,000 mg daily in four divided doses. Special precautions. Hydrocortisone must be given concomitantly to prevent adrenal insufficiency, particularly if used in breast cancer. Suggested dose is 100 mg daily in divided doses for 2 weeks, then 40 mg daily in divided doses.

Toxicity

1. *Myelosuppression and other hematologic effects:* Leukopenia and thrombocytopenia are rare and if they occur, they resolve rapidly when the drug is stopped.
2. *Nausea, vomiting and other gastrointestinal effects:* Occasional and usually mild.
3. *Mucocutaneous effects:* A morbilliform rash is commonly seen during the first week of treatment, but it usually disappears within one week.
4. *Hormonal effects:*
   a. Adrenal insufficiency is common without replacement; hydrocortisone is administered in patients with normal adrenal glands.
   b. Hypothyroidism is uncommon.
   c. Masculinization is possible.
5. *Neurologic effects:*
   a. Lethargy is common. Although usually mild and transient, it is occasionally severe.
   b. Vertigo, nystagmus and ataxia are occasional.
6. *Miscellaneous effects:*
   a. Facial flushing is uncommon
   b. Periorbital edema is uncommon
   c. Cholestatic jaundice is rare
   d. Fever is uncommon.

ANASTROZOLE

Other name: Arimidex.

Decreases estrogen biosynthesis by selective inhibition of aromatase (estrogen synthetase) (Figs 2.2 and 2.3).

Primary Indications

1. Carcinoma of the breast (advanced) as first-line treatment in women with hormone receptor-positive or unknown cancers.

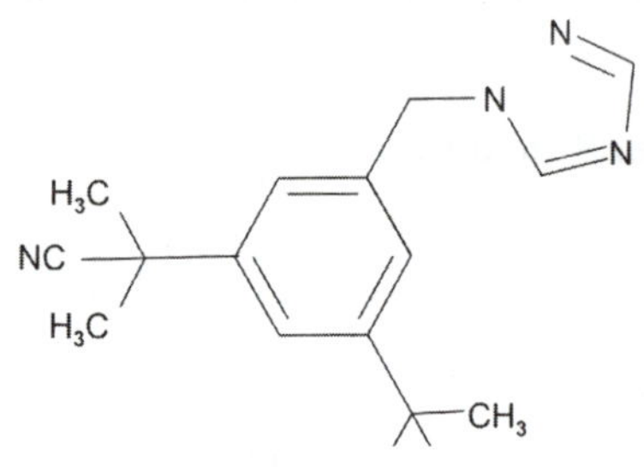

Fig. 2.2: Chemical structure of anastrozole

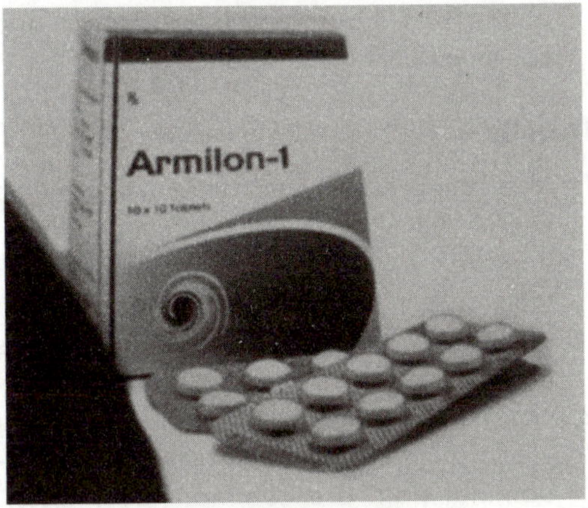

Fig. 2.3: Anastrozole 1 mg tablets

2. Carcinoma of the breast after progression in patients previously responsive to tamoxifen therapy.

   Usual dosage and schedule. 1 mg PO daily.

Special Precautions

Potential hazard to fetus if given during pregnancy.

Toxicity

1. *Myelosuppression and other hematologic effects:* No dose-related myelosuppression. Thromboembolic events are uncommon (3–4%).
2. *Nausea, vomiting, and other gastrointestinal effects:* Nausea is occasional; vomiting is uncommon. Diarrhea and constipation are occasional.
3. *Mucocutaneous effects:* Rash is uncommon. Hot flushes are common (25–30%) vaginal dryness and leukorrhea are uncommon.
4. *Miscellaneous effects:* These include the following:
   a. Asthenia is common.
   b. Musculoskeletal pain is occasional.
   c. Headache and dizziness are occasional.
   d. Arthralgia is occasional.
   e. Peripheral edema and weight gain are occasional (lower than with megestrol).
   f. Dyspnea and cough are occasional.
   g. Hypercalcemia is rare.
   h. Uterine bleeding appears less commonly than with tamoxifen.
   i. Osteoporosis and fractures are more common than with tamoxifens.

ARSENIC TRIOXIDE

Other name: Trisenox.

Mechanism of Action

Although the mechanism is incompletely understood, effects of arsenic trioxide include morphologic changes and DNA fragmentation characteristic of apoptosis and alteration of the fusion protein PML-RAR-a.

Primary Indication

Acute promyelocytic leukemia that is refractory to retinoid and anthracycline therapy and has (15;17) translocation or PML-RAR-a gene expression.

Usual Dosage and Schedule

1. Induction 0.15 mg/kg IV daily until marrow remission.
   Maximum of 60 doses.
2. Consolidation, 0.15 mg/kg IV daily for 25 doses over a period of up to 5 weeks. Consolidation is started 3 to 6 weeks after completion of induction therapy.

Special Precautions

1. Tachycardia and prolonged QT interval are common. This may lead to complete atrioventricular block with fatal ventricular arrhythmia. Electrolyte (including magnesium) abnormalities should be corrected prior to initiation of therapy and patients with prolonged QT intervals should have measures taken to reduce this prolongation prior to treatment with arsenic trioxide. A QT value greater than 500 msec during therapy is an indication to suspend arsenic trioxide treatment and to initiate measures to correct other risk factors that may be contributing to the prolongation of the QT.
2. Acute promyelocytic leukemic differentiation syndrome, similar to that observed with retinoic acid, may be seen and is potentially fatal. This syndrome consists of fever, dyspnea, weight gain, pulmonary infiltrates and pleural or pericardial effusions with or without leukocytosis. High-dose corticosteroids (e.g. dexamethasone 10 mg bid) should be started at the first signs of this syndrome and continued until it has subsided.

Toxicity

1. *Myelosuppression and other hematologic effects:* Anemia, thrombocytopenia and neutropenia are occasional. Leukocytosis is common, disseminated intravascular coagulation is occasional and may be severe. Infections and neutropenic fever are occasional.
2. *Nausea, vomiting and other gastrointestinal effects:* Nausea, vomiting, diarrhea and abdominal pain are common (over 50%). Gastrointestinal bleeding with or without diarrhea is occasional (8%). Constipation, anorexia and other abdominal distress are occasional.
3. *Mucocutaneous effects:* Sore throat is common (40%). Dermatitis, pruritus and ecchymosis are also common. More severe mucocutaneous reactions including local exfoliation, urticaria, and oral blistering are occasional to uncommon. Epistaxis is common (25%). Eye irritation and injection are occasional.
4. *Miscellaneous effects:*
   a. Tachycardia and prolonged QT interval are common. This may lead to complete atrioventricular block with fatal ventricular arrhythmia.
   b. Acute promyelocytic leukemic differentiation syndrome, similar to that seen with retinoic acid, may be seen. This consists of fever, dyspnea, weight gain, pulmonary infiltrates, and pleural or pericardial effusions with

or without leukocytosis. This syndrome may be fatal.

c. Headache and insomnia are common. Edema and pleural effusion are common (though not commonly serious) and general weight gain is occasional. Drug hypersensitivity is uncommon. Injection site edema, erythema and pain are occasional.
d. Hypokalemia, hypomagnesemia and hyperglycemia are common (45–50%). Hyperkalemia is occasional to common (18%), as are elevated transaminases, hypocalcemia and hypoglycemia.
e. Cough and dyspnea are common (over 50%). Pleural effusion, hypoxia, wheezing, and asymptomatic auscultatory findings are occasional to common (8–20%).
f. Renal failure is occasional.

ASPARAGINASE

Other names: L-asparaginase, Elspar, Kidrolase, Pegaspargase.

Mechanism of Action

Hydrolysis of serum asparagine occurs, which deprives leukemia cells of the required amino acid and inhibits protein synthesis.

Normal cells are spared because they generally, have the ability to synthesize their own asparagine. Pegaspargase is a chemically modified formulation of asparaginase in which the L-asparaginase is covalently conjugated with monomethoxypolyethylene glycol.

This modification increases its half-life in the plasma by a factor of 4 to about 5.7 days and reduces its recognition by the immune system, which allows the drug to be used in patients previously hypersensitive to native L-asparaginase.

Primary Indication

Acute lymphocytic leukemia, primarily for induction therapy.

Usual Dosage and Schedule

Both schedules are usually used in combination with other drugs.

The schedules listed are only two of many acceptable dosing schedules.

1. L-asparaginase, 6,000 to 18,500 IU/m^2 IV daily for up to 14 days (Fig. 2.4).
2. Pegaspargase, 2,500 IU/m^2 IM (or IV) once every 14 days in patients who have developed hypersensitivity to native forms of L-asparaginase.

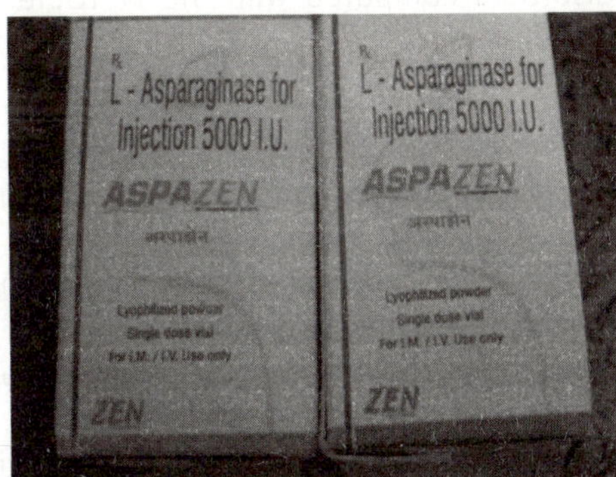

Fig. 2.4: L-asparaginase injection

Special Precautions

Asparaginase is contraindicated in patients with pancreatitis or a history of pancreatitis. Asparaginase is contraindicated in patients who have had significant hemorrhagic events associated with prior L-asparaginase therapy. Pegaspargase is also contraindicated in patients who have had previous serious allergic reactions such as generalized urticaria, bronchospasm, laryngeal edema, hypotension, or other unacceptable adverse reactions to prior pegaspargase.

1. Be prepared to treat anaphylaxis at each administration of the drug. Epinephrine, antihistamines, corticosteroids and life-support equipment should be readily available.
2. Administration of the drug concurrently with or immediately before vincristine may increase vincristine toxicity.
3. The IM route is preferred for pegaspargase because of a lower incidence of hepatotoxicity, coagulopathy, and gastrointestinal and renal disorders compared with the IV route of administration.

Toxicity

1. *Myelosuppression and other hematologic effects:* Occasional.
2. *Nausea, vomiting, and other gastrointestinal effects:* Occasional and usually mild.
3. *Mucocutaneous effects:* No toxicity occurs except as a sign of hypersensitivity.
4. *Anaphylaxis:* Mild to severe hypersensitivity reactions, including anaphylaxis, occur in 20 to 30 percent of patients. Such reaction is less likely to occur during the first few days of treatment. It is particularly common with intermittent schedules or repeat cycles. If the patient develops hypersensitivity to the Escherichia coli-derived anzyme (Elspar), Erwinia-derived asparaginase may be safely substituted because the two enzyme preparations are not cross-reactive. Note that hypersensitivity may also develop to Erwinia derived asparaginase, and continued preparedness to treat anaphylaxis must be maintained.

   If administered IM, asparaginase should be given in an extremity so that a tourniquet can be applied to slow the systemic release of asparaginase in case anaphylaxis occurs.

   Approximately 30 percent patients previously sensitive to L-asparaginase will have a hypersensitivity reaction to pegaspargase, whereas only 10 percent of those who were not hypersensitive to the native form will have a hypersensitivity reaction to the polyethylene glycol—modified drug.
5. *Miscellaneous effects:* These include the following:
   a. Mild fever and malaise are common and occasionally progress to severe chills and malignant hyperthermia.
   b. Hepatotoxicity is common and occasionally severe. Abnormalities observed include, elevations of serum glutamic oxaloacetic transaminase (SGOT), alkaline phosphatase and bilirubin, depressed levels

of hepatic derived clotting factors and albumin and hepatocellular fatty metamorphosis.

c. Renal failure is rare.

d. Pancreatic endocrine and exocrine dysfunction often with manifestations of pancreatitis, occasionally occurs.
   Nonketotic hyperglycemia is uncommon.

e. CNS effects (depression, somnolence, fatigue, confusion, agitation, hallucinations, or coma) are seen occasionally.
   They are usually reversible following discontinuation of the drug.

CAPECITABINE

Other name: Xeloda (Fig. 2.5).

Mechanism of Action

An orally administered prodrug that is converted to fluorouracil intracellularly. When this is converted to the active nucleotide, 5-fluoro-2-deoxyuridine monophosphate, it inhibits the enzyme thymidylate synthetase and blocks DNA synthesis. The triphosphate may also be mistakenly incorporated into RNA, which interferes with RNA processing and protein synthesis.

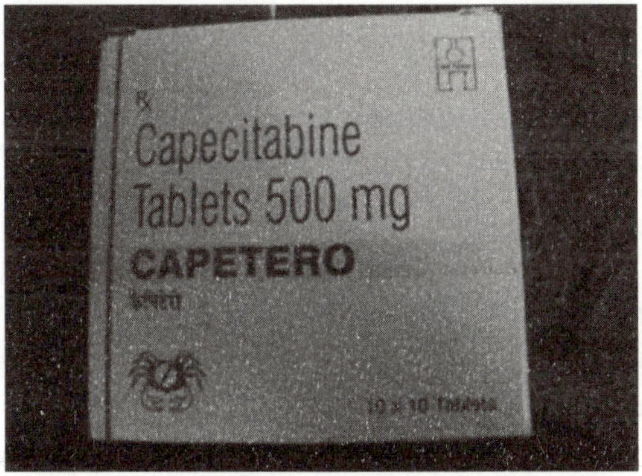

Fig. 2.5: Capecitabine tablet

Primary Indications

1. Metastatic breast cancer that is resistant to anthracycline and paclitaxel—containing chemotherapy regimens. May also be used in patients in whom anthracyclines are contraindicated.
2. Colorectal carcinoma, particularly in situations where continuous infusion of fluorouracil might have been used.
3. Pancreatic carcinoma.

Usual Dosage and Schedule

Generally taken with water, twice daily (about 12 hours between doses) within 30 min after a meal.

1. 1,250 mg/m^2 PO twice daily for 2 weeks, followed by a 1-week rest, given as 3-week cycles.
2. 1,000 to 1,250 mg/m^2 PO twice daily for 2 weeks, in combination with docetaxel 75 mg/m^2 IV over 1 hour once every 3 weeks. Two weeks of treatment are followed by a 1 week rest to complete the 3-week cycle.
3. 800 to 825 mg/m^2 PO twice daily for 5 or 7 days a week as a radiosensitizer for the duration of radiotherapy unless toxicity prohibits continuation.

Special Precaution

Patients with moderate renal impairment (Ccr=30 to 50 ml/min) require a 25 percent dosage reduction. Diarrhea may be severe and require fluid and electrolyte replacement. Incidence and severity may be worse in patients 80 years of age or older. Therapy may need to be interrupted and subsequent doses decreased for severe or repeated toxicity. Increase in prothrombin time (PT) and international normalized ratio (INR) may be seen in patients previously stable on oral anticoagulants. Monitor PT/INR more frequently when patient is on capecitabine.

Toxicity

1. *Myelosuppression and other hematologtic effects:* Common, but when used as a single agent, these usually are mild to moderate, with anemia predominating. Neutropenia is common when used in combination and may be associated with neutropenic fever.
2. *Nausea, vomiting and other gastrointestinal effects:* Both nausea (45%) and vomiting (35%) are common but usually not severe. Diarrhea is common (55%) in up to 15 percent of patients, it is severe to life-threatening. Gastrointestinal motility disorders including ileus may be seen and necrotizing enterocolitis has been reported. Abdominal pain is occasional to common.

   Anorexia is occasional to common (26%), hyperbilirubinemia is common (48%) but only occasionally severe or life-threatening.
3. *Mucocutaneous effects:* Hand and foot syndrome is common (54%) and may be severe. Dermatitis is also common (27%), as is stomatitis, but it is uncommon that these are severe. Eye irritation and increased lacrimation are occasional.
4. *Miscellaneous effects:* These include the following:
   a. Fatigue is common
   b. Paresthesias are occasional
   c. Fever is occasional
   d. Headache or dizziness is occasional
   e. Cardiotoxicity is possible, as with any fluorinated pyrimidine.
5. Hand and foot syndrome and diarrhea may be ameliorated by celecoxib 200 mg PO bid.

CARBOPLATIN

Other names: Paraplatin, CBDCA.

Mechanism of Action

Covalent binding to DNA.

Primary Indication

Ovarian, endometrial and lung cancers and other cancers in which cisplatin is active.

Usual Dosage and Schedule

Area-under-the-curve (AUC) dosing (Calvert formula) is generally preferred.

1. Target AUC is commonly 4 to 6, depending on previous treatment and other drugs to be

used. Administration dose (mg)= (target AUC) × ([creatinine clearance] +25).

Administration dose is given by IV infusion over 15 to 60 min and repeated every 3 to 4 weeks.

2. 300 to 400 mg/m^2 IV by infusion over 15 to 60 min or longer, repeated every 3 to 4 weeks.
3. Higher doses up to 1,600 mg/m^2 divided over several days have been used followed by stem cell rescue (e.g. bone marrow transplantation).

Special Precaution

Much less renal toxicity than cisplatin, so there is no need for a vigorous hydration schedule or forced diuresis. If AUC dosing is not used, reduce dose to 250 mg/m^2 for creatinine clearance of 41 to 59 ml/min dose has to L.

Toxicity Profiles of Platinum Analogs in Clinical Use

Cisplatin, Carboplatin and Oxaliplatin

1. Myelosuppression nephrotoxicity neurotoxicity ototoxicity nausea and vomiting.
2. Anaphylactic-like reactions to carboplatin have been reported and may occur within minutes of carboplatin administration. Epinephrine, corticosteroids and antihistamines have been employed to alleviate symptoms.

Toxicity

1. *Myelosuppression and other hematologic effects:* Anemia, granulocytopenia and thrombocytopenia are common and dose limiting. Red blood cell transfusions or erythropoietin may be required. Thrombocytopenia may be delayed (days 18–28).
2. *Nausea, vomiting, and other gastrointestinal effects:* Nausea and vomiting are common, but vomiting (65%) is not as frequent or as severe as with cisplatin and can be controlled with combination antiemetic regimens. Liver function abnormalities are common. Gastrointestinal pain is occasional.
3. *Mucocutaneous effects:* Alopecia is uncommon, mucositis is rare.
4. *Renal tubular abnormalities:* Elevation in serum creatinine or blood urea nitrogen occurs occasionally. More common is electrolyte loss with decreases in serum sodium, potassium, calcium and magnesium.
5. *Miscellaneous effects:*
   a. Peripheral neuropathies and central neurotoxicity is uncommon.
   b. Allergic reactions are uncommonly seen. These include rash, urticaria, pruritus and rarely bronchospasm and hypotension.
   c. Cardiovascular effects (cardiac failure, embolism, cerebrovascular accidents) are uncommon.
   d. Hemolytic uremic syndrome is rare.

CARMUSTINE

Other names: BCNU, BiCNU, Gliadel wafer (surgically implantable, biodegradable polymer wafer that releases impregnated carmustine from the hydrophobic matrix after implantation).

Mechanism of Action

Alkylation and carbamoylation by carmustine metabolites interfere with the synthesis and function of DNA, RNA and proteins.

Carmustine is lipid-soluble and easily enters the brain.

Primary Indications

A. *Systemic therapy:*
   1. Hodgkin's and Non-Hodgkin's lymphomas
   2. Brain tumors
   3. Multiple myeloma
   4. Melanoma.

B. *Implantable carmustine-impregnated wafer:*
   1. Glioblastoma multiforme.

Usual Dosage and Schedule

A. *Systemic therapy:*
   1. 200 to 240 mg/m^2 IV as a 30 to 45 min infusion every 6 to 8 weeks. Dose often is divided and given over 2 to 3 days. Some recommend limiting the cumulative dose to 1,000 mg/m^2 to limit pulmonary and renal toxicity.
   2. Higher doses of up to 600 mg/m^2 have been used with stem cell rescue (e.g. bone marrow or peripheral blood stem cell transplantation).

B. *Implantable carmustine-impregnated wafer:*
   1. Up to 8 wafers, each containing 7.7 mg of carmustine, are applied to the resection cavity surface after removal of the tumor.

Special Precaution

For systemic therapy, due to delayed myelosuppression and other hematologic effects (3–6 weeks), do not administer drug more often than every 6 weeks. Await a return of normal platelet and granulocyte counts before repeating therapy. Amphotericin B may enhance the potential for renal toxicity, bronchospasm and hypotension.

Toxicity

Systemic Therapy

1. *Myelosuppression and other hematologic effects:* Delayed and often biphasic, with the nadir at 3 to 6 weeks; it may be cumulative with successive doses. Recovery may be protracted for several months. High-dose therapy requires stem cell rescue.
2. *Nausea, vomiting and other gastrointestinal effects:* Effects beginning 2 hours after therapy and lasting upto 4 to 6 hours are common.
3. *Mucocutaneous effects:*
   a. Facial flushing and a burning sensation at the IV site may be due to alcohol used to reconstitute the drug, this is common with rapid injection.

b. Hyperpigmentation of skin after accidental contact is common.

4. *Miscellaneous effects:*
   a. Hepatotoxicity is uncommon but can be severe.
   b. Pulmonary fibrosis is uncommon at low doses, but its frequency increases at doses higher than 1,000 mg/m^2.
   c. Secondary neoplasia is possible.
   d. Renal toxicity is uncommon at doses of less than 1,000 mg/m^2.
   e. With high-dose therapy, encephalopathy, hepatotoxicity, and pulmonary toxicity are common and dose limiting. Hepato veno-occlusive disease also occurs (occasional).

Implantable Carmustine Impregnated Wafer

Limited toxicity beyond that expected from craniotomy is seen. Serious intracranial infection was seen in 4 percent of patients compared with 1 percent of placebo-treated patients. Brain edema not responsive to steroids may also be seen in a similar percentage of patients. Abnormal wound healing may occur. Remnants of the wafer may be seen for many months after implantation.

CETUXIMAB

Other names: Epidermal growth factor receptor (EGFr) antibody, C225, Erbitux.

Mechanism of Action

Epidermal growth factor receptor antibody that blocks the ligandbinding site and inhibits proliferation of cells. It is thought potentially most useful in those tumors that overexpress epidermal growth factor receptor.

Primary Indications

1. Carcinoma of head and neck
2. Lung cancer.

Usual Dosage and Schedule

400 mg/m^2 IV loading dose administered over 2 hours on day 1. Then 250 mg/m^2 IV maintenance doses administered over 1 hour weekly thereafter. May be administered in combination with other agents.

Special Precaution

Severe anaphylactoid reactions may occur.

Toxicity

1. *Myelosuppression and other hematologic effects:* Leukopenia and anemia are occasional.
2. *Nausea, vomiting and other gastrointestinal effects:* Nausea, is occasional.
3. *Miscellaneous effects:* These include the following:
   a. Asthenia is common.
   b. Allergic or hypersensitivity reactions are occasional but may be severe.
   c. Chills are occasional.
   d. Human antichimeric antibodies (HACAs) are uncommon.

CISPLATIN

Other names: Cis-Diamminedichloroplatinum (II), DDP, CDDP, Platinol.

Mechanism of Action

Similar to alkylating agents with respect to binding and crosslinking strands of DNA.

Primary Indications

Usually used in combination with other cytotoxic drugs.

1. Testis, ovary, endometrial, cervical, bladder, head and neck, gastrointestinal and lung carcinomas.
2. Soft tissue and bone sarcomas.
3. Non-Hodgkin's lymphoma.

Usual Dosage and Schedule

1. 40 to 120 mg/m^2 IV on day 1 as infusion every 3 weeks (Fig. 2.6).
2. 15 to 20 mg/m^2 IV on days 1 to 5 as infusion every 3 to 4 weeks.

Special Precautions

Do not administer if serum creatinine level is more than 1.5 mg/dl. Irreversible renal tubular damage may occur if vigorous diuresis is not maintained, particularly with higher doses (higher than 40 mg/m^2), and with additional concurrent nephrotoxic drugs such as the aminoglycosides. At higher doses, diuresis with mannitol with or without furosemide plus vigorous hydration are mandatory.

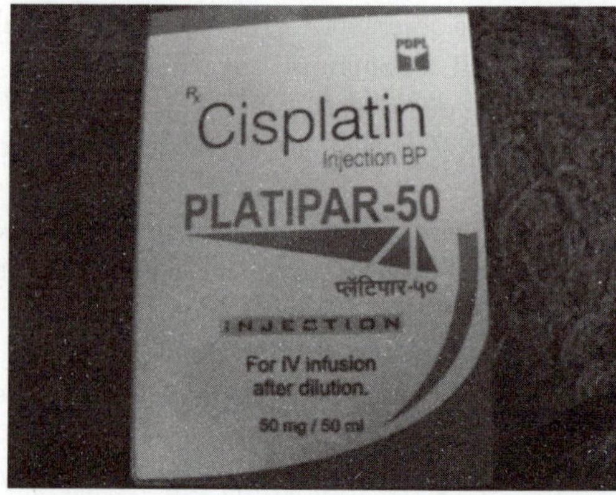

Fig. 2.6: Cisplatin injection

1. An acceptable method for hydration in patients without cardiovascular impairment for cisplatin doses up to 80 mg/m^2 is as follows.
   a. Have patient void, and begin infusion of 5 percent dextrose in half-normal saline with KCi 20 mEq/l and $MgSO_4$ 1 g/l (8 mEq/l); run at 500 ml/hr for 1.5 to 2.0 l.
   b. After 1 hour of infusion give 12.5 g of mannitol by IV push.
   c. Immediately thereafter, start the cisplatin (mixed in normal saline at 1 mg/ml) and infuse over 1 hour through the sidearm of the IV line while continuing the hydration.
   d. Give additional mannitol (12.5 – 50.0 g by IV push) if necessary to maintain urinary output of 250 ml/hr over the duration of the hydration. If patient gets more than 1 l behind on urinary output or signs or symptoms of congestive heart failure develop, 40 mg of furosemide may be given.

2. For doses of more than 80 mg/m^2, a more vigorous hydration is recommended.
   a. Have patient void, and begin infusion of 5 percent dextrose in half-normal saline with KCi 20 mEq/l and $MgSO_4$ 1 g/l (8 mEq/l); run at 500 ml/hr for 2.5 to 3.0 l.
   b. After 1 hour of infusion, give 25 g of mannitol by IV push.
   c. Continue hydration.
   d. After 2 hours of hydration, if urinary output is at least 250 ml/hr, start the cisplatin (mixed in normal saline at 1 mg/ml) and infuse over 1 to 2 hours (1 mg/m^2/min) through the sidearm of the IV line while continuing the hydration.
   e. Give additional mannitol (12.5 – 50 g by IV push) if necessary to maintain urinary output of 250 ml/hr over the duration of the hydration. If patient gets more than 1 l behind on urinary output or signs or symptoms of congestive heart failure develop, 40 mg of furosemide may be given.
3. For patients with known or suspected cardiovascular impairment (ejection fraction under 45%), a less vigorous rate of hydration may be used, provided the dose of cisplatin is limited (e.g. less than 60 mg/m^2). An alternative is to give carboplatin. Long-term use of cisplatin can lead to cisplatin resistance (Fig 2.7).

Toxicity

1. *Myelosuppression and other hematologic effects:* Mild-to-moderate, depending on the dose. Relative lack of myelosuppression and other hematologic effects allows cisplatin to be used in full doses with more myelo-suppressive drugs. Anemia is common and may have a hemolytic component. Anemia often is amenable to epoetin therapy.
2. *Nausea, vomiting and other gastrointestinal effects:* Severe and often intractable vomiting regularly begins within 1 hour of starting cisplatin and lasts 8 to 12 hour. Prolonged

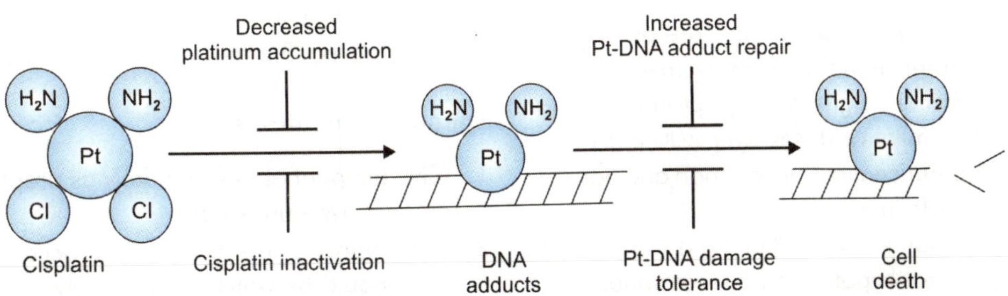

Fig. 2.7: Resistance with cisplatinum

nausea, vomiting and other gastrointestinal effects occur occasionally.

These effects may be minimized by the use of a combination antiemetic regimen, e.g. dexamethasone ondansetron or granisetron, and lorazepam.

3. *Mucocutaneous effects:* None.
4. *Renal tubular damage:* Acute reversible and occasionally irreversible nephrotoxicity may occur, particularly if adequate attention is not given to achieving sufficient hydration and diuresis. Nephrotoxic antibiotics increase risk of acute renal failure.
5. *Ototoxicity:* High-tone hearing loss is common, but significant hearing loss at vocal frequencies occurs only occasionally. Tinnitus is uncommon.
6. *Severe electrolyte abnormalities:* These abnormalities, e.g. marked hyponatremia, hypomagnesemia, hypocalcemia, and hypokalemia, may be seen up to several days after treatment.
7. *Anaphylaxis:* May occur after several doses. Responds to epinephrine, antihistamines, and corticosteroids.
8. *Miscellaneous effects:* These are as follows:
   a. Peripheral neuropathies are clinically significant signs and symptoms common at cumulative doses over 300 mg/m^2.
   b. Hyperuricemia is uncommon and parallels renal failure.
   c. Autonomic dysfunction with symptomatic postural hypotension is occasional.

CLADRIBINE

Other names: 2-Chlorodeoxyadenosine, Leustatin.

Mechanism of Action

Deoxyadenosine analog with high cellular specificity for lymphoid cells. Resistant to effect of adenosine deaminase.

Accumulates in cells as triphosphate, is incorporated into DNA and inhibits DNA repair enzymes and RNA synthesis. Also results in NAD depletion. Effect is independent of cell division.

Primary Indications

1. Hairy-cell leukemia
2. Chronic lymphocytic leukemia
3. Waldenström's macroglobulinemia
4. Possibly other lymphoid neoplasms.

Usual Dosage and Schedule

1. 0.09 mg/kg (3.33 mg/m^2) IV daily as a continuous 7-day infusion.
2. 0.14 mg/kg (5.2 mg/m^2) IV as a 2-hour infusion daily for 5 days.
3. 0.14 mg/kg (5.2 mg/m^2) SC daily for 5 days.

Special Precautions

1. Give allopurinol 300 mg daily as prophylaxis against hyperuricemia.
2. Opportunistic infections occur occasionally and should be watched for closely.

Toxicity

1. *Myelosuppression and other hematologic effects:* Moderate granulocyte suppression is common. Marrow suppression with leukopenia and thrombocytopenia may be prolonged for over a year. Serious infection is common. Profound suppression of CD4 and CD8 counts is common and often prolonged for over 1 year. Opportunistic infections including herpes, fungus, and Pneumocystis infection may occur and should be watched for. Some routinely use prophylaxis against one or more of these infections, including acyclovir 400 mg bid and trimethoprim-sulfamethoxazole 1 double strength tablet twice daily on 2 or 3 days a week.
2. *Nausea, vomiting and other gastrointestinal effects:* Mild nausea with decrease in appetite is common, but no vomiting is expected.
3. *Mucocutaneous effects:* Rash is common.
4. *Miscellaneous effects:*
   a. Fever, possibly due to release of pyrogens from tumor cells, is common.
   b. Headache, dizziness, insomnia, fatigue, myalgia and arthralgia are occasional.
   c. Edema and tachycardia are occasional.
   d. Cough, shortness of breath and abnormal breath sounds are occasional.

CORTICOSTEROIDS

Other names: Prednisone, dexamethasone (Decadron), and others.

Mechanism of Action

Unknown but apparently related to the presence of glucocorticoid receptors in tumor cells. Mediated in part by bcl-2 gene and promotion of apoptotic cell death.

Primary Indications

1. Acute and chronic lymphocytic leukemia
2. Hodgkin's and Non-Hodgkin's lymphomas
3. Multiple myeloma
4. Carcinoma of the breast
5. Cerebral edema or spinal cord injury (compression)
6. Nausea and vomiting from chemotherapy.

Usual Dosage and Schedule

1. Prednisone: Dose varies with neoplasm and combination.

   Typical regimen, except for acute lymphocytic leukemia, is as follows:
   a. 40 mg/m^2 PO days 1 to 14 every 4 weeks or
   b. 100 mg/m^2 PO days 1 to 5 every 4 weeks.
2. Prednisone: For acute lymphocytic leukemia, 40 to 50 mg/m^2 PO daily for 28 days.
3. Dexamethasone: For cerebral edema or spinal cord injury, 10 mg IV push; then 16 to 32 mg PO daily. As signs and symptoms are controlled, gradually reduce to lowest effective dose.

Special Precaution

Monitor for hyperglycemia.

Toxicity

1. *Myelosuppression and other hematologic effects:* None.
2. *Nausea, vomiting and other gastrointestinal effects:* No acute nausea or vomiting. Epigastric pain, extreme hunger and occasional peptic ulceration with bleeding may occur even with short courses. Antacids or inhibitors of acid secretion are recommended as prophylaxis.
3. *Mucocutaneous effects:* Acne; increased risk for oral, rectal and vaginal thrush. Thinning of skin and striae develop with continuous use.
4. *Suppression of adrenal-pituitary axis:* May lead to adrenal insufficiency when corticosteroids are withdrawn. This problem is not common with intermittent schedules.
5. *Metabolic effects:* Potassium depletion, sodium and fluid retention, diabetes, increased appetite, loss of muscle mass, myopathy, weight gain, osteoporosiss and development of cushingoid features. Their frequency depends on dose and duration of therapy.
6. *Miscellaneous effects:* These include the following:
   a. CNS effects, including euphoria, depression and sleeplessness, are common and may progress to dementia or frank psychosis.
   b. Increased susceptibility to infection is common.
   c. Subcapsular cataracts in patients are uncommon but have been seen even when used for prophylaxis and treatment of drug-induced emesis.

CYCLOPHOSPHAMIDE

Other names: CTX, Cytoxan Neosar.

Mechanism of Action

Metabolism of cyclophosphamide by hepatic microsomal enzymes produces active alkylating metabolites. Cyclophosphamide's primary effect is probably on DNA (Fig. 2.8).

Primary Indications

1. Breast, lung, ovary, testis and bladder carcinomas
2. Bone and soft tissue sarcomas
3. Hodgkin's and Non-Hodgkin's lymphomas
4. Acute and chronic lymphocytic leukemias
5. Waldenstrom's macroglobulinemia
6. Neuröblastoma and Wilms' tumor of childhood

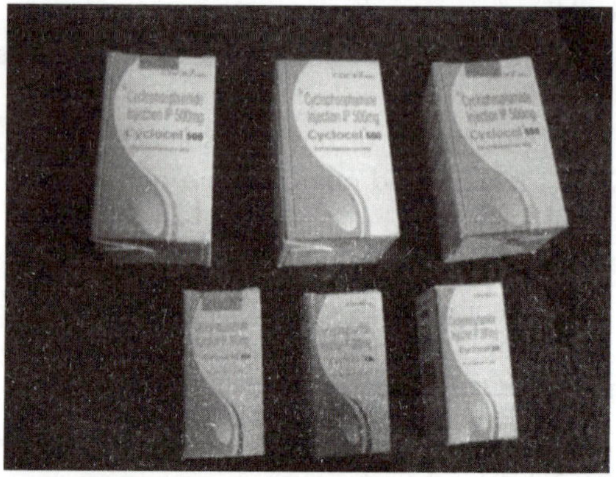

Fig. 2.8: Cyclophosphamide injection 500 mg and 200 mg

7. Gestational trophoblastic neoplasms
8. Multiple myeloma.

Usual Dosage and Schedule

1. 1,000 to 1,5000 mg/m^2 IV every 3 to 4 weeks or
2. 400 mg/m^2 PO days 1 to 5 every 3 to 4 weeks or
3. 60 to 120 mg/m^2 PO daily.
4. High-dose regimens (4–7 g/m^2 divided over 4 days) are investigational and should be used only with some kind of stem cell rescue (e.g. bone marrow transplantation) and mesna bladder protection.

Special Precaution

Give dose in the morning, maintain ample fluid intake, and have patient empty bladder several times daily to diminish the likelihood of cystitis.

Toxicity

1. *Myelosuppression and other hematologic effects:* Dose limiting. Platelets are relatively spared. Nadir is reached about 10 to 14 days after IV dose with recovery by days 21.
2. *Nausea, vomiting and other gastrointestinal effects:* Frequent with large IV doses; less common after oral doses. Symptoms begin several hours after treatment and are usually over by the next day.
3. *Mucocutaneous effects:* Reversible alopecia is common, usually starting after 2 to 3 weeks. Skin and nails may become darker. Mucositis is uncommon.
4. *Bladder damage:* Hemorrhagic or non-hemorrhagic cystitis may occur in 5 to 10 percent of patients treated. It is usually reversible with discontinuation of the drug, but it may persist and lead to fibrosis or death. Frequency is diminished by ample fluid intake and morning administration of the drug. Mesna will protect from this effect.
5. *Miscellaneous effects:* These include the following:
   a. Immunosuppression is common.
   b. Amenorrhea and azoospermia are common.
   c. Inhibition of antidiuretic hormone is of significance only with very large doses.
   d. Interstitial pulmonary fibrosis is rare.
   e. Secondary neoplasia is possible.
   f. Acute and potentially fatal cardiotoxicity occurs with high-dose therapy. Abnormalities include pericardial effusion, congestive heart failure, decreased electrocardiographic voltage and fibrin microthrombi in cardiac capillaries with endothelial injury and hemorrhagic necrosis.

CYTARABINE

Other names: Cytosine arabinoside, are -C, Cytosar-U, DepoCyt (cytarabine, liposomal for intrathecal use only) (Fig. 2.9).

Mechanism of Action

A pyrimidine analog antimetabolite that when phosphorylated to arabinosyl-cytosine triphosphate

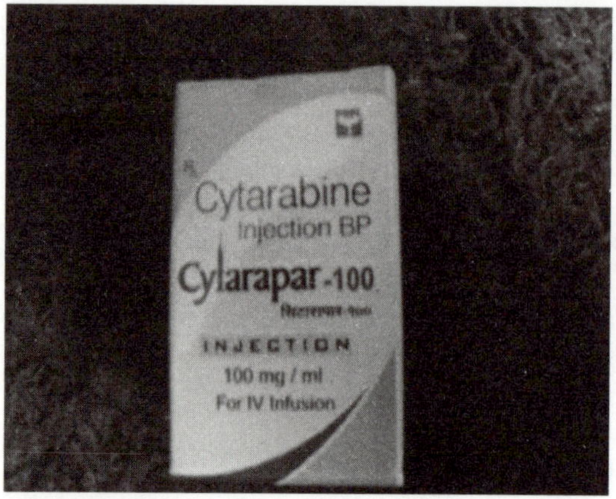

Fig. 2.9: Cytarabine injection

(ara-CTP) is a competitive inhibitor of DNA polymerase.

Primary Indications

1. Acute nonlymphocytic leukemia.
2. Non-Hodgkin's lymphoma (leukemia).
3. Meningeal lymphoma or leukemia.

Usual Dosage and Schedule

1. *Induction:* 100 mg/m^2 IV daily as a continuous infusion for 5 to 7 days (in combination with other drugs).
2. *Maintenance:* 100 mg/m^2 SC every 12 hours for 4 or 5 days every 4 weeks (with other drugs).
3. *Intrathecally:*
   a. 40 to 50 mg/m^2 of cytarabine, unencapsulated, every 4 days in preservative-free buffered isotonic diluent.
   b. 50 mg of cytarabine liposomal, repeated in 14 to 28 days.
4. *High-dose* (tolerated poorly by patient over 70 years of age).
   a. *Induction:* 21 to 3 g/m^2 IV over 1 to 2 hours every 12 hours for up to 12 doses.
   b. *Consolidation:* 3 g/m^2 IV over 3 hours every 12 hours on days 1, 3 and 5.

Special Precautions

1. None for standard doses. When administering high-doses, give in 1to 3 hours infusion. Longer infusion enhances toxicity.
2. CNS toxicity is increased in patients with a decreased creatinine clearance.
3. Cytarabine liposomal (Depo Cyt) should be used only intrathecally.

Toxicity (Standard Dose Only)

1. *Myelosuppression and other hematologic effects:* Dose-limiting leukopenia and thrombocytopenia occur, with nadir at 7 to 10 days after treatment has ended and with recovery during the following 2 weeks, depending on the degree of suppression. Megaloblastosis is common.
2. *Nausea, vomiting and other gastrointestinal effects:* Common, particularly if the drug is given as a push or rapid infusion.
3. *Mucocutaneous effects:* Stomatitis is seen occasionally.
4. *Miscellaneous effects:* These include the following:
   a. Flu-like syndrome with fever, arthralgia and sometimes occasional rash.

b. Transient mild hepatic dysfunction is occasional.

Toxicity (High-Dose)

1. *Myelosuppression and other hematologic effects:* Universal.
2. *Nausea, vomiting and other gastrointestinal effects:* Nausea, vomiting and diarrhea are common.
3. *Mucocutaneous effects:* Occasional to common mucositis.
4. *Neurotoxicity:* Cerebellar toxicity is common, particularly in the elderly, but is usually mild and reversible. However, on occasion it has been severe and permanent or fatal.
5. *Conjunctivitis:* Hydrocortisone 2 drops OU qid for 10 days may ameliorate or prevent keratitis.
6. *Hepatic toxicity with cholestatic jaundice:* Uncommon.

DACARBAZINE

Other names: Imidazole carboxamide, DIC, DTIC-Dome (Fig. 2.10).

Mechanism of Action

Uncertain but probably interacts with preformed macromolecules by alkylation. Inhibits DNA, RNA, and protein synthesis.

Primary Indications

1. Melanoma
2. All soft tissue sarcomas
3. Hodgkin's lymphoma.

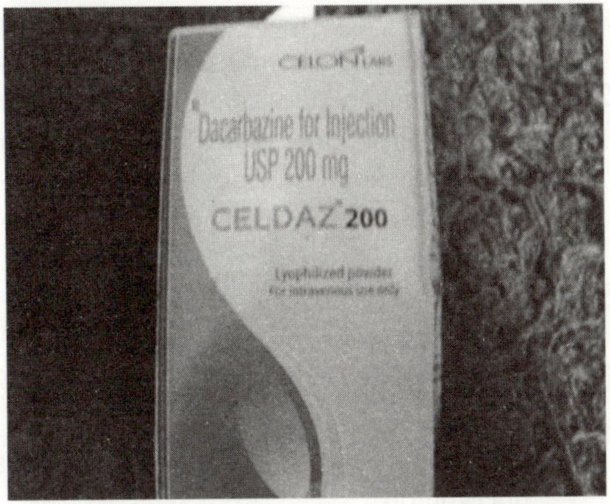

Fig. 2.10: Dacarbazine injection 200 mg vial

Usual Dosage and Schedule

1. 150 to 250 mg/m^2 IV push or rapid infusion on days 1 to 5 every 3 to 4 weeks or
2. 400 to 500 mg/m^2 IV push or rapid infusion on days 1 and 2 every 3 to 4 weeks or
3. 200 mg/m^2 IV daily as a continuous 96-hours infusion.

Special Precautions

1. Administer cautiously to avoid extravasation, as tissue damage may occur.
2. Venous pain along the injection site may be reduced by diluting dacarbazine in 100 to 200 ml of 5 percent dextrose in water and infusing over 30 min rather than injecting rapidly. Ice application may also reduce pain.

Toxicity

1. *Myelosuppression and other hematologic effects:* Mild-to-moderate.

This factor allows dacarbazine to be used in full doses with other myelosuppressive drugs.

2. *Nausea, vomiting and other gastrointestinal effects:* Common and severe but decrease in intensity with each subsequent daily dose. Onset is within 1 to 3 hours, with duration up to 12 hours.
3. *Mucocutaneous effects:*
   a. Moderately severe tissue damage if extravasation occurs.
   b. Alopecia is uncommon.
   c. Erythematous or urticarial rash is uncommon.
4. *Miscellaneous effects:* These include the following:
   a. Flue-like syndrome with fever, myalgia and malaise lasting for several days is uncommon.
   b. Hepatic toxicity is uncommon.

DACTINOMYCIN

Other name: Actinomycin D, act-D and Cosmegen.

Mechanism of Action

Binds to DNA and inhibits DNA-dependent RNA synthesis.

Inhibition of topoisomerase II.

Primary Indications

1. Gestational trophoblastic neoplasms
2. Wilms' tumor, childhood rhabdomyosarcoma, and Ewing's sarcoma.

Usual Dosage and Schedule

1. Children 0.40 to 0.45 mg/m^2 (up to a maximum of 0.5 mg) IV daily for 5 days every 3 to 5 weeks.
2. Adults.
   a. 0.40 to 0.45 mg/m^2 IV on days 1 to 5 every 2 to 3 weeks.
   b. 0.5 mg IV daily for 5 days every 3 to 5 weeks.

Special Precautions

1. Administer by slow IV push through the sidearm of a running IV infusion, being careful to avoid extravasation, which causes severe soft tissue damage.
2. If given at or about the time of infection with chickenpox or herpes zoster, a severe generalized disease may occur that sometimes results in death.

Toxicity

1. *Myelosuppression and other hematologic effects:* May be dose limiting and severe. They begin within the first week of treatment, but the nadir may not be reached for 21 days.
2. *Nausea, vomiting and other gastrointestinal effects:* Severe vomiting often occurs during the first few hours after drug administration and lasts up to 24 hours.
3. *Mucocutaneous effects:*
   a. Erythema, hyperpigmentation, and desquamation of the skin with potentiation

by previous or concurrent radiotherapy are common.

b. Oropharyngeal mucositis is potentiated by previous or concurrent radiotherapy.
c. Alopecia is common.
d. Moderately severe tissue damage occurs with extravasation.

4. *Miscellaneous effects:* These include the following:
   a. Mental depression is rare.
   b. Hepatoveno-occlusive disease is worse with higher doses and shorter schedules, e.g. single dose of 2.5 mg versus 5 days at 0.5 mg/day.

DAUNORUBICIN, LIPOSOMAL

Other name: Daunoxome.

Mechanism of Action

Daunorubicin, liposomal, which is designed to be protected from removal by the reticuloendothelial system, has a prolonged circulation time compared with unprotected drug. The agent penetrates tumor tissue and releases the strand breakage mediated by anthracycline effects on topoisomerase II, DNA intercalation and DNA polymerase inhibition.

Primary Indication

Advanced Kaposi's sarcoma, associated with human immunodeficiency virus (HIV).

Usual Dosage and Schedule

40 mg/m^2 IV over 60 min every 2 weeks.

Special Precautions

1. Must be diluted to a concentration of 1 mg/ml with 5 percent dextrose for injection. Liposomal daunorubicin should be considered as an irritant and care should be taken to avoid extravasation.
2. Do not give if the patient has significantly impaired cardiac function.
3. Do not exceed a lifetime cumulative dose of 550 mg/m^2 (400 mg/m^2 if the patient was given prior chest radiotherapy).

   Patients with HIV may experience a decrease in left ventricular ejection fraction and congestive heart failure at lower doses than those without.
4. Reduce or hold dose in patients with impairment of liver function. A 25 percent dose reduction is recommended if the serum bilirubin is 1.2 to 3 mg/dl. One-half the normal dose is recommended in patients with serum bilirubin concentration greater than 3 mg/dl.

Toxicity

Effects that are a result of liposomal daunorubicin have been somewhat difficult to determine with certainty because most patients have been on several other agents that may cause marrow or other toxicity.

1. *Myelosuppression and other hematologic effects:* Common and dose-related. May be severe.
2. *Nausea, vomiting and other gastrointestinal effects:* Nausea, vomiting and diarrhea are common.
3. *Mucocutaneous effects:* Alopecia is occasional. Stomatitis is occasional.
4. *Miscellaneous effects:* These include the following:
   a. Cardiac events including cardiomyopathy or congestive heart failure may occur and are dose-dependent.
   b. Acute infusion-associated reactions with back pain, flushing and tightness in the chest and throat, alone or in combination, have occurred in approximately 14 percent of patients treated with liposomal daunorubicin. They usually occur with the first infusion and are not likely to occur later if the first infusion is given without a reaction. They generally occur during the first 5 min of the infusion and subside with interruption of the infusion. Some patients tolerate restarting at a lower rate of infusion. Most patients are able to continue therapy.
   c. Fatigue is common.
   d. Fever is common.
   e. Pain at the injection site is likely after extravasation.

DOCETAXEL

Other name: Taxotere.

Mechanism of Action

Enhanced formation and stability of microtubules. Antineoplastic effect may result from national tubules or altered tubulin-microtubule equilibrium arrest is seen and is associated with accumulated polymicrotubules.

Primary Indications

1. Carcinoma of the breast
2. Nonsmall cell lung cancer.

Usual Dosage and Schedule

1. 60 to 100 mg/m^2 as a 1 hour infusion every 3 weeks. Methasone 8 mg PO bid for 3 days starting 1 day prior to docetaxel should be given before each course of docetaxel to limit the frequency and severity of hypersensitivity reactions and to reduce the severity of fluid retention.
2. 35 mg/m^2 as a 1hour infusion weekly. Dexamethasone 8 mg PO bid. One day before and 10 mg IV 30 min before should be given before weeks 1 and 2 of docetaxel administration to limit the frequency and severity of hypersensitivity reactions. If there are no hypersensitivity reactions in the first 2 weeks, the oral doses given the day prior to docetaxel may be eliminated.

Special Precautions

1. Severe hypersensitivity reactions with flushing and hypotension with or without dyspnea occur in about 1 percent of patients (even when premedication is used).

2. Should be used with caution in patients with bilirubin above upper limit of normal or other abnormal liver function tests (greater than 1.5 times the upper limit of normal) because of more profound neutropenia.

Toxicity

1. *Myelosuppression and other hematologic effects:* Severe (grade 4) neutropenia is common and dose-related. Many patients have neutropenic fever.
2. *Nausea, vomiting and other gastrointestinal effects:* Nausea with or without vomiting is common but brief; severe episodes are uncommon. Mild diarrhea is common; severe diarrhea is rare.
3. *Mucocutaneous effects:* Mild mucositis is common; severe mucositis is uncommon. Alopecia is common. Mild-to-moderate cutaneous reactions such as maculopapular eruptions are common; severe reactions that may be associated with desquamation or bullous eruptions occur only occasionally if systemic prophylaxis is used. Mild-to-moderate nail changes are common, but severe onycholysis is uncommon.
4. *Hypersensitivity reactions:* Mild-to-moderate hypersensitivity reactions with flushing, hypotension (or rarely hypertension) with or without dyspnea, and drug fever are occasional with use of the prophylactic regimen recommended. Severe hypersensitivity reactions are uncommon.
5. *Miscellaneous effects:* These include the following:
   a. Fluid retention syndrome is common and cumulative (more commonly after four courses); can be reduced to occasional frequency (6%) by prophylactic steroids; may limit continuing therapy. May be associated with both pleural and pericardial effusions.
   b. Mild and reversible dysesthesias or paresthesias are common; more severe sensory neuropathies are uncommon.
   c. Reversible increases in transaminase, alkaline phosphatase and bilirubin.
   d. Local reaction comprises of reversible peripheral phlebitis.
   e. Fatigue, weakness (asthenia), and myalgia are common, arthralgia is occasional.
   f. Excessive tear formation secondary to anatomic narrowing of nasolacrimal duct is occasional to common.

DOXORUBICIN

Other names: ADR, Adriamycin, Rubex, Hydroxyl-daunorubicin (Fig. 2.11).

Mechanism of Action

DNA strand breakage mediated by anthracycline effects topoisomerase II, DNA intercalation, and DNA polymerase inhibition.

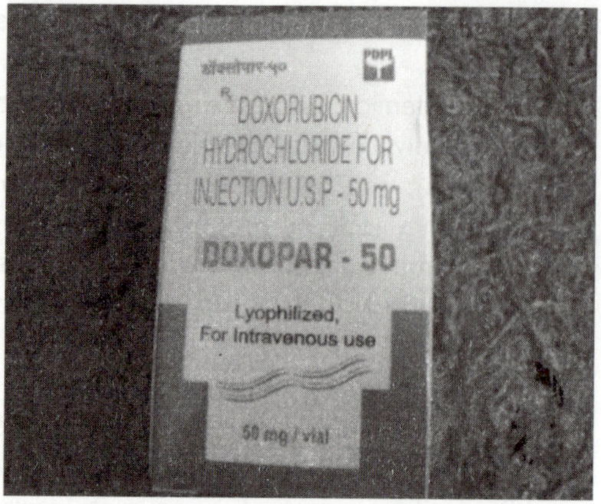

Fig. 2.11: Doxorubicin 200 mg

Primary Indications

1. Breast, bladder, liver, lung, prostate, stomach and thyroid carcinomas
2. Bone and soft tissue sarcomas
3. Hodgkin's and non-Hodgkin's lymphomas
4. Multiple myeloma
5. Acute lymphocytic and acute nonlymphocytic leukemias
6. Wilms' tumor, neuroblastoma and rhabdomyosarcoma of childhood.

Usual Dosage and Schedule

1. 60 to 75 mg/m^2 IV every 3 weeks (or as 96-hours continuous infusion).
2. 30 mg/m^2 IV on days 1 and 8 every 4 weeks (in combination with other drugs).
3. 9 mg/m^2 IV daily for 4 days as a continuous infusion (in myeloma).
4. 15 to 20 mg/m^2 IV weekly.
5. 50 to 60 mg instilled into the bladder weekly for 4 weeks, then every 4 weeks for 6 cycles.

Special Pre cautions

1. Administer over several minutes into the sidearm of a running IV infusion (except when given as a continuous infusion), taking care to avoid extravasation.
2. Do not give if patient has significantly impaired cardiac function (ejection fraction less than 45%), angina pectoris, cardiac arrhythmia or recent myocardial infarction.
3. Do not exceed a lifetime cumulative dose of 550 mg/m^2 (450 mg/m^2 if patient was given prior chest radiotherapy or concomitant cyclophosphamide) unless there are known risk modifiers such as continuous infusion, weekly dosing, or cardioprotective dexrazoxane and serial measurements of cardiac ejection fraction show minimal change and adequate function.
4. Reduce or hold dose if patient has impaired liver function.
   a. For serum bilirubin of 1.2 to 3.0 mg/dl, give one-half the normal dose.
   b. For serum bilirubin of more than 3.0 mg/dl, give one-fourth the normal dose.

Toxicity

1. *Myelosuppression and other hematologic effects:* Dose limiting for most patients. Nadir white blood cell and platelet counts occur at 10 to 14 days; recovery by day 21.

2. *Nausea, vomiting and other gastrointestinal effects:* Mild-to-moderate in about one-half of patients.
3. *Mucocutaneous effects:*
   a. Stomatitis that is dose-dependent.
   b. Alopecia beginning 2 to 5 weeks from start of therapy with recovery following completion of therapy is common.
   c. Recall of skin reaction due to prior radiotherapy is common.
   d. Severe local tissue damage possibly progressing to skin ulceration and necrosis, if SC extravasation occurs is common.
   e. Hyperpigmentation of skin overlying veins used for drug injection in which chemical phlebitis has occurred is common.
4. *Cardiac effects:* Potentially irreversible congestive heart failure may occur owing to cardiomyopathy. The incidence is highly dependent on the lifetime cumulative dose, which should not exceed 550 mg/m^2. This limit is lower (450 mg/m^2) if patient has received prior chest radiotherapy or is taking cyclophosphamide concomitantly. Weekly schedule and 96-hours infusions are less cardiotoxic and higher cumulative doses may be tolerable. Congestive heart failure may be predicated by serial measurement of left ventricular function or endomyocardial biopsy. Discontinue drug if there is clinical congestive heart failure or if the ejection fraction falls on the radionuclide angiogram:
   a. To less than 45 percent or
   b. To less than 50 percent if the total decrease is 10 percent or more (e.g. falls from 59 – 49%). If repeat ejection fraction determination shows return of function, drug may be cautiously restarted, but ejection fraction determination should be done before each dose. Transient electrocardiographic changes are common and are not usually serious.
5. *Miscellaneous effects:* These include the following:
   a. Red urine caused by drug and its metabolities is common.
   b. Chemical phlebitis and phlebosclerosis of veins used for injection are common, particularly if a vein is used repeatedly.
   c. Fever, chills and urticaria are uncommon.

DOXORUBICIN, LIPOSOMAL

Other name: Doxil.

Mechanism of Action

Doxorubicin, liposomal, which is designed to be protected from removal by the reticuloendothelial system, has a prolonged circulation time compared with unprotected drug. The agent penetrates tumor tissue and releases the active ingredient doxorubicin. The active drug causes DNA strand breakage mediated by anthracycline effects on topoisomerase II, DNA intercalation, and DNA polymerase inhibition.

Primary Indications

1. Advanced Kaposi's sarcoma, associated with HIV

2. Ovarian carcinoma
3. Multiple myeloma.

Usual Dosage and Schedule

1. 20 mg/m^2 IV infusion at a rate of 1 mg/min for 5 the first dose, then over 30 min for subsequent doses every 2 to 3 weeks for Kaposi's sarcoma.
2. 40 to 50 mg/m^2 IV infusion at a rate of 1 mg/min for the first dose, then over 1 hour every 4 weeks for ovarian carcinoma.
3. 40 mg/m^2 IV infusion at a rate of 1 mg/min for the first dose, then over 1 hour every 4 weeks for multiple myeloma, together with vincristine and dexamethasone.

Special Precautions

1. Must be diluted in 250 ml of 5 percent dextrose for injection. Liposomal doxorubicin is not a vesicant but should be considered as an irritant.
2. Initial doses should be given at a rate of 1 mg/min to avoid infusion reactions.

Toxicity

Effects that are a result of liposomal doxorubicin have been somewhat difficult to determine with certainly because most patients have been on several other agents that may cause marrow or other toxicity. Some of the toxic effects are as follows:

1. *Myelosuppression and other hematologic effects:* Common and dose-related. May be severe.
2. *Nausea, vomiting and other gastrointestinal effects:* Nausea and vomiting are common at the higher doses. Constipation is occasional. Diarrhea is occasional. Anorexia is occasional.
3. *Mucocutaneous effects:* Palmar-Plantar erythrodysesthesia is common at the higher doses and is occasionally severe. May be reduced by celecoxib 100 to 200 mg PO bid. Stomatitis is common. Alopecia is occasional. Rash is occasional to common.
4. *Miscellaneous effects:* These include the following:
   a. Cardiac events, including cardiomyopathy or congestive heart failure, occur in 5 to 10 percent of patients treated. This is dose-dependent and not adequately tested, but appears to be less common than with unincapsulated drug.
   b. Acute infusion-associated reactions with flushing, shortness of breath, facial swelling, headache, chills, back pain, tightness in the chest and throat, or hypotension, alone or in combination, have occurred in approximately 7 percent of patients treated with liposomal doxorubicin. They usually occur with the first infusion and are not likely to occur later if the first infusion is given without a raction. Most resolve over the course of several hours to a day.
   c. Asthenia is occasional.
   d. Fever is occasional.
   e. Pain at the inmnjection site is likely after extravasation.

EPIRUBICIN

Other names: Ellence, 4- Epi-doxorubicin, EPI (Fig. 2.12).

Mechanism of Action

DNA strand breakage, mediated by anthracycline effects on topoisomerase II.

Primary Indications

1. Carcinomas of the breast, esophagus, lung, ovary and stomach
2. Hodgkin's and non-Hodgkin's lymphoma
3. Soft tissue sarcomas.

Usual Dosage and Schedule

70 to 90 mg/m^2 IV every 3 weeks administered through the sidearm of a freely flowing IV infusion.

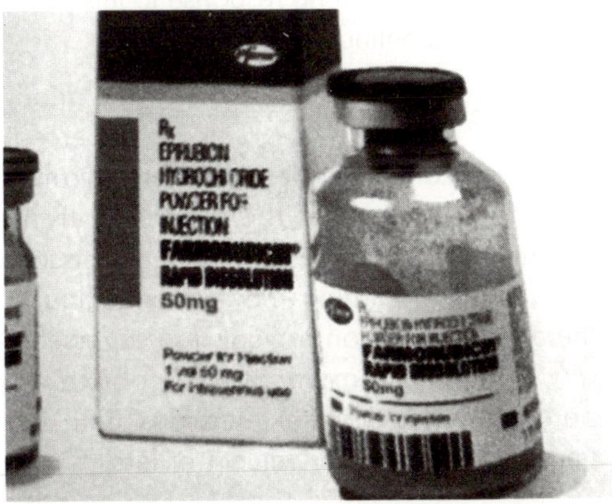

Fig. 2.12: Epirubicin 50 mg

Special Precautions

1. Take care to avoid extravasation.
2. Do not exceed a lifetime cumulative dose of 900 mg/m^2 (use a lesser dose for patients with prior chest radiotherapy or prior anthracycline or anthracenedione therapy).
3. Reduce or hold dose if patient has impaired liver function.

For serum bilirubin of 1.2 to 3.0 mg/dl, give one-fourth the normal dose.

1. *Myelosuppression and other hematologic effects:* Dose- limiting leukopenia with recovery by day 21.
2. *Nausea, vomiting and other gastrointestinal effects:* Nausea and vomiting are common. Diarrhea and abdominal pain are occasional.
3. *Mucocutaneous effects:*
   a. Stomatitis that is dose-dependent.
   b. Alopecia, beginning approximately 10 days after the first treatment, with regrowth when cessation of drug treatment occurs, is common but not universal (25–50%).
   c. Flushes, skin and nail hyperpigmentation, photosensitivity and hypersensitivity to irradiated skin (radiation recall reaction) have been observed.
   d. Severe local tissue damage possibly progressing to skin ulceration and necrosis, if SC extravasation occurs, is common.
4. *Cardiac effects:*
   a. Potentially irreversible congestive heart failure may occur owing to cardiomyopathy. The incidence depends on the lifetime

dose, which should not exceed 900 mg/m^2. This limit is lower if patient has received prior chest radiotherapy or prior anthracycline or anthracenedione therapy. Congestive heart failure may be predicted by serial measurement of left ventricular function or endomyocardial biopsy.

b. Transient electrocardiographic changes are similar in type and frequency to those observed after doxorubicin.

5. *Miscellaneous effects:*
   a. Red-orange urine for 24 hours after injection owing to drug and its metabolites is common.
   b. Urticaria and anaphylaxis have been reported in patients treated with epirubicin; signs and symptoms of these reactions may vary from skin rash and pruritus to fever, chills and shock.

EPOETIN

Other names: Recombinant human erythropoietin (rHuEPO), EPO, Epoetin-alfa, Epogen, Procrit.

Mechanism of Action

Epoetin-alfa is a recombinant glycoprotein that contains 165 amino acids in a sequence identical to that of endogenous human erythropoietin. It has the same biologic activity, inducing erythropoiesis by stimulating the division and differentiation of committed erythroid progenitor cells.

Primary Indications

1. Anemia from chemotherapy in patients with nonmyeloid malignancies
2. Anemia associated with malignancy, as in multiple myeloma or anemia of chronic disease
3. Anemia associated with chronic renal failure
4. Anemia associated with zidovudine therapy in HIV-infected patients.

Usual Dosage and Schedule

1. Starting dose is 150 U/kg SC three times a week. The dose may be escalated to 300 U/kg SC three times a week, after a 4 to 8 week trial at the initial dose, in patients who have not responded satisfactorily.
2. Alternative dose is 40000 U SC once weekly. If there is no response after 4 to 8 weeks, the dose may be increased to 60000.

   USC once weekly. If no response to this dose, it should be discontinued.

Special Precautions

1. Contraindicated in patients with uncontrolled hypertension or known hypersensitivity to albumin or mammalian cell derived products.
2. Iron supplementation may be beneficial if there is any question of body iron stores. If at any time the hematocrit rises above 40 percent, hold epoetin injections until the hematocrit falls to 36 percent or less.

Toxicity

1. *Myelosuppression and other hematologic effects:* The therapeutic effect is an increase in hemoglobin, and no myelosuppression is to be expected. Rarely, it may induce pure red cell aplasia with associated neutralizing antierythropoietin antibodies.
2. *Nausea and vomiting:* None.
3. *Mucocutaneous effects:* Rare rashes or hives.
4. *Miscellaneous effects:* These are as follows:
   a. Improved energy level, activity level, and self-rated quality of-life scores occur in patients receiving therapy.
   b. Edema is occasional.
   c. Diarrhea is occasional.
   d. A rise in blood pressure occurs in about 25 percent of patients. Hypertension may rarely occur in association with a significant increase in hematocrit; the risk is greatest in patients with pre-existing hypertension. Chest pain is uncommon; edema is occasional.
   e. Seizures are rare.
   f. Influenza-like syndrome is rare to uncommon. Fever alone is occasional.
   g. Thrombotic complications are uncommon.

ESTROGENS

Other names: Diethylstilbestrol (DES), Chlorotrianisene (TACE), Diethylstilbestrol diphosphate (Stiplphostrol) and others.

Mechanism of Action

Suppression of testosterone production via negative feedback on hypothalamus.

Primary Indication

Prostate carcinoma.

Usual Dosage and Schedule

1. DES 1 to 3 mg PO daily.
2. Chlorotrianisene 12 to 25 mg PO daily.
3. Diethylstilbestrol diphosphate 500 to 1000 mg IV daily for 5 to 7 days, then 250 to 500 mg IV one or two times weekly.

Special Precautions

1. Acute filuid retention and pulmonary edema are possible, particularly with high-dose IV therapy.
2. Hypercalcemia may occur with initial therapy.

Toxicity

1. *Myelosuppression and other hematologic effects:* None.
2. *Nausea, vomiting and other gastrointestinal effects:* Nausea with possible vomiting is common at the beginning of therapy but diminishes or stops with continued treatment. Severity may be lessened by beginning treatment with doses lower than those recommended. Diarrhea is uncommon.
3. *Mucocutaneous effects:* Darkening of nipples is common.
4. *Miscellaneous effects:* These are as follows:
   a. Peripheral edema due to sodium retention is common, but congestive heart failure occurs in fewer than 5 percent of patients.
   b. Any patient taking estrogens may be at higher risk than normal for

thromboembolism. An increase in cardiovascular deaths has been seen in male patients given DES at 5 mg daily for prostate carcinoma.

c. Increased bone pain, tumor pain and local disease flare are associated with both good tumor response and tumor progression.
d. Feminization occurs in male patients.

ETOPOSIDE

Other names: Epipodophyllotoxin, VP-16, VP-16-213, VePesid, Etopophos (etoposide phosphate) (Fig. 2.13).

Mechanism of action

Interaction with topoisomerase II produces single-strand breaks in DNA. It arrests cells in late S or G2 phase.

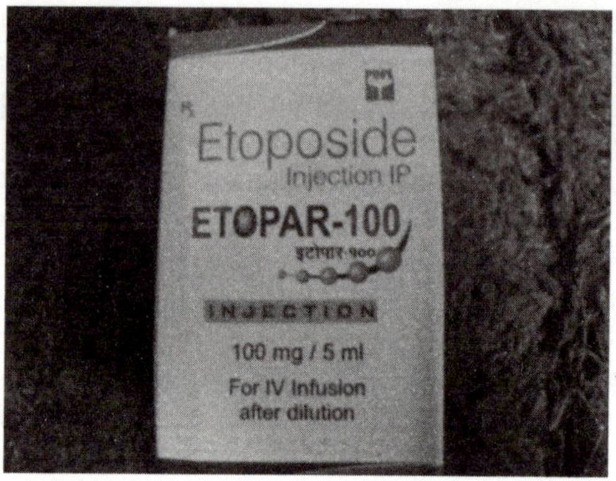

Fig. 2.13: Etoposide injection

Primary Indications

1. Small cell anaplastic and nonsmall cell lung carcinomas
2. Stomach carcinoma
3. Germ cell cancers
4. Lymphomas
5. Acute leukemia
6. Neuroblastoma.

Usual Dosage and Schedule

1. 120 mg/m^2 IV on days 1 to 3 every 3 weeks.
2. 50 to 100 mg/m^2 IV on days 1 to 5 every 2 to 4 weeks.
3. 125 to 140 mg/m^2 IV on days 1, 3 and 5 every 3 to 5 weeks.
4. 50 mg/m^2 PO daily for 21 days. Repeat after 1 to 2 weeks of rest.
5. High-dose therapy (750–2,400 mg/m^2) is investigational and should be used only with progenitor cell rescue (e.g. bone marrow or peripheral blood stem cell transplantation).

Special Precautions

1. Administer etoposide as a 30 to 60 min infusion to avoid severe hypotension. Monitor blood pressure during infusion. Etoposide phosphate may be administered as a 5-min bolus infusion.
2. Take care to avoid extravasation.
3. Etoposide must be diluted in 20 to 50 volumes (100–250 ml) of isotonic saline before use.

Etoposide phosphate vials (100 mg) may be reconstituted in 5 to 10 ml (water, saline, or dextrose) to a concentration of 10 or 20 mg/ml.

4. Decrease dose by 50 percent for bilirubin levels of 1, 5 to 3 mg/dl, decrease by 75 percent for bilirubin levels of 3 to 5 mg/dl, discontinue drug if bilirubin level is above 5 mg/dl.
5. Decrease dose by 25 percent for creatinine clearance rate of less than 30 ml/min.

Toxicity

1. *Myelosuppression and other hematologic effects:* Dose-limiting leukopenia and less severe thrombocytopenia have a nadir at 16 days with recovery by days 20 to 22.
2. *Nausea, vomiting and other gastrointestinal effects:* Usually mild to moderate nausea and vomiting in about one-third of patients receiving standard doses, common with high-dose therapy. Anorexia is common. Diarrhea is uncommon.
3. *Mucocutaneous effects:*
   a. Alopecia is common.
   b. Stomatitis is uncommon with standard-doses and common with high-dose therapy.
   c. Painful rash may occur with high-dose therapy.
   d. Chemical phlebitis is occasional.
4. *Miscellaneous effects:*
   a. Hepatotoxicity is rare
   b. Peripheral neurotoxicity is rare
   c. Allergic reaction is rare
   d. Hemorrhagic cystitis may occur with high-dose therapy.

FILGRASTIM

Other names: Granulocyte colony-stimulating factor, G-CSF, Neupogen (Figs 2.14 and 2.15).

Mechanism of Action

Recombinant human G-CSF. Promotes growth and differentiation of myeloid progenitor cells. May improve survival and funetion of granulocytes.

Primary Indications

1. Prophylaxis of granulocytopenia secondary to intensive chemotherapy.

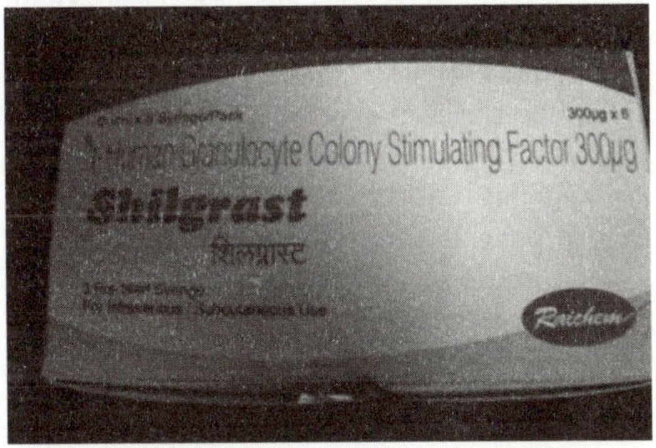

Fig. 2.14

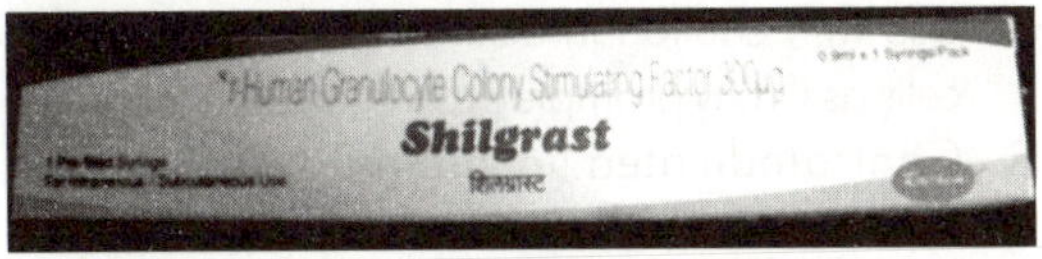

Fig. 2.15

Figs 2.14 and 2.15: Filgrastim 300 µg

2. Treatment of granulocytopenia secondary to chemotherapy.
3. Granulocytopenia from primary marrow disorders such as idiopathic neutropenia and aplastic anemia and myelodysplastic syndrome.
4. Granulocytopenia associated with AIDS and its therapy.

Usual Dosage and Schedule

1. *Adjunct to chemotherapy:* Commonly 200 to 400 μg/m² (5–10 μg/kg) SC daily, starting no sooner than 24 hours and no later than 4 days after the last dose of chemotherapy, for 10 to 20 days until the neutrophil count exceeds 10,000/Ml after the expected nadir. Because of cost factors, vial size, and comparability of effect with "ballpark" doses, some physicians choose to treat patients weighing less than 75 kg with 300 μg daily and patients weighing more than 75 kg with 480 μg daily.
2. *Other purposes:* 40 to 500 mg/m² SC, IM, or IV daily. Dose and duration are dependent on the purpose of administration.

Special Precautions

1. Use with caution in disorders of myeloid stem cells as it may promote growth of leukemic cells.
2. Contraindicated in patients with known hypersensitivity to *E. coli*-derived proteins.

Toxicity

1. *Myelosuppression and other hematologic effects:* None (leukocytosis).
2. *Nausea, vomiting and other gastrointestinal effects:* Rare to uncommon.
3. *Mucocutaneous effects:* Exacerbation of pre-existing dermatologic conditions is occasional; pyoderma gangrenosum is rare.
4. *Miscellaneous effects:* Usually mild and short-lived.
   a. Bone pain, musculoskeletal symptoms such as cramps and back or leg pain are common.
   b. Splenomegaly with prolonged use. Rarely has been associated with splenic rupture.
   c. Exacerbation of pre-existing inflammatory or autoimmune disorders is rare.
   d. Mild elevation of lactate dehydrogenase and alkaline phosphatase.
   e. Allergic-type reactions may occur, including urticaria and anaphylaxis.
   f. Adult respiratory distress syndrome has been reported in neutropenic patients.

FLUDARABINE

Other names: FAMP, Fludara.

Mechanism of Action

Inhibition of DNA polymerase and ribonucleotide reductase.

Primary Indications

1. Chronic lymphocytic leukemia
2. Macroglobulinemia
3. Indolent lymphomas
4. Acute leukemia (in combination).

Usual Dosage and Schedule

25 mg/m^2 IV as a 30 min inusion daily for 5 days. Other dose schedules, usually less intensive, have been used, often in combinations with other drugs. Repeat every 4 weeks.

Special Precautions

1. If there is the potential for tumorlysis syndrome, administer allopurinol and ensure good hydration and close clinical monitoring.
2. Transfusion-associated graft-versus-host disease may be seen. Therefore, prior irradiation of blood products for transfusion in patients at risk is recommended.
3. Reduce dose by 20 percent for Ccr 30 to 70 ml/m; do not treat if Ccr <30 ml/m.

Toxicity

1. *Myelosuppression and other hematologic effects:*
   Granulocytopenia and thrombocytopenia are common, and may be severe, cumulative, and prolonged infection, particularly pneumonia, is common during early courses and uncommon after the sixth course.
2. *Nausea, vomiting and other gastrointestinal effects:* Common (30%) but not usually severe. Diarrhea is occasional.
3. *Mucocutaneous effects:* Occasional mucositis, rash, no alopecia.
4. *Neurotoxicity:* Uncommon at usual dosage. Somnolence or fatigue, paresthesias and twitching of extremities may be seen.
   Severe neurologic symptoms including visual disturbances have been common at higher doses than those recommended.
5. *Immunosuppression:* Common. Usually seen as a depression in CD4 and CD8 lymphocyte counts. Opportunistic infections may result, and many recommend pneumocystic pneumonia prophylaxis until the CD4 lymphopenia resolves.
6. *Miscellaneous effects:*
   a. Abnormal liver or renal function is rare
   b. Severe pulmonary toxicity is occasional
   c. Edema is occasional
   d. Tumorlysis syndrome is rare.

FLUOROURACIL

Other names: 5-FU, Adrucil, Efudex, Fluoroplex, 5-fluorouracil.

Mechanism of action

A pyrimidine antimetabolite that, when converted to the active nucleotide, inhibits the enzyme thymidylate synthetase and thereby blocks DNA synthesis.

Primary Indications

1. Breast, colorectal, anal, stomach, pancreas, esophagus, liver, head and neck and bladder carcinomas.
2. Actinic keratosis; basal and squamous cell carcinomas of skin (topically).

Usual Dosage and Schedule

1. *Systemic:*
   a. 500 mg/m^2 IV on days 1 to 5 every 4 weeks or
   b. 450 to 600 mg/m^2 IV weekly.
   c. 200 to 400 mg/m^2 daily as a continuous IV infusion.
   d. 1,000 mg/m^2 daily for 4 days as a continuous IV infusion every 3 to 4 weeks.
   e. Leucovorin 20 mg/m^2 IV is followed by fluorouracil 425 mg/m^2 IV. The combination is given daily for 5 days. Courses are repeated every 4 weeks.
2. *Intracavitary:* 500 to 1,000 mg for pericardial effusion; 2,000 to 3,000 mg for pleural or peritoneal effusions.
3. *Intraarterial (liver):* 800 to 1,200 mg/m^2 as a continuous infusion on days 1 to 4, followed by 600 mg/m^2 as a continuous infusion on days 5 to 21.
4. *Topically:* Apply solution or cream twice daily. Use only 5 percent strength for carcinomas.

Special Precautions

1. Reduce dose in patients with compromised liver function.
2. For intraarterial infusion, add 5,000 U of heparin to 1 L of 5 percent dextrose in water together with the daily dose of fluorouracil. The catheter position should be checked with dye injection every few days to ensure that it has not moved and that the hepatic artery has not thrombosed. Ulcer-like pain or other significant gastrointestinal symptoms are indications to discontinue intraarterial therapy, as hemorrhage or perforation may occur.
3. Precipitation may occur when leucovorin and fluorouracil are mixed in the same bag.

Toxicity

1. *Myelosuppression and other hematologic effects:* Dose limiting with a nadir at 10 to 14 days after the last dose and recovery by 21 days.
2. *Nausea, vomiting and other gastrointestinal effects:* Nausea and vomiting may occur but are not usually severe. Diarrhea is common with higher doses, continuous infusion, or when used in combination with leucovorin and irinotecan. Esophagitis and proctitis may also occur.
3. *Mucocutaneous effects:* Some of them are as follows:
   a. Stomatitis is an early sign of severe toxicity. It progresses from soreness and erythema to frank ulceration, which becomes hemorrhagic in a small number of patients.
   b. Partial alopecia is uncommon.
   c. Hyperpigmentation of skin over face, hands, and the veins used for infusion is occasional.

   d. Maculopapular rash is uncommon.
   e. Sun exposure tends to increase skin reactions.
   f. "Hand and foot syndrome" with painful erythematous desquamation and fissures of palms and soles is common with continuous infusion and occasional with other schedules or combinations.
4. *Miscellaneous effects:* These include the following:
   a. Neurotoxicity including headache, minor visual disturbances and cerebellar ataxia is rare.
   b. Increased lacrimation is uncommon.
   c. Cardiac toxicity including arrhythmias, angina, ischemia, and sudden death is rare. It may be more common with continuous infusion and previous history of coronary artery disease.
   d. Hypertriglyceridemia when given in combination with levamisole.

FLUTAMIDE

Other name: Eulexin.

Mechanism of Action

Competitive inhibitor of androgens at the cellular androgen receptor in the prostate cancer cells.

Primary Indication

Carcinoma of the prostate, most often in combination with luteinizing hormone-releasing hormone agonists.

Usual Dosage and Schedule

250 mg PO every 8 hours.

Special Precaution

Serum transaminase levels should be measured prior to starting treatment with flutamide. Flutamide is not recommended in patients whose serum transaminase valuses exceed twice the upper limit of normal.

Toxicity

1. *Myelosuppression and other hematologic effects:* None.
2. *Nausea, vomiting and other gastrointestinal effects:* Nausea and vomiting are uncommon to occasional. Diarrhea, flatulence and mild abdominal pain are common.
3. *Mucocutaneous effects:* Mild skin rash is occasional.
4. *Miscellaneous effects:* These include the following:
   a. Secondary pharmacologic effects including breast tenderness, breast swelling, hot flashes, impotence, and loss of libido are common but reversible after cessation of therapy.
   b. Elevated liver function tests are uncommon; liver failure is rare but may be preceded by flu-like symptoms or right upper quadrant pain and tenderness.
   c. Hypertension is occasional.
   d. Adverse cardiovascular events are similar to those seen with orchiectomy.

FULVESTRANT

Other name: Faslodex.

Mechanism of Action

An estrogen receptor antagonist that binds to the estrogen receptor in a competitive manner. It down regulates the estrogen receptor protein in human breast cancer cells. This is associated with a dose-related decrease in the expression of the progesterone receptor and a decrease in the Ki67 labeling index, a marker for cell proliferation. *In vitro* demonstration of reversible inhibition of the growth of tamoxifen-resistant as well as estrogen-sensitive human breast cancer cell lines.

Primary Indication

Hormone receptor-positive metastatic breast cancer in postmenopausal women with disease progression following antiestrogen therapy. (There are no efficacy data for premenopausal women with advanced breast cancer).

Usual Dosage and Schedule

250 mg IM (into the buttock[s]) as either a single 5 ml injection or two concurrent 2.5 ml injections, repeated once monthly.

Special Precaution

Safety has not been evaluated in patients with moderate to severe hepatic impairment.

Toxicity

1. *Myelosuppression and other hematologic effects:* Anemia is rare.
2. *Nausea, vomiting and other gastrointestinal effects:* Nausea is common; vomiting, constipation, diarrhea, and anorexia are occasional.
3. *Mucocutaneous effects:* Rash and increased sweating are occasional.
4. *Miscellaneous effects:*
   a. For the body as a whole, headache, back pain, abdominal pain, injection site pain and pelvic pain are occasional. Occasional patients also experience a flu-like syndrome or fever.
   b. Vasodilation is occasional (18%).
   c. Dizziness, insomnia, paresthesias, depression and anxiety are uncommon to occasional.
   d. Pharyngitis, dyspnea and increased cough are occasional.

GEFITINIB

Other names: Iressa, ZD1839 (Fig. 2.16).

Mechanism of Action

Selectively inhibits tyrosine kinase activity of the epidermal growth factor receptor (EGFR). Epidermal growth factor receptor tyrosine kinase inhibition by gefitinib impairs epidermal growth factor-stimulated autophosphorylation and thus blocks growth signals within the cell.

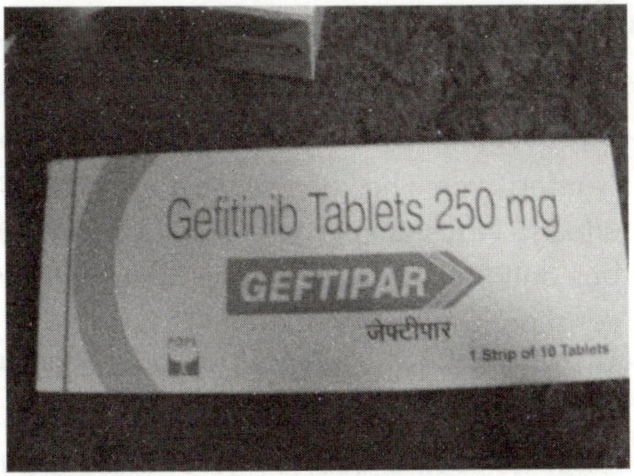

Fig. 2.16: Gefitinib tablet

Primary Indication

Carcinoma of the lung, 2, other carcinomas expressing EGFR.

Usual Dosage and Schedule

1. 250 to 500 mg daily.
2. 250 to 500 mg daily for 14 consecutive days every 4 weeks.

Special Precaution

Diarrhea may be dose limiting and require discontinuation of the drug.

Toxicity

1. *Myelosuppression and other hematologic effects:* Uncommon, except for anemia, which is occasional and not dose-related.
2. *Nausea, vomiting and other gastrointestinal effects:* Nausea, vomiting and diarrhea are common. Diarrhea may be dose limiting. Anorexia, constipation and abdominal pain are also common but usually not severe.
3. *Mucocutaneous effects:* Acne-like or folliculitis-type rash is common, usually appearing by day 14; frequency and severity are dose-related. May be associated with dry skin and itching. Rash usually does not worsen with continued treatment and resolves within a week of discontinuation of the drug. Dry mouth and conjunctivitis are occasional.
4. *Miscellaneous effects:*
   a. Dyspnea is occasional to common
   b. Asthenia is common
   c. Headache is occasional
   d. Somnolence is occasional
   e. Elevated hepatic transaminases are occasional but may be severe (grade 3 or 4).

GEMCITABINE

Other name: Gemzar (Fig. 2.17).

Mechanism of Action

After being metabolized intracellularly to the active diphosphate and triphosphate nucleotides, gemcitabine, a cytidine analog, inhibits ribonucleotide reductase and competes with deoxycytidine triphosphate for incorporation into DNA.

Primary Indications

1. Carcinoma of the pancreas, locally advanced or metastatic

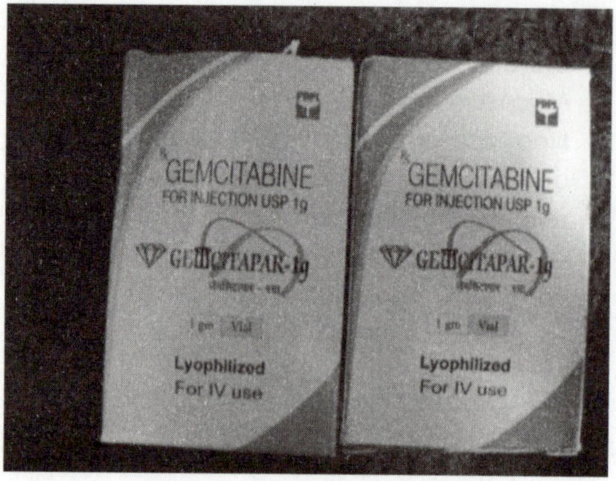

Fig. 2.17: Gemcitabine injection 1 g

2. Nonsmall cell carcinoma of the lung
3. Carcinomas of the breast, bladder and ovary.

Usual Dosage and Schedule

1. 1,000 mg/m^2 IV over 30 min once weekly for up to 7 weeks when used as a single agent. After 1 week of rest, subsequent cycles are given once weekly for 3 consecutive weeks out of 4.
2. 1,000 to 1,250 mg/m^2 IV over 30 min once weekly for 2 or 3 successive weeks during each 3 to 4 week cycle, when used in combination in lung cancer.

Special Precaution

Prolongation of infusion time beyond 60 min increases toxicity.

Toxicity

1. *Myelosuppression and other hematologic effects:* Myelosuppression is dose-related and common.
2. *Nausea, vomiting, and other gastrointestinal effects:* Nausea and vomiting are common but only occasionally severe. Diarrhea and constipation are occasional to common.
3. *Mucocutaneous effects:* Rash, alopecia, and mucositis are occasional.
4. *Miscellaneous effects:* Some of these are as follows:
   a. Transient elevations of serum transaminases and alkaline phosphatase are common
   b. Mild proteinuria and hematuria are common
   c. Hemolytic-uremic syndrome is rare (0.25%)
   d. Fever without documented infection is common
   e. Mild paresthesias are occasional
   f. Dyspnea is occasional.

HYDROXYUREA

Other names: Hydrea, Mycocel (Fig. 2.18).

Mechanism of Action

Interferes with DNA synthesis, at least in part by inhibiting the enzymatic conversion of ribonucleotides to deoxyribonucleotides.

Primary Indications

1. Head and neck carcinomas.

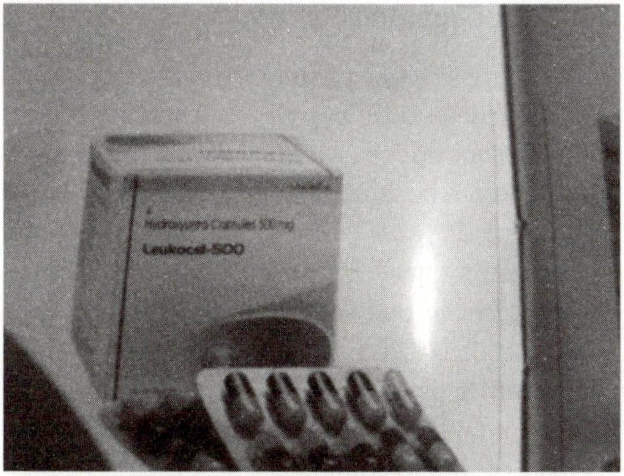

Fig. 2.18: Hydroxyurea 500 mg capsules

2. Chronic granulocytic (myelogenous) leukemia, acute lymphocytic and acute nonlymphocytic leukemia with high blast counts.
3. Essential thrombocythemia.
4. Polycythemia rubra vera.
5. Prevention of retinoic acid syndrome in acute promyelocytic leukemia.

Usual Dosage and Schedule

1. 800 to 2,000 mg/m^2 PO as a single or divided daily dose or
2. 3,200 mg/m^2 PO as a single dose every third day (not for leukemias).

Special Precaution

The daily dose must be adjusted for blood count trends. Be careful not to change dose too often because there is a delay in response.

Toxicity

1. *Myelosuppression and other hematologic effects:* Occurs at doses of more than 1,600 mg/m^2 daily by day 10. Recovery is usually prompt. Increased red cell mean corpuscular volume is common.
2. *Nausea, vomiting and other gastrointestinal effects:* Nausea is common at high doses. Other gastrointestinal symptoms are uncommon.
3. *Mucocutaneous effects:* Stomatitis is rare. Maculopapular rash may be seen. Inflammation of mucous membrane caused by radiation may be exaggerated.
4. *Miscellaneous effects:* Some of these are as follows:
   a. Temporary renal function impairment or dysuria is uncommon
   b. CNS disturbances are rare
   c. May be leukemogenic.

IFOSFAMIDE

Other name: Ifex (Fig. 2.19).

Mechanism of Action

Metabolic activation by microsomal liver enzymes produces biologically active intermediates that attack nucleophilic sites, particularly on DNA.

Primary Indications

1. Testicular and lung cancers
2. Bone and soft tissue sarcomas
3. Lymphoma.

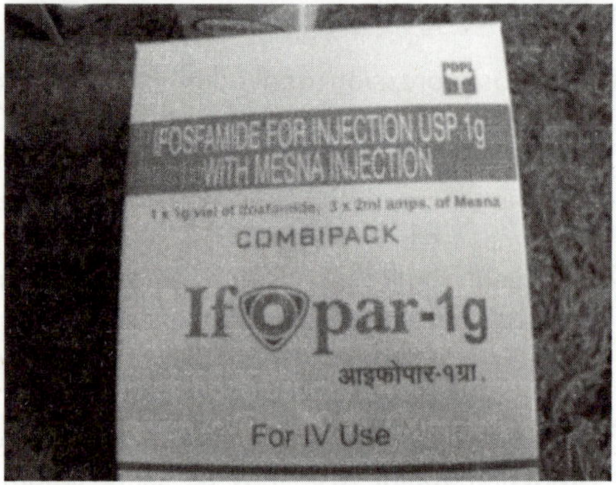

Fig. 2.19: Ifosfamide injection

Special Precaution

Must be used with mesna to prevent hemorrhagic cystitis. Mesna dose is at least 20 percent of the ifosfamide dose (on a weight basis), administered just prior to (or mixed with) the ifosfamide dose and again at 4 and 8 hours after the ifosfamide to detoxify the urinary metabolites that cause the hemorrhagic cystitis. Higher doses of ifosfamide may require higher doses and longer durations of mesna.

Neither mesna nor its only metabolite, mesna disulfide, affects ifosfamide or its antineoplastic metabolites. Mesna disulfide is reduced in the kidney to a free thiol compound, which then reacts chemically with urotoxic metabolites resulting in their detoxification. Vigorous hydration is also required with a minimum of 2 l of oral or IV hydration daily. Administer as a slow IV infusion over a period of at least 30 min.

Usual Dosage and Schedule

1. 12 g/m^2 IV over 30 min or more daily for 5 consecutive days every 3 or 4 weeks, usually with other agents. Mesna 120 mg/m^2 is given just before ifosfamide, then mesna 1,200 mg/m^2 as a daily continuous infusion is given until 16 hours after the last dose of ifosfamide.
2. 3.6 g/m^2 IV daily as a 4 hours infusion for 2 consecutive days, usually with other agents. Mesna is given at a dose of 750 mg/m^2 IV just prior to and at 4 and 8 hours after the start of the ifosfamide.
3. Higher dosage schedules have been used experimentally with up to 14 g/m^2 being used per course over a 6 day period, with equal or greater doses of mesna.

Toxicity

1. *Myelosuppression and other hematologic effects:* Dose limiting. Platelets are relatively spared. Granulocyte nadirs are commonly reached at 10 to 14 days and recovery is seen by day 21. Thrombocytopenia may be seen with higher doses.
2. *Nausea, vomiting and other gastrointestinal effects:* Common without standard antiemetics.
3. *Mucocutaneous effects:* Alopecia is common; mucositis is rarely seen at standard doses; dermatitis is rare.
4. *Hemorrhagic cystitis:* Common and dose limiting unless a uroprotective agent such as mesna is used. With mesna, the incidence of hemorrhagic cystitis is 5 to 10 percent, and

gross hematuria is uncommon. Increasing the duration of mesna may alleviate the problem during subsequent cycles.

5. *Miscellaneous effects:*
   a. CNS toxicity (somnolence, confusion, depressive psychosis, hallucinations, disorientation and uncommonly seizures, cranial nerve dysfunction, or coma) is occasional with doses in the lower range and more common with larger doses.
   b. Infertility is common in men and women, as with other alkylating agents.
   c. Renal impairment is occasional to common. Fanconi syndrome is dependent on dose. May be associated with severe acidosis.
   d. Liver dysfunction is uncommon.
   e. Phlebitis is uncommon.
   f. Fever is rare.
   g. Peripheral neuropathy with high-dose therapy is uncommon.

IMATINIB MESYLATE

Other names: Gleevec, STI-571 (signal transduction inhibitor 571) (Fig. 2.20).

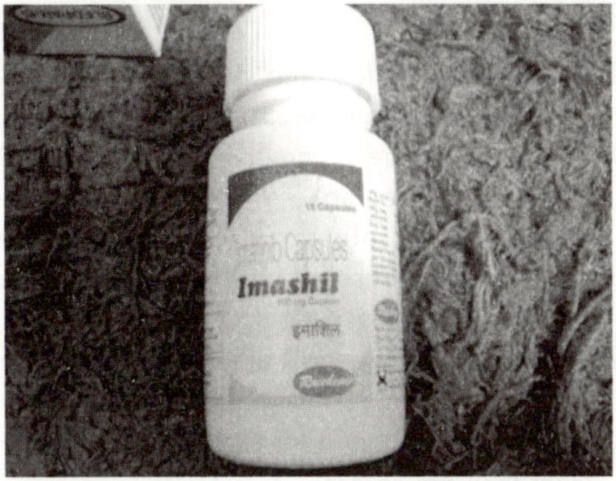

Fig. 2.20: Imashil

Mechanism of Action

Inhibitor of the constitutively activated Bcr- Abl tyrosine kinase that is created as a consequence of the (9;22) chromosomal translocation and is required for the transforming function and excess proliferation seen in chronic myelogenous leukemia. It also inhibits platelet-derived growth factor receptor tyrosine kinase and c-Kit tyrosine kinase, the latter of which is activated in gastrointestinal stromal tumors.

Primary Indications

1. Chronic myelogenous leukemia (newly diagnosed) in chronic phase; after failure of interferon-a; or in the accelerated or the blast phase of the disease.
2. Gastrointestinal stromal tumor.

Usual Dosage and Schedule

1. 400 to 600 mg PO daily in the chronic phase of chronic myelogenous leukemia or gastrointestinal stromal tumors.
2. 600 to 800 mg PO daily in the accelerated phase or blast crisis.

Special Precaution

None.

Toxicity

1. *Myelosuppression and other hematologic effects:* Moderate neutropenia and thrombocytopenia are common in all phases, but severe neutropenia or thrombocytopenia is uncommon unless patients are in the accelerated phase or blast crisis of chronic myelogenous leukemia.
2. *Nausea, vomiting and other gastrointestinal effects:* Nausea, vomiting abdominal pain and diarrhea are common, but it is uncommon that they are severe.
3. *Mucocutaneous effects:* Skin rash is common; pruritus and petechiae are occasional.
4. *Miscellaneous effects:* These include the following:
   a. Fluid retention and edema are common. Pleural effusion and ascites are uncommon.
   b. Musculoskeletal pain or cramps, arthralgia, headache, fever and fatigue are common, but it is uncommon that they are severe or life-threatening.
   c. Dyspnea and cough are occasional.
   d. Elevated liver function tests or serum creatinine are uncommon to rare. Rare cases of severe hepatotoxicity have been seen.

INTERFERON-α

Other names: Roferon-A (interferon alpha-2a, recombinant alpha A interferon), Intron A (interferon alpha-2h, recombinant alpha-2 interferon).

Mechanism of Action

Believed to involve direct inhibition of tumor cell growth and modulation of the immune response of the host, including activation of natural killer cells, modulation of antibody production and induction of major histocompatibility antigens.

Primary Indications

1. Chronic myelogenous leukemia
2. Melanoma (both as adjuvant and metastatic disease therapy)
3. Non-Hodgkin's lymphoma (low grade), mycosis fungoides
4. Multiple myeloma
5. Hairy-cell leukemia
6. Renal-cell carcinoma
7. Other carcinomas in combination with chemotherapy (e.g. fluorouracil in colon carcinoma)
8. Kaposi's sarcoma, associated with HIV
9. Condyloma acuminatum (intralesional)
10. Chronic hepatitis B and C.

Usual Dosage and Schedule

1. 3 to 10 $\times$ 10^6 IU IM or SC in various schedules. Daily dosing is often used for several weeks or months, followed by three-times-a-week dosing.
2. As adjuvant therapy for high-risk melanoma, 20×10^6 IU/m^2 IV 5 consecutive days weekly for 4 weeks, then 10 $\times 10^6$ IU/ m^2 SC three times weekly for 48 weeks.

3. For HIV- related Kaposi's sarcoma, 30×10^6 IU/m^2 SC or IM three times weekly, with dose modifications based upon toxicity.

   Investigationally, doses have been higher (up to 50×10^6 IU/m^2 per dose), usually IV at doses higher than 10×10^6 IU/m^2.

Special Precaution

May cause or aggravate life-threatening or fatal neuropsychiatric, autoimmune, ischemic, and infectious disorders. Patients with persistently severe or worsening signs or symptoms of these conditions should be withdrawn from therapy.

Toxicity

1. *Myelosuppression and other hematologic effects:* Common but usually mild to moderate and transient, even with continued therapy. Higher doses may be associated (25% of patients receiving the recommended adjuvant therapy for melanoma) with granulocyte counts of under 750/IU and consequent increased risk for infection.
2. *Nausea, vomiting, and other gastrointestinal effects:* Anorexia and nausea are common, occurring in up to two-thirds of all patients, but vomiting is only occasional. Diarrhea and loose stools are occasional to common.
3. *Mucocutaneous effects:* Rash, dryness, or inflammation of the oropharynx, dry skin or pruritus and partial alopecia are occasional to common.
4. *Flu-like syndrome:* Syndrome with fatigue, fever, chills, sweating, myalgias, arthralgias, and headache is common to universal with greater severity at higher doses. Tends to diminish with continuing therapy and acetaminophen.
5. *Neurologic effects:* Some of these are:
   a. Occasional paresthesias or numbness in peripheral nervous system.
   b. CNS toxicity is uncommon at lower doses, but with higher doses, there is an increased likelihood of problems including headache, dizziness, somnolence, anxiety, depression (including suicidal behavior), confusion, hallucinations, cerebellar dysfunction and emotional lability.
6. *General systemic effects:* Fatigue, anorexia, and weight loss are common with chronic administration.
7. *Cardiovascular effects:* Mild hypotension is common but rarely symptomatic. Rarely to uncommonly seen are symptoms like hypertension, chest pain, arrhythmias and other cardiovascular disorders.
8. *Respiratory effects:* Dyspnea and cough are occasional at higher doses.
9. *Infectious effects:* Exacerbation of herpetic eruptions and nonherpetic cold sores is uncommon.
10. *Miscellaneous effects:* Leg cramps, insomnia, urticaria, hot flashes and coagulation disorders are uncommon. Visual problems including blurring, diplopia, dry eyes, nystagmus and photophobia are uncommon. Retinopathy, usually asymptomatic, is rare.

11. *Metabolic effects and laboratory abnormalities:*
    a. Elevated liver enzymes are common.
    b. Mild proteinuria and increase in serum creatinine are occasional.
    c. Hypercalcemia is occasional.
    d. Hypothyroidism and hyperthyroidism with or without antithyroid antibodies.
    e. Hypertriglyceridemia is rare.
12. Antibody development: Antibody development (binding and neutralizing) occurs more readily with interferon alpha-2a than with interferon alpha-2b. The significance of this is not clear, though it may be associated with the development of clinical resistance in some patients.

IRINOTECAN

Other names: Camptosar, CPT-11.

Mechanism of Action

Irinotecan, a semisynthetic water-soluble derivative of camptothecin, is a prodrug for the lipophilic metabolite SN-38, a potent inhibitor of topoisomerase I, which is an enzyme essential for effective replication and transcription. It binds to the topoisomerase I-DNA cleavable complex, preventing religation after cleavage by topoisomeraseI (Fig. 2.21).

Primary Indication

Carcinoma of the colon or rectum, either in combination with fluorouracil and leucovorin as primary therapy of metastatic disease or as a single agent after failure of fluorouracil-based therapy.

Usual Dosage and Schedule

1. 125 mg/m^2 IV over 90 min weekly for 4 weeks followed by a 2-week rest to complete one cycle when used either as a single agent or in combination with fluorouracil and leucovorin.
2. 180 mg/m^2 IV over 90 min every 2 weeks when used with leucovorin (over 2 hours) plus bolus fluorouracil followed by a 22 hours infusion of fluorouracil.
3. For severe or worse diarrhea (7 stools or more over pretreatment), doses should be held. When the diarrhea has improved (7 stools or less over pretreatment), treatment may be restarted with doses modified downward by 25 to 30 mg/m^2 during the current and subsequent cycles if there was an increase in stools or 7 to 9 per day and by 50 to 60 mg/m^2 if there was an increase in stools of 10 or more. Doses are also held during treatment and reduced in the same and subsequent cycles for severe netropenia (absolute neutrophil count under 1,000).

Special Precautions

1. Both early and late diarrhea may occur. That which occurs within 24 hours (a cholinergic effect) should be treated with atropine 0.25 to 1 mg IV. Late diarrhea should be treated promptly with loperamide (up to 2 mg every 2 hours until

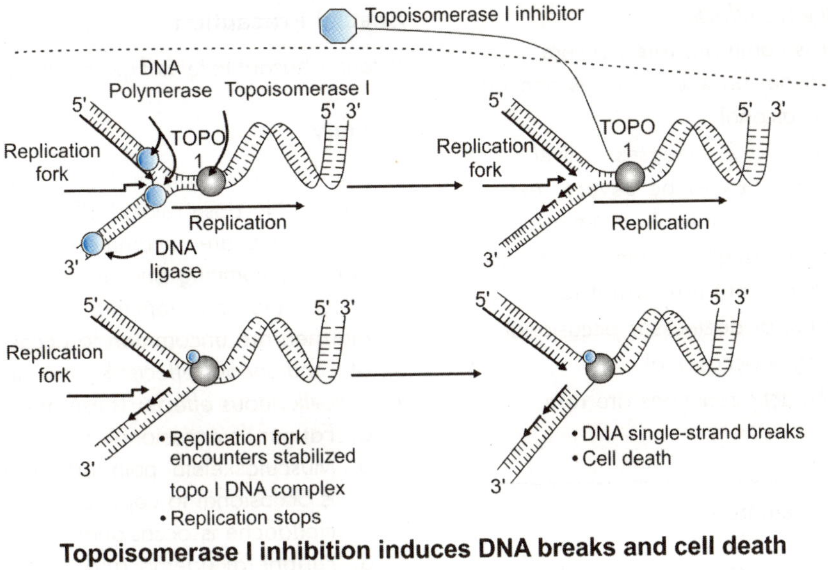

Fig. 2.21: Mechanism of action of Irinotecan

the patient is diarrhea-free for 12 hours) and prompt fluid and electrolyte replacement as indicated, if the diarrhea becomes severe (increase of seven or more stools per day) or there is dehydration or postural hypotension.

2. Consideration should be given to antibiotic therapy such as with an oral fluoroquinolone, particularly if the patient is neutropenic.
3. A vascular syndrome characterized by sudden unexpected thromboembolic events has also been described.

Toxicity

1. *Myelosuppression and other hematologic effects:* Neutropenia is common and often severe, particularly in combination therapy; anemia and thrombocytopenia are common but not usually (<5%) severe.
2. *Nausea, vomiting and other gastrointestinal effects:* Nausea and vomiting are common and are occasionally severe. Early diarrhea is common but is not usually (<5%) severe. Late diarrhea is common (85%) and is occasionally severe (15%) to life-threatening (5–10%). Abdominal cramping is common, occasionally severe. Anorexia is common.
   Constipation and dyspepsia are occasional. Ileus, colitis, or toxic megacolon are seen rarely.
3. *Mucocutaneous effects:* Alopecia and mucositis are common. Rash and sweating occur occasionally.

4. *Miscellaneous effects:*
   a. Fever is common, rarely severe
   b. Headache, back pain, chills and edema are occasional
   c. Grade 1 to 2 increases in liver function abnormalities to be severe, except in patients with known liver metastasis
   d. Dyspnea, cough, or rhinitis is occasional to common but usually not severe
   e. Insomnia or dizziness is occasional
   f. Flushing is occasional
   g. Anaphylactic reactions are rare.

LETROZOLE

Other name: Femara.

Mechanism of Action

Decreases estrogen biosynthesis by selective inhibition of aromatase (estrogen synthetase) in peripheral tissues.

Primary Indication

Carcinoma of the breast, advanced or metastatic, that is hormone receptor positive or unknown in postmenopausal women as firstline treatment or in hormone-responsive postmenopausal women with progression following antiestrogen therapy.

Usual Dosage and Schedule

2.5 mg PO daily.

Special Precaution

Potential hazard to fetus if given during pregnancy.

Toxicity

1. *Myelosuppression and other hematologic effects:* No dose-related effect. Thromboembolic events are uncommon to rare.
2. *Nausea, vomiting and other gastrointestinal effects:* Nausea, vomiting, constipation and diarrhea are uncommon to occasional.
3. *Mucocutaneous effects:* Rash is uncommon.
4. *Miscellaneous effects:* These are as follows:
   a. Fatigue is occasional
   b. Musculoskeletal pain (arthralgia or bone) is occasional to common
   c. Headache is occasional
   d. Peripheral edema and weight gain are occasional (lower than with megestrol)
   e. Dyspnea and cough are uncommon to occasional
   f. Hot flushes are occasional
   g. Hypercalcemia is rare.

LUTEINIZING HORMONE—RELEASING HORMONE ANALOGS

Other names: Leuprolide (Lupron, Lupron depot, Viadur), goserelin (Zoladex depot), triptorelin pamoate (Trelstar depot).

Mechanism of Action

Initial release of follicle-stimulating hormone and luteinizing hormone from the anterior pituitary, followed by diminution of gonadotropin secretion owing to desensitization of the pituitary to gonadotropin-releasing hormone and consequent decrease in the respective gonadal hormones. May also have direct effects on cancer cells, at least in cancer of the breast, in which gonado-tropin releasing hormone-binding sites have been demonstrated.

Primary Indications

1. Metastatic prostate carcinoma
2. Breast carcinoma in premenopausal and perimenopausal women with metastatic disease (goserelin).

Usual Dosage and Schedule

1. Leuprolide depot 7.5 mg IM monthly, 22.5 mg IM every 3 months, or 30 mg IM every 4 months
2. Goserelin depot, 3.6 mg implant for breast carcinoma
3. Triptorelin depot 3.75 mg IM monthly.

Special Precaution

Worsening of symptoms may occur during the first few weeks.

Toxicity

Some of the toxic reactions are as follows:

1. *Myelosuppression and other hematologic effects:* Rare if at all.
2. *Nausea, vomiting, and other gastrointestinal effects:* Anorexia, nausea, vomiting, and constipation are uncommon.
3. *Mucocutaneous effects:* Erythema and ecchymosis at the injection site, rash, hair loss and itching are uncommon.
4. *Cardiovascular effects:* Congestive heart failure, hypertension and thrombotic episodes are uncommon. Peripheral edema is occ-asional.
5. *Miscellaneous effects:* These are as follows:
    a. Dizziness, pain, headache, and paresthesias are uncommon.
    b. Hot flashes are common; decreased libido is common; gynecomastia with or without tenderness is uncommon; impotence is occasional to common.
    c. Bone pain, or "flare" is common on initiation of therapy in patients with bony metastasis. This can be minimized by pretreating with flutamide or another androgen antagonist in men with prostate cancer.
    d. Hypersensitivity reactions with rare angioneurotic edema and anaphylaxis have been reported.

MELPHALAN

Other names: Phenylalanine mustard, L-sarcolysin, L-PAM. Alkeran (Fig. 2.22).

Mechanism of Action

Alkylating agent with primary effect on DNA. Amino acid-type structure may result in cellular transport that is different from other alkylating agents.

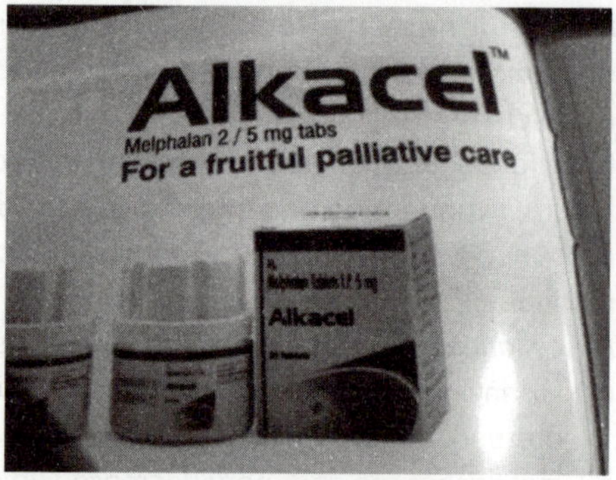

Fig. 2.22: Melphalan tablet

Primary Indications

1. Multiple myeloma
2. Breast and ovarian carcinomas.

Usual Dosage and Schedule

1. 8 mg/m^2 PO on days 1 to 4 every 4 weeks or
2. 10 mg/m^2 PO on days 1 to 4 every 6 weeks or
3. 3 to 4 mg/m^2 PO daily for 2 to 3 weeks, then 1 to 2 mg/m^2 PO daily for maintenance.
4. High-dose regimens of 140 to 200 mg/m^2 IV have been used, followed by stem cell rescue (e.g. bone marrow transplantation).
5. 16 mg/m^2 IV every 2 weeks × 4, then every 4 weeks.

Special Precautions

1. Myelosuppression and other hematologic effects may be delayed and prolonged up to 4 to 6 weeks.
2. Reduce IV dose by 50 percent for creatinine levels higher than 1.5 times normal.

Toxicity

1. *Myelosuppression and other hematologic effects:* Dose limiting; nadir at days 14 to 21.
2. *Nausea, vomiting, and other gastrointestinal effects:* Nausea, vomiting and diarrhea are uncommon at standard doses but common with high-dose regimens.
3. *Mucocutaneous effects:* Alopecia, dermatitis, and stomatitis are uncommon at standard doses; alopecia and mucositis are common with high-dose regimens.
4. *Miscellaneous effects:*
   a. Acute nonlymphocytic leukemia and myelodysplasia are rare but well-documented.
   b. Pulmonary fibrosis is rare.

MERCAPTOPURINE

Other names: 6-Mercaptopurine, 6-MP, Purinethol.

Mechanism of Action

A purine antimetabolite that, when converted to the nucleotide, inhibits the formation of nucleotides necessary for DNA and RNA synthesis.

Primary Indication

Acute lymphocytic and juvenile chronic granulocytic (myelogenous) leukemias.

Usual Dosage and Schedule

1. 100 mg/m^2 PO daily if used alone
2. 50 to 90 mg/m^2 PO daily if used with methotrexate.

Special Precautions

1. Decrease dose by 75 percent when used concurrently with allopurinol.
2. Increase interval between doses or reduce dose in patients with renal failure.

Toxicity

1. *Myelosuppression and other hematologic effects:* Common but mild at recommended doses.
2. *Nausea, vomiting and other gastrointestinal effects:* Nausea and vomiting are uncommon. Diarrhea is rare.
3. *Mucocutaneous effects:* Stomatitis may be seen with very large doses. Dry scaling rash is uncommon.
4. *Miscellaneous effects:*
   a. Intrahepatic cholestasis and mild focal centrolobular necrosis with Jaundice are uncommon.
   b. Hyperuricemia with rapid leukemia and cell lysis is common.
   c. Fever is uncommon.

MESNA

Other name: Mesnex.

Mechanism of Action

Mesna disulfide is reduced in the kidney to a free thiol compound, which then reacts chemically with urotoxic metabolites of ifosfamide, resulting in their detoxification.

Primary Indication

Prophylaxis for ifosfamide-induced hemorrhagic cystitis.

Usual Dosage and Schedule

Mesna dose is at least 20 percent of the ifosfamide dose (on a weight [mg] basis), administered just prior to (or mixed with) the ifosfamide dose and again at 4 and 8 hours after the ifosfamide to detoxify the urinary metabolites that cause the hemorrhagic cystitis. Higher doses of ifosfamide may require higher doses and longer durations of mesna.

Special Precaution

Contraindicated if patient is sensitive to thiol compounds. Does not prevent or ameliorate any adverse effects of ifosfamide other than hemorrhagic cystitis. Neither mesna nor its only metabolite, mesna disulfide, affects ifosfamide or its antineoplastic metabolites.

Toxicity

1. *Myelosuppression and other hematologic effects:* None.

2. *Nausea, vomiting and other gastrointestinal effects:* Nausea, vomiting and diarrhea are occasional. Nausea and vomiting more commonly from ifosfamide.
3. *Mucocutaneous effects:* Bad taste in the mouth is common.
4. *Miscellaneous effects:* These include the following:
   a. Headache, fatigue and limb pain are occasional
   b. Hypotension and allergic reaction are uncommon to rare
   c. Gives false-positive test for urinary ketones.

METHOTREXATE

Other names: Amethopterin, MTX, Mexate, Trexall (Fig. 2.23).

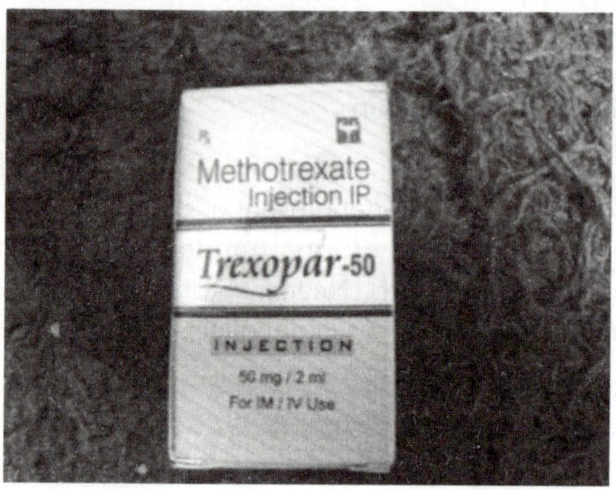

Fig. 2.23: Methotrexate injection 50 mg

Mechanism of Action

Inhibition of dihydrofolate reductase, which results in a block of the reduction of dihydrofolate to tetrahydrofolate. This blockage in turn inhibits the formation of thymidylate and purines and arrests DNA (predominantly), RNA, and protein synthesis.

Primary Indications

1. Breast, head and neck, gastrointestinal, lung and gestational trophoblastic carcinomas
2. Osteosarcomas (high-dose methotrexate)
3. Acute lymphocytic leukemia
4. Meningeal leukemia or carcinomatosis
5. Non-Hodgkin's lymphoma.

Usual Dosage and Schedule

1. *Gestational trophoblastic carcinoma:* 15 to 30 mg PO or IM on days 1 to 5 every 2 weeks.
2. *Other carcinomas:* 40 to 80 mg/m^2 IV or PO two to four times monthly with a 7 to 14 day interval between doses.
3. *Acute lymphocytic leukemia:* 15 to 20 mg/m^2 PO or IV weekly (together with mercaptopurine).
4. *Osteogenic sarcoma:* Up to 12 g/m^2 with leucovorin rescue (high-dose methotrexate). This usage requires an on-site monitoring of methotrexate levels and a high degree of expertise to administer safely.
5. *Intrathecally:* 12 mg/m^2 (not more than 20 mg) twice weekly.

Special Precautions

1. High-dose methotrexate (over 80 mg/m^2) should be administered only by individuals experienced in its use and at institutions where serum methotrexate levels can be readily measured.
2. Intrathecal methotrexate must be mixed in buffered physiologic solution containing no preservative.
3. Avoid aspirin, sulfonamides, tetracycline, phenytoin, and other protein-bound drugs that may displace methotrexate and cause an increase in free drug.
4. Oral anticoagulants, e.g. warfarin, may be potentiated by methotrexate; therefore prothrombin time should be followed carefully.
5. Oral antibiotics may decrease methotrexate absorption; penicillin and nonsteroidal antiinflammatory drugs decrease clearance of methotrexate.
6. Monitor use with theophylline.
7. In patients with renal insufficiency, it may be necessary to markedly reduce the dose or discontinue methotrexate therapy.
8. Do not give if patient has an effusion because of "reservoir" effect.

Toxicity

1. *Myelosuppression and other hematologic effects:* Occurs commonly, with nadir at 6 to 10 days after a single IV dose. Recovery is rapid.
2. *Nausea, vomiting and other gastrointestinal effects:* Occasional at standard doses.
3. *Mucocutaneous effects:*
   a. Mild stomatitis is common and a sign that maximum tolerated dose has been reached. Higher doses may result in confluent or hemorrhagic stomal ulcers and bloody diarrhea.
   b. Erythematous rashes, urticaria and skin pigment changes are uncommon.
   c. Mild alopecia is frequent.
4. *Miscellaneous effects:*
   a. Acute hepatocellular injury is uncommon at standard doses
   b. Hepatic fibrosis is uncommon but seen at low chronic doses
   c. Pneumonitis is rare
   d. Polyserositis is rare
   e. Renal tubular necrosis is rare at standard doses
   f. Convulsions and a Guillain-Barrê-like syndrome following intrathecal therapy are uncommon.

MITOMYCIN

Other names: Mitomycin C, Mutamycin (Fig. 2.24).

Mechanism of Action

Alkylation and cross-linking by mitomycin metabolites interfere with structure and function of DNA.

Primary Indication

Bladder (intravesical), esophagus, stomach, anal and pancreas carcinomas.

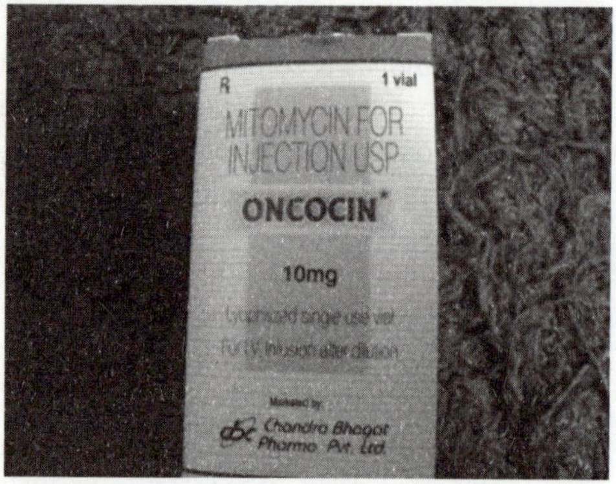

Fig. 2.24: Mitomycin injection

Usual Dosage and Schedule

1. 20 mg/m^2 IV on day 1 every 4 to 6 weeks or
2. 2 mg/m^2 IV on days 1 to 5 and 8 to 12 every 4 to 6 weeks.
3. 10 mg/m^2 IV on day 1 every 8 weeks in combination with fluorouracil and doxorubicin for stomach and pancreatic carcinomas.
4. 30 to 40 mg instilled into the bladder weekly for 4 to 8 weeks. then monthly for 6 months.

Special Precaution

Administer as slow push or rapid infusion through the sidearm of a rapidly running IV infusion, taking care to avoid extravasation.

Toxicity

1. *Myelosuppression and other hematologic effects:* Serious, cumulative and dose limiting. Nadir is reached usually by 4 weeks but may be delayed. Recovery is often prolonged over many weeks and occasionally the cytopenia never disappears.
2. *Nausea, vomiting and other gastrointestinal effects:* Nausea and vomiting are common at higher doses, but severity is usually mild-to-moderate.
3. *Mucocutaneous effects:*
   a. Stomatitis and alopecia are common.
   b. Cellulitis at injection site if extravasation occurs is common.
4. *Miscellaneous effects:* These include the following:
   a. Renal toxicity is uncommon
   b. Pulmonary toxicity is uncommon but may be severe
   c. Fever is uncommon
   d. Secondary neoplasia is possible
   e. Hemolytic-uremic syndrome is rare.

MITOXANTRONE

Other names: Novantrone, dihydroxyanthracene-dione, DHAD, DHAQ.

Mechanism of Action

DNA strand breakage mediated by anthracenedione effects on topoisomerase II.

Primary Indications

1. Acute nonlymphocytic leukemia
2. Carcinoma of the breast or ovary
3. Non-Hodgkin's and Hodgkin's lymphoma.

Usual Dosage and Schedule

1. 12 to 14 mg/m^2 IV as a 5 to 30 min infusion once every 3 weeks for solid tumors.
2. 12 mg/m^2 IV as a 5 to 30 min infusion daily for 3 days for acute nonlymphocytic leukemia.

Special Precaution

Rarely causes extravasation injury if infiltrated. Cardiotoxicity probably less than with doxorubicin; but prior anthracycline, chest irradiation, or underlying cardiac diease increases the risk.

Toxicity

1. *Myelosuppression and other hematologic effects:* Universal.
2. *Nausea, vomiting and other gastrointestinal effects:* Nausea and vomiting are common but less frequent and less severe than with doxorubicin. Diarrhea is uncommon.
3. *Mucocutaneous effects:* Alopecia is common, but its frequency and severity are less than with doxorubicin. Mucositis is occasional.
4. *Cardiac toxicity:* Probably less than with doxorubicin; there is no clear maximum dose, though the risk appears to increase at 125 mg/m^2 cumulative dose.
5. *Miscellaneous effects:*
   a. Local erythema and swelling with transient blue discoloration if extravasated, but rarely leads to severe skin damage.
   b. Green or blue discoloration of urine.
   c. Phlebitis is uncommon.

OCTREOTIDE

Other names: Sandostatin, Sandostatin LAR Depot.

Mechanism of Action

Somatostatin analog that inhibits release of polypeptide hormones, particularly in the pancreas and gut. Slows gastrointestinal transit time. Promotes water and electrolyte absorption, reflecting change from overall secretory to absorptive state.

Primary Indications

1. Carcinoid tumors.
2. Vasoactive intestinal peptide tumors and other amine precursor uptake and decarboxylation tumors.
3. Chemotherapy induced diarrhea.
4. Acromegaly.

Usual Dosage and Schedule

100 to 1,500 mg/day SC in two to four divided doses. Doses are usually started at the lower end and titrated upward to the best symptomatic improvement. If patients respond favorably to the rapid-acting SC injections, may be maintained on Sandostatin LAR Depot in a dose of 20 mg given IM intragluteally at 4-week intervals. Caution should be used in treating for more than 3 months.

Special Precaution

Lower doses indicated if severe renal dysfunction (creatinine level under 5 mg/dl).

Toxicity

1. *Myelosuppression and other hematologic effects:* None.
2. *Nausea, vomiting and other gastrointestinal effects:* Nausea, abdominal discomfort, bloating and diarrhea are common, particularly early in early therapy. Vomiting is only occasionally seen. Decreased gallbladder contractility and decreased bile secretion may result in biliary abnormalities.

   Gallstones develop in less than 2 percent if treatment is for 1 month or less but can be seen in 25 percent, if treatment is for 1 year or more. Ascending cholangitis and pancreatitis are uncommon to rare.
3. *Mucocutaneous effects:* Local site reactions are occasional; other effects are rare.
4. *Endocrine effects:* Hypoglycemia or hyperglycemia is uncommon; hypothalamic pituitary dysfunction is rare.
5. *Cardiovascular effects:* Bradycardia and other conduction abnormalities occur in up to 25 percent of patients with acromegaly who are treated with octreotide.

OXALIPLATIN

Other name: Eloxatin (Fig. 2.25).

Mechanism of Action

Similar to alkylating agents with respect to binding and crosslinking strands of DNA, forming DNA adducts and thereby inhibiting DNA replication and transcription. Primary indication is carcinoma of the colon and rectum.

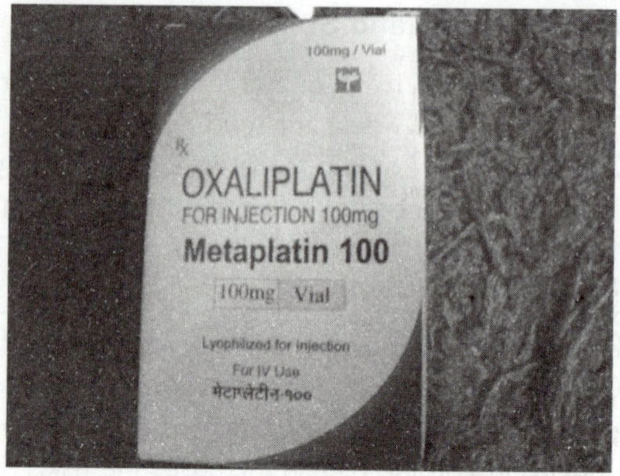

Fig. 2.25: Oxaliplatin injection

Usual Dosage and Schedule

1. *Single agent:* 130 mg/m^2 as a 2 hours infusion every 3 weeks or 85 mg/m^2 as a 3 hours infusion every 2 weeks.
2. *Combination therapy:* 85 to 100 mg/m^2 as a 2-h infusion every 2 weeks in combination with fluorouracil (often as a continuous infusion).

Special Precaution

Acute neurosensory and neuromotor symptoms may develop with the infusion. Laryngospasm may be minimized by avoiding cold drinks or food for a few days following treatment. Chronic neurosensory symptoms are dose limiting.

Toxicity

1. *Myelosuppression and other hematologic effects:* Low-grade myelosuppression is common, but grade 3 or 4 granulocytopenia,

thrombocytopenia, or anemia is uncommon (about 5%). Hemolytic anemia is rare.

2. *Nausea, vomiting and other gastrointestinal effects:* Nausea, vomiting and diarrhea are common but not commonly severe.

   These may be worsening of cholinergic syndrome when given with irinotecan.
3. *Mucocutaneous effects:* Alopecia is uncommon. Stomatitis is increased when used with fluorouracil.
4. *Miscellaneous effects:* These include the following:
   a. Neurotoxicity consisting of paresthesias and cold induced dysesthesias in the stocking glove or perioral distribution is common as acute transient change that begins with the infusion and lasts for less than 1 week. Chronic sensory neuropathy, fine motor disturbance, and ataxia are occasional to common with cumulative dosing (cumulative dose dependent) and may last for months. It is occasionally grade 3 to 4.
   b. Laryngospasm may develop during or within 2 hr of the, **Taxanes**: Comparative pharmacokinetic and toxicologic characteristics.

Characteristic of Paclitaxel and Docetaxel

Differentiating features of paclitaxel and docetaxel are given in Table 2.2.

PACLITAXEL

Other name: Taxol (Fig. 2.26).

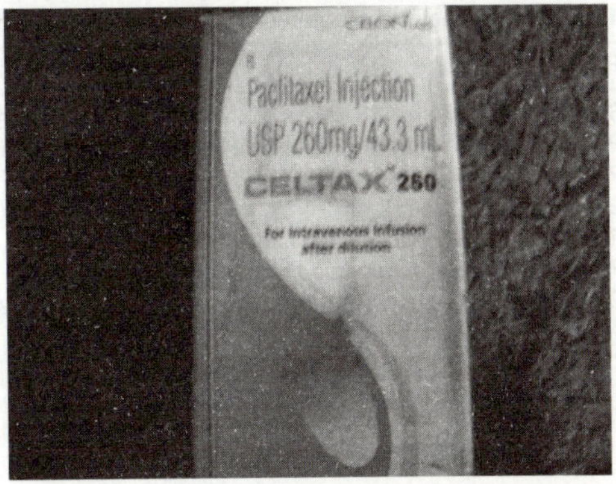

Fig. 2.26: Paclitaxel injection

Mechanism of Action

Enhanced formation and stabilization of microtubules.

Antineoplastic effect may result from nonfunctional tubules or altered tubulin-microtubule equilibrium. Mitotic arrest is seen and is associated with accumulated polymerized microtubules (Fig. 2.27).

Primary Indications

1. Carcinomas of the ovary, breast, lung, head and neck, bladder, and cervix
2. Melanoma
3. Kaposi's sarcoma, AIDS-related.

Usual Dosage and Schedule

1. 135 to 200 mg/m^2 as a 24 hours infusion every 3 weeks.
2. 135 to 225 mg/m^2 as a 3 hours infusion every 3 weeks.

Table 2.2: Characteristic features of paclitaxel and docetaxel

Paclitaxel	*Docetaxel*
Standard adult dose: 135 (24-hr infusion), 175-225 (3-hr infusion)	75-100 (1-hr infusion)
Pharmacokinetic behavior: Saturable elimination and distribution	Triphasic
Plasma half-life: 10-20 hr	10-20 hr
Clearance: 20-25 L/hr2	36 L/hr
Primary route: Hepatic metabolism and biliary elimination	Hepatic metabolism and biliary elimination
Principal toxicity: Neutropenia	Neutropenia
Other toxicities: Alopecia, neurotoxicity, myalgia, hypersensitivity reactions, asthemia	Alopecia, skin and nail toxiciC ty, asthenia, mylgia, fluid retention, neurotoxicity, hypersensitivity reactions

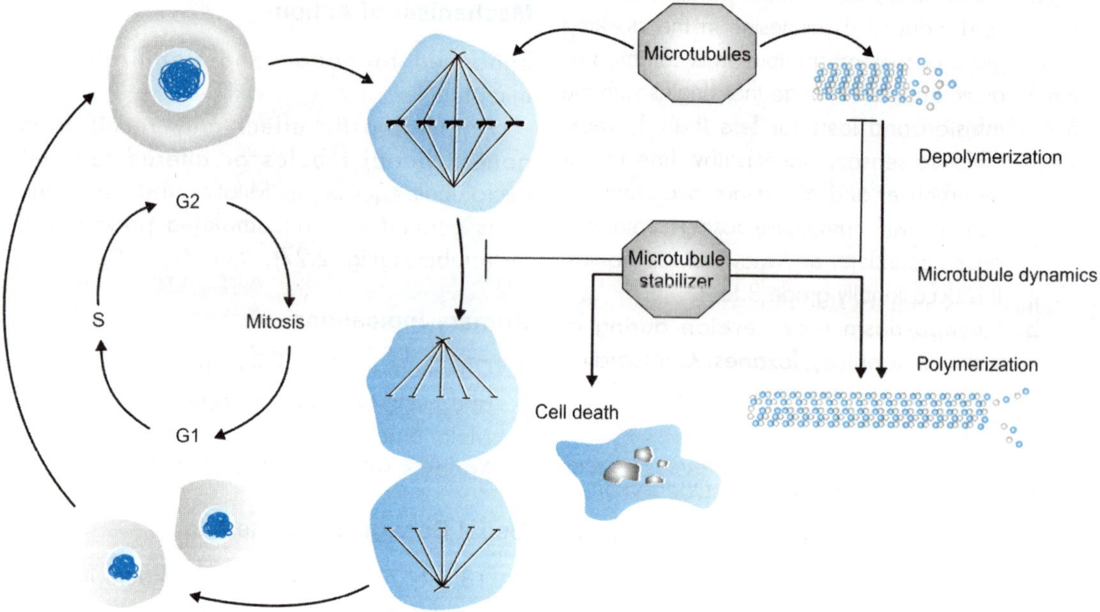

Fig. 2.27: Microtubule dynamics as a target of cancer therapy: How does it works?

3. 100 mg/m^2 as a 3 hours infusion every 2 weeks for the treatment of AIDS-related Kaposi's sarcoma.
4. 80 to 100 mg/m^2 as a 1 hour weekly infusion.
5. 200 mg/m^2 as a 1 hour infusion every 3 weeks.

Special Precaution

Anaphylactoid reactions with dyspnea, hypotension (or occasionally hypertension), bronchospasm, urticaria, and erythematous rashes may occur as a result of the paclitaxel itself or the Cremophor vehicle required to make paclitaxel water-soluble. Such reaction is minimized but not totally prevented by pretreatment with antihistamines and corticosteroids and by prolonging the infusion rate (to 24 hours). Paclitaxel must be filtered with a 0.2 mm in-line filter.

Standard Pretreatment Regimen

1. Dexamethasone 20 mg IV for doses greater than 100 mg/m^2 and 10 mg IV for doses less than or equal to 100 mg/m^2 30 to 60 min prior to treatment.
2. Diphenhydramine 50 mg IV 30 to 60 min before treatment.
3. Histamine H_2-receptor antagonist IV 30 to 60 min before treatment (e.g. cimetidine 300 mg).

Toxicity

1. *Myelosuppression and other hematologic effects:* Granulocytopenia is universal and dose limiting; thrombocytopenia is common; anemia is occasional.
2. *Nausea, vomiting, and other gastrointestinal effects:* Common but usually not severe.
3. *Mucocutaneous effects:* Alopecia is universal; mucositis is occasional at recommended doses.
4. *Hypersensitivity reactions:* Dyspnea, hypotension (or occasionally hypertension), bronchospasm, urticaria and erythematous rashes are occasionally seen, despite precautions.
5. *Miscellaneous effects:*
   a. Sensory neuropathy is common (30–35%) and may progressively worsen with time. Recovery may take months to years
   b. Hepatic dysfunction is uncommon
   c. Diarrhea is occasional and mild
   d. Myalgias and arthralgias are common (25%)
   e. Seizures are rare
   f. Abnormal electrocardiogram is occasional. If clinically significant bradycardia occurs, stop drug. Restart at slower rate when stable.

PAMIDRONATE

Other name. Aredia.

Mechanism of Action

A bisphosphonate that inhibits osteoclastic resorption of bone and calcium release induced by tumor cytokines.

Primary Indications

1. Hypercalcemia associated with malignancy
2. Osteolytic bone metastases of breast cancer
3. Osteolytic and osteoporotic bone lesions of multiple myeloma
4. Paget's disease.

Usual Dosage and Schedule

1. *Multiple myeloma:* 90 mg IV as a 4 hours infusion every month
2. *Breast cancer:* 90 mg IV as a 2 hours infusion every 3 to 4 weeks
3. *Hypercalcemia of malignancy:* 60 to 90 mg IV as a 4 to 24 hours infusion. May be repeated every 1 to 8 weeks, as needed.

Special Precaution

Potential for renal tubular damage, particularly if infused more rapidly. Renal clearance parallels creatinine clearance, but adverse effects do not appear to be worse with decreased clearance when given on a monthly basis. Serum electrolytes and renal function should be monitored closely.

Toxicity

1. *Myelosuppression and other hematologic effects:* Rare.
2. *Nausea, vomiting and other gastrointestinal effects:* Abdominal pain, anorexia, constipation, nausea and vomiting are uncommon to occasional.
3. *Mucocutaneous effects:* Infusion site reaction is occasional.
4. *Miscellaneous effects:* Some of them include:
   a. Fatigue is occasional.
   b. Laboratory abnormalities are occasional (hypocalcemia, hypokalemia, hypomagnesemia, and hypophosphatemia, particularly at 90 mg dose).
   c. Uveitis, iritis, scleritis and episcleritis are rare.
   d. Bone pain and generalized pain are occasional.
   e. Renal tubular damage is uncommon.

PEGFILGRASTIM

Other names: Neulasta, Pegylated G-CSF.

Mechanism of Action

Pegfilgrastim is recombinant granulocyte-stimulating factor (GCSF) that is conjugated to polyethylene glycol. This delays renal clearance and increases the serum half-life from about 3.5 to about 15 to 80 hours after a single SC injection. Promotes growth and differentiation of myeloid progenitor cells. May improve survival and function of granulocytes.

Primary Indication

Prophylaxis of granulocytopenia and associated infection in patients who are at high-risk from chemotherapy for nonmyeloid malignancies.

Usual Dosage and Schedule

6 mg SC once (usually on day 2) for each 21 or 28 day chemotherapy cycle. Should not be given between 14 days before and 24 hours after each chemotherapy cycle.

Special Precautions

1. Use with caution in disorders of myeloid stem cells as it may promote growth of leukemic cells.
2. The fixed dose formulation should not be used in infants, children and others weighing less than 45 kg.

Toxicity

1. *Myelosuppression and other hematologic effects:* None (leukocytosis).
2. *Nausea, vomiting and other gastrointestinal effects:* Rare to uncommon.
3. *Mucocutaneous effects:* Exacerbation of pre-existing dermatologic conditions is occasional; pyoderma gangrenosum is possible.
4. *Miscellaneous effects:* Usually mild and short lived.
   a. Bone pain, musculoskeletal symptoms such as cramps and back or leg pain are common.
   b. Splenomegaly with prolonged use is possible. Splenic rupture has been reported with the parent compound filgrastim.
   c. Exacerbation of pre-existing inflammatory or autoimmune disorders is rare.
   d. Mild elevation of lactate dehydrogenase and alkaline phosphatase.
   e. Allergic type reactions may occur, as they have been seen with the parent compound filgrastim.
   f. Adult respiratory distress syndrome has been reported in neutropenic patients receiving filgrastim and is possible with pegfilgrastim.

PORFIMER

Other name: Photofrin.

Mechanism of Action

Photosensitizing agent. Cellular damage occurs as a result of light-induced radical reactions, including superoxide and hydroxyl radicals.

Primary Indications

1. Obstructive esophageal cancers.
2. Completely or partially obstructing endobronchial nonsmall cell lung cancer.
3. Microinvasive endobronchial nonsmall cell lung cancer in patients for whom surgery and radiotherapy are not indicated.

Usual Dosage and Schedule

2 mg/kg as a slow IV injection over 3 to 5 min. This is followed by illumination with laser light 40 to 50

hours following injection of porfimer. A second course may be given after a minimum of 30 days.

Special Precautions

1. Contraindicated in patients with porphyria and tracheoesophageal or bronchoesophageal fistulas.
2. Contraindicated if tumor is eroding into a major blood vessel.
3. Patients must avoid exposure of skin and eyes to direct sunlight or bright indoor light for 30 days to minimize severe photosensitivity reactions. Sunscreens are of no value.

Toxicity

1. *Myelosuppression and other hematologic effects:* No marrow suppression, but anemia is common.
2. *Nausea, vomiting are occasional to common:* Other gastrointestinal effects including abdominal pain and constipation are occasional.
3. *Cutaneous effects:* Photosensitivity reaction is occasional to common, particularly if extravasation occurs at injection site, see special precautions above.
4. *Miscellaneous effects:*
   a. Atrial fibrillation is occasional. Hypertension, hypotension and tachycardia are occasional.
   b. Occasional cough, dyspnea, pleural effusion, pneumonia and respiratory insufficiency have been seen.
   c. Ocular discomfort may be seen, particularly from bright light.
   d. Anxiety, anorexia, confusion and insomnia are occasional.
   e. Occasional asthenia, back pain, chest pain and other pain. (Chest pain probably results from inflammatory response within area of treatment).

PROCARBAZINE

Other name: Matulane.

Mechanism of Action

Uncertain but appears to affect preformed DNA, RNA, and protein.

Primary Indications

1. Hodgkin's and non-Hodgkin's lymphomas
2. Brain tumors
3. Melanoma.

Usual Dosage and Schedule

60 to 100 mg/m^2 PO daily for 7 to 14 days every 4 weeks (in combination with other drugs).

Special Precaution

Many food and drug interactions are possible. Their clinical significance is described below:

Drug or Food Possible Result

1. Ethanol Disulfiram-like reactions: nausea, vomiting, visual disturbances, headache

2. Sympathomimetics, hypertensive crisis, tremors, tricyclic antidepressants, excitation, angina, cardiac tyramine-rich foods palpitations (Cheese, wine, bananas)
3. CNS depressants additive depression.

Toxicity

1. *Myelosuppression and other hematologic effects:* Pancytopenia is dose limiting. Recovery may be delayed.
2. *Nausea, vomiting and other gastrointestinal effects:* Nausea is frequent during first few days until tolerance develops.
   Diarrhea is uncommon but may be severe.
3. *Mucocutaneous effects:* These include the following:
   a. Stomatitis is uncommon
   b. Alopecia, pruritus and drug rash are uncommon.
4. *CNS effects:* Paresthesias, neuropathies, headache, dizziness, depression, apprehension, nervousness, insomnia, nightmares, hallucinations, ataxia, confusion, convulsions and coma have been reported with varying frequency.
5. *Miscellaneous effects:* These include the following:
   a. Secondary neoplasia is possible. Acute leukemia and lung cancer have been reported. Risk for lung cancer is increased by smoking
   b. Visual disturbances are rare
   c. Postural hypotension is rare
   d. Hypersensitivity reactions are rare
   e. Has strong potential for teratogenesis.

PROGESTINS

Other names: Medroxyprogesterone acetate (Provera, Depo-Provera), hydroxyprogesterone caproate (Delalutin), megestrol acetate (Megace).

Mechanism of Action

Mechanisms for antitumor effects or for appetite stimulation are not clear.

Primary Indications

1. Appetite stimulation.
2. Endometrial and breast carcinomas.

Usual Dosage and Schedule

1. *As an appetite stimulant:* Megestrol acetate 160 to 800 mg PO daily.
2. *As an antineoplastic agent:* Megestrol acetate 80 to 320 mg PO daily; medroxyprogesterone acetate 1,000 to 1,500 mg IM weekly or 400 to 800 mg PO twice weekly; hydroxyprogesterone caproate 1,000 to 1,500 mg IM weekly.

Toxicity

1. *Myelosuppression and other hematologic effects:* None.
2. *Nausea, vomiting and other gastrointestinal effects:* Rare.
3. *Mucocutaneous effects:* Mild alopecia and skin rash are uncommon.

4. *Miscellaneous effects:* These include the following:
   a. Mild fluid retention is occasional to common
   b. Mild liver function abnormalities are occasional; intrahepatic cholestasis may occur
   c. Menstrual irregularities are common
   d. Improved appetite and weight gain are common.

RITUXIMAB

Other name: Rituxan.

Mechanism of Action

Rituximab is a genetically engineered chimeric (murine and human) monoclonal antibody directed against the CD20 antigen found on the surface of normal cells and in high copy number on malignant B lymphocytes (but not stem cells). The Fab domain of rituximab binds to the CD20 antigen on B lymphocytes and B-cell non-Hodgkin's lymphomas, and the Fc domain recruits immune effector functions to mediate B-cell lysis (Fig. 2.28).

Primary Indications

1. Non-Hodgkin's B-cell lymphoma that is low grade or follicular, CD20 positive and refractory to conventional therapy.
2. Non-Hodgkin's B-cell lymphoma other than low grade or follicular, often in combination or sequence with other therapy.

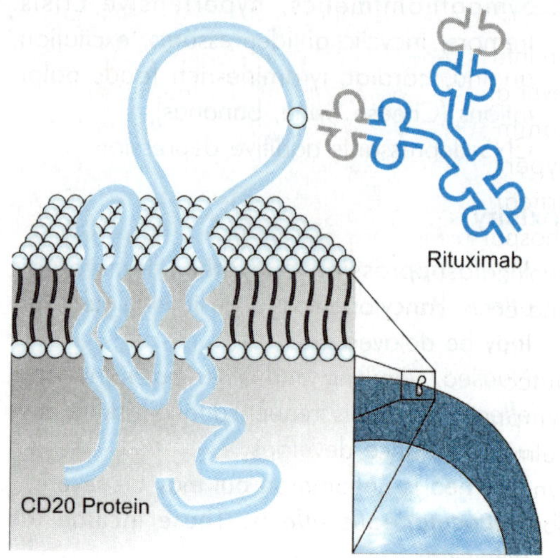

Fig. 2.28: Rituximab: Mechanism of action

Usual Dosage and Schedule

375 mg/m^2 given as a slow IV infusion, initially at a rate of 50 mg/hr. If hypersensitivity or other infusion-related events do not occur, escalate in 50 mg/hr increments to a maximum of 400 mg/hr. Usually takes 4 to 6 hr to infuse initial therapy. Interrupt or slow the infusion rate for reducing infusion related events. Repeat the dose once weekly for 4 to 8 doses. Premedication with acetaminophen and diphenhydramine may attenuate infusionrelated symptoms. Corticosteroids should not be used for premedication.

Special Precaution

An infusion-related set of symptoms consisting of fever and chills, with or without true rigors, occur commonly during the first infusion. Other hypersensitivity symptoms including nausea, urticaria, fatigue, headache, pruritus, bronchospasm, dyspnea, sensation of tongue or throat swelling, rhinitis, vomiting, hypotension, flushing, and pain at disease sites may also be seen.

Rarely infusion-related events result in fatal outcomes. Fatal reactions have followed a symptom complex that includes hypoxia, pulmonary infiltrates, acute respiratory distress syndrome, myocardial infarction, ventricular fibrillation and cardiogenic shock. Hypersensitivity reactions generally start within 30 to 120 min of starting the infusion. Most will resolve with slowing or interruption of the infusion and with supportive care, including IV saline, diphenhydramine, and acetaminophen. Severe reactions will additionally require aggressive cardiorespiratory support including oxygen, epinephrine, vasopressor, corticosteroids and bronchodilators and may preclude additional teatment with rituximab. The rate of infusion events decreases from 80 percent during the first infusion to 40 percent during subsequent infusions.

Toxicity

1. *Myelosuppression and other hematologic effects:* Uncommon. However, B-cell depletion occurs in 70 to 80 percent of patients, with decreased immunoglobulins in a minority of patients. Infectious events occur in about 30 percent of patients treated with rituximab, but only uncommonly are they severe.
2. *Nausea, vomiting and other gastrointestinal effects:* Nausea is common (23%) but rarely severe. Vomiting and diarrhea are occasional.
3. *Mucocutaneous effects:* Pruritus, rash, urticaria, and night sweats are occasional. Severe mucocutaneous reactions including Stevens-Johnson syndrome, lichenoid dermatitis, vesiculobullous dermatitis and toxic epidermal necrolysis are rare but have been reported from 1 to 13 weeks following rituximab exposure.
4. *Miscellaneous effects:*These include the following:
   a. Infusion-related hypersensitivity reactions (may include fever, chills, headache, myalgia, weakness, nausea, urticaria, pruritus, throat irritation, rhinitis, dizziness and hypertension) are common, but usually resolve with interruption or slowing the rate of infusion and administration of supportive therapy; see special precautions above.
   b. Myalgia and arthralgia are occasional. Rarely, a serum sickness-like reaction may be seen that requires corticosteroid therapy.
   c. Hypotension is occasional but rarely severe. Chest pain, bronchospasm, tachycardia, edema and postural hypotension are uncommon. Severe angioedema, arrhythmia, and angina are rare.
   d. Renal failure, possibly requiring dialysis, has been seen, particularly in association

with tumorlysis syndrome in patients with high tumor cell burden.

SARGRAMOSTIM

Other names: Granulocyte-macrophage colony-stimulating factor, GM-CSF, Leukine.

Mechanism of Action

Promotes growth and differentiation of myeloid progenitor cells.

May improve survival and function of granulocytes, eosinophils, monocytes and macrophages. Induces release of secondary cytokines (interleukin-1 and tumor necrosis factor).

Primary Indications

1. Myeloid reconstitution after peripheral blood or bone marrow progenitor cell transplantation.
2. Neutrophil recovery following chemotherapy in acute myelogenous leukemia.
3. Mobilization of peripheral blood progenitor cells.
4. Granulocytopenia from primary marrow disorders such as myelodysplastic syndrome and aplastic anemia.
5. Granulocytopenia associated with AIDS and its therapy.

Usual Dosage and Schedule

1. Myeloid reconstitution after autologous stem cell transplantation 250 µg/m² IV daily as a 2 hours infusion beginning 2 to 4 hours after the autologous stem cell infusion and not less than 24 hours after the last dose of chemotherapy or less than 12 hours after the last dose of radiotherapy. Continue for 21 days or until the absolute neutrophil count reaches 20000/µl.
2. Bone marrow transplantation failure or engraftment delay. 250 µg/m² daily for 14 days as 2 hours IV infusion. If no marrow recovery, may be repeated in 7 days at same or higher dose (500 µg/m²). Dose and duration are dependent on the response.
3. Mobilization of peripheral blood progenitor cells. The recommended dose is 250 µg/m²/day administered IV over 24 hours or SC once daily. Dosing should continue at the same dose through the period of peripheral blood progenitor cell collection.
4. Neutrophil recovery following chemotherapy in acute myelogenous leukemia 250 µg/m²/day administered IV over a 4 hours period starting 4 days following the completion of induction chemotherapy and continuing until the absolute neutrophil count is greater than 1,500 cells/µl for 3 consecutive days or a maximum of 42 days.
5. Aplastic anemia, myelodysplastic syndrome, and AIDS. Doses may be much lower (50 to 100 µg/m² SC or IM daily).

Special Precaution

Flushing, tachycardia, dyspnea, and nausea occur commonly with the first dose of IV therapy; do not infuse over less than 2 hours; longer infusion may help.

Toxicity

1. *Myelosuppression and other hematologic effects:* None (leukocytosis).
2. *Nausea, vomiting and other gastrointestinal effects:* Occasional.
3. *Mucocutaneous effects:* Rash is uncommon; exacerbation of pre-existing dermatologic conditions is occasional; mild local reactions at injection site are common.
4. *Miscellaneous effects:* Usually mild and short-lived at standard doses, but with increasing dose may be more severe. Some of them are:
   a. Bone pain, musculoskeletal symptom such as cramps, and back or leg pain are common.
   b. Pericarditis, fluid retention and venous thrombosis are dose-related but uncommon at standard doses.
   c. Flu-like symptoms (fever, chills, aches, headache) are occasional at standard doses and common at higher doses.

SURAMIN

Mechanism of Action

Glycosaminoglycan agonist-antagonist that blocks the binding of growth factors to their receptors. Growth factors affected, include platelet-derived growth factor, transforming growth factor-B, and heparin-binding growth factor-2 (also known as basic fibroblast growth factor). Inhibits DNA polymerases, reverse transcriptase, and other proteins. Also inhibits glycosaminoglycan metabolism.

Primary Indications

1. Prostate carcinoma that is hormone refractory.
2. High-grade gliomas.

Usual Dosage and Schedule

A loading dose of 1,000 mg/m^2 is infused over 2 hours on day 1. One hour infusions of 400, 300, 250, and 200 mg/m^2 are given on days 2,3,4 and 5, respectively, followed by 275 mg/m^2 infusions twice a week for 2 weeks (days 8,11,15 and 19) and once weekly thereafter through week 12. This dosing regimen is designed to achieve a sustained suramin plasma concentration of 100 to 300 μg/ml. Various other schedules are used to achieve a similar plasma level.

Special Precautions

1. Measurement of plasma levels has been advocated in many studies to achieve the narrow concentration that is therapeutic and not prohibitively toxic. Therapy should be held if the plasma concentration exceeds 300 μg/ml.
2. Due to adrenal suppression, patients require hydrocortisone 25 mg in the morning and 15 mg at bedtime.
3. Prothrombin time should be followed closely as coagulopathy may develop.

Toxicity

1. *Myelosuppression and other hematologic effects:* Common but usually not severe.

2. *Nausea, vomiting and other gastrointestinal effects:* Uncommon.
3. *Mucocutaneous effects:* Transient erythematous rash is common.
4. *Adrenocortical insufficiency:* Common.
5. *Neurotoxicity:* Paresthesias are seen commonly and severe polyradiculopathy occurs occasionally. Motor weakness may be seen following termination of therapy. The degree of toxicity appears to be related to the plasma suramin level, with acute serious reactions uncommon at plasma levels of less than 350 μg/ml.
6. *Miscellaneous effects:*
   a. Vortex keratopathy with photophobia, tearing, and blurred vision are common.
   b. Liver function abnormalities are common but reversible.
   c. Coagulopathy is occasional with elevations of the prothrombin time, partial thromboplastin time and thrombin time, with increased risk of spontaneous bleeding.
   d. Proteinuria is common; decrease in creatinine clearance is occasional.
   e. Malaise, fatigue, and lethargy are common after 2 to 4 months of therapy.

TAMOXIFEN

Other name: Nolvadex.

Mechanism of Action

Tamoxifen is a selective estrogen receptor modulator that inhibits estrogen effects by competing with estrogen for binding on the cytosol estrogen receptor protein in cancer cells. This complex is probably transported into the nucleus, where it affects nucleic acid function. It also has effects on cellular growth factors, epidermal growth factors, and transforming growth factors—a and b (Fig. 2.29).

Primary Indications

1. *Breast carcinoma*
   a. Metastatic tumors in postmenopausal or premenopausal women with estrogen receptor—positive (or unknown) tumors.
   b. Adjuvant therapy in women with estrogen receptor—positive (or progesterone receptor—positive) tumors after primary therapy. Optimal duration of therapy for most women is probably limited to 5 years.
   c. Breast cancer prevention in very high-risk women.

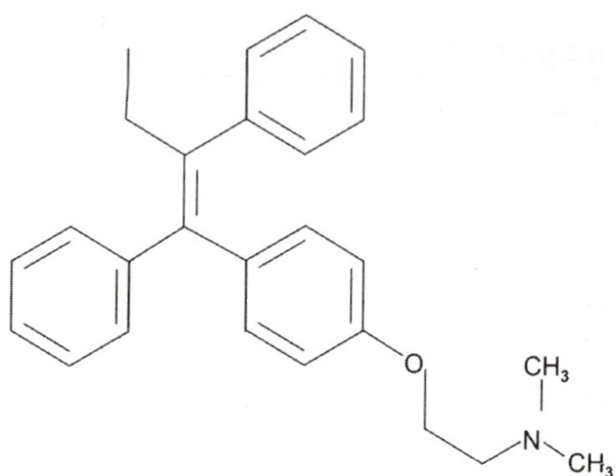

Fig. 2.29: Structure of tamoxifen

2. *Melanoma*, in combination with other drugs (controversial).

Usual Dosage and Schedule

1. 20 mg PO as single daily dose
2. 10 mg PO twice daily.

Special Precautions

1. Hypercalcemia may be seen during initial therapy.
2. Not recommended as primary cancer preventive agent for most women except under auspices of a controlled clinical trial.

Toxicity

1. *Myelosuppression and other hematologic effects:* Uncommon and mild.
2. *Nausea, vomiting, and other gastrointestinal effects:* Nausea occurs early in the course of therapy in up to 20 percent of patients but abates rapidly as therapy is continued. Diarrhea is occasional.
3. *Mucocutaneous effects:* Cataracts and other eye toxicities have been observed, but effects due to drug are uncommon. Skin rash and pruritus vulvae are uncommon. May cause increase or marked decrease in vaginal secretions and result in difficult or painful intercourse.
4. *Miscellaneous effects:* These include the following:
   a. Hot flashes are common.
   b. Vaginal bleeding and menstrual irregularity are uncommon to occasional.
   c. Lassitude, headache, leg cramps and dizziness are uncommon.
   d. Peripheral edema is occasional.
   e. Increased bone pain, tumor pain, and local disease flare (associated both with good tumor response as well as with tumor progression) are occasional.
   f. Slowed progression of osteoporosis.
   g. Reduction in serum cholesterol with favorable changes in lipid profile.
   h. Thromboembolic phenomena are rare.
   i. Liver function test abnormalities are occasional.
5. *Carcinogenesis:* Uterine carcinomas are rare (two to four times the predicted incidence in adjuvant trials). Uterine sarcomas are very rare.

TEMOZOLOMIDE

Other name: Temodar (Fig. 2.30).

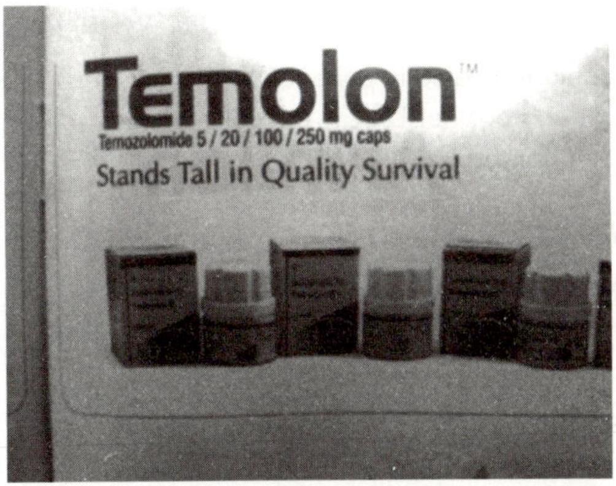

Fig. 2.30: Temozolomide

Mechanism of Action

Undergoes rapid conversion to the reactive substituted imidazole carboxamide MTIC. This compound is believed to be active primarily through alkylation (methylation) of DNA at the O6 and N7 positions of guanine.

Primary Indications

1. Anaplastic astrocytoma that is refractory to nitrosoureas
2. Other gliomas
3. Metastatic carcinomas to the brain.

Usual Dosage and Schedule

1. 150 to 200 mg/m^2 PO on an empty stomach daily for 5 days every 28 days
2. 75 mg/m^2 PO on an empty stomach daily during radiation therapy for up to 7 weeks.

Special Precautions

Contraindicated in patients with a hypersensitivity to dacarbazine (DTIC), because both drugs are metabolized to MTIC.

Toxicity

1. *Myelosuppression and other hematologic effects:* Some myelosuppression is common, but only occasionally is it severe.
2. *Nausea, vomiting and other gastrointestinal effects:* Nausea, vomiting, and constipation are common but only occasionally severe. Occasionally patients may also develop abdominal pain or anorexia.
3. *Mucocutaneous effects:* Rash and pruritus are occasional.
4. *Miscellaneous effects:* These include the following:
   a. Headache, fatigue, asthenia and fever are common (20–65%).
   b. Peripheral edema is occasional.
   c. Neurologic symptoms are common on temozolomide, but it is difficult to distinguish whether the symptoms are from the drug or from the disease. Common findings are convulsions, hemiparesis, dizziness, abnormal coordination, amnesia, and insomnia. Occasional findings are paresthesias, somnolence, paresis, incontinence, ataxia, dysphasia, gait abnormality, myalgias and confusion. Diplopia or other visual abnormalities are occasional.
   d. Anxiety and depression are occasional.

THALIDOMIDE

Other name: Thalomid (Fig. 2.31).

Mechanism of Action

Multiple potential mechanisms, including inhibition of vascular endothelial growth factor, inhibition of tumor necrosis factor-α, direct inhibition of G1 growth and promotion of apoptosis, and expansion of natural killer cells and costimulation of T cells.

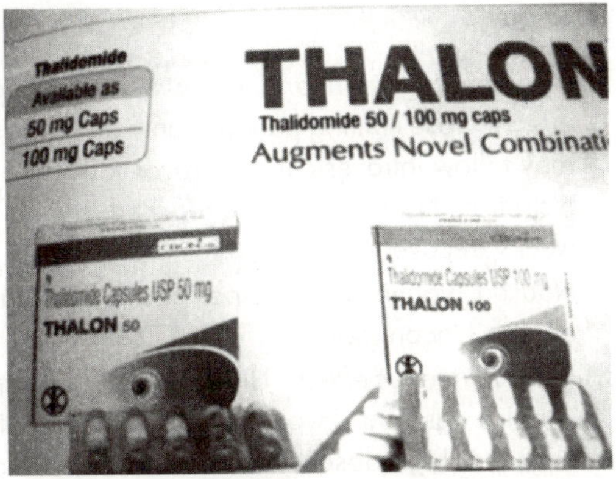

Fig. 2.31: Thalidomide capsules

Primary Indications

1. Multiple myeloma
2. Myelodysplastic syndrome.

Usual Dosage and Schedule

A starting dose of 50 to 100 mg once daily in the evening. The dose is escalated weekly by 50 to 100 mg until the maximum dose specified is reached, commonly up to 400 mg daily.

Special Precaution

Severe and life-threatening birth defects, primarily phocomelia, can be caused by taking even a single 50 mg dose. For this reason, special precautions must be taken to ensure that female patients are not pregnant when the drug is started and that both female and male patients practice strict birth control measures.

Toxicity

1. *Myelosuppression and other hematologic effects:* None to minimal myelosuppression. Occasional deep venous thrombosis.
2. *Nausea, vomiting and other gastrointestinal effects:* Constipation is common.
3. *Mucocutaneous effects:* Macular rash, usually involving the trunk, is common. Alopecia is uncommon. Rare severe or life-threatening epidermal damage.
4. *Miscellaneous effects:* These include the following:
   a. Dose-dependent somnolence and dizziness are common. Tolerance usually develops to the sedative effects. Dizziness may be related to hypotension and can be minimized by adequate hydration and avoidance of rapid postural changes.
   b. Peripheral neuropathy is common (25%) with chronic therapy. Occasional patients develop myalgia, tremor or muscle spasms.
   c. Fatigue is common.
   d. Headache is occasional.
   e. Edema is occasional to common.
   f. Hypothyroidism is occasional.
   g. Birth defects (see special precautions above).
   h. Hypercoagulability with deep venous thrombosis is occasional.

THIOTEPA

Other names: Triethylenethiophosphoramide, Thioplex.

Mechanism of Action

Alkylating agent similar to mechlorethamine.

Primary Indications

1. Superficial papillary carcinoma of urinary bladder
2. Malignant peritoneal, pleural, or pericardial effusions
3. Carcinoma of breast and ovary
4. Neoplastic meningeal infiltrates.

Usual Dosage and Schedule

1. 12 mg/m^2 IV bolus every 3 weeks in combination with vinblastine and doxorubicin for breast cancer.
2. 30 to 60 mg in 40 to 50 ml of water instilled into the bladder and retained for 1 hour. Dose is repeated weekly for 3 to 6 weeks, then every 3 weeks for five cycles.
3. 25 to 30 mg/m^2 in 50 to 100 ml of saline solution as a single intracavitary injection. Dose may be repeated as tolerated by blood counts.
4. 10 to 15 mg intrathecally.
5. High-dose therapy with 500 to 1,000 mg/m^2 over 3 days has been used followed by stem cell rescue (e.g. bone marrow transplantation).

Special Precaution

Dose should be reduced in patients with impaired renal function, as the drug is excreted primarily in the urine.

Toxicity

1. *Myelosuppression and other hematologic effects:* Dose limiting pancytopenia and sepsis may follow intravesical or intracavitary administration. Nadir counts are reached in 1 to 2 weeks; recovery by 4 weeks is usual.
2. *Nausea, vomiting and other gastrointestinal effects:* Uncommon.
3. *Mucocutaneous effects:* Uncommon. Thiotepa is not a vesicant. Hyperpigmentation of skin occurs at high doses.
4. *Miscellaneous effects:* These include the following:
   a. Local pain, dizziness, headache and fever are uncommon
   b. Secondary neoplasms are possible
   c. Amenorrhea and azoospermia are common
   d. CNS effects occur with high-dose therapy.

TOPOTECAN

Other name: Hycamptin.

Mechanism of Action

Topotecan, a semisynthetic derivative of camptothecin, is a potent inhibitor of topoisomerase I, an enzyme essential for effective replication and transcription. It binds to the topoisomerase I-DNA cleavable complex, preventing religation after cleavage by topoisomerase I.

Primary Indications

1. Ovarian carcinoma
2. Small cell and nonsmall cell lung carcinoma.

Usual Dosage and Schedule

Chemotherapy Book for 124 or Oncologist 1.5 mg/m^2 IV as a 30-min infusion daily × 5, every 3 weeks.

Toxicity

1. *Myelosuppression and other hematologic effects:* Leukopenia is universal and dose limiting. Anemia and thrombocytopenia are common and occasionally severe.
2. *Nausea, vomiting and other gastrointestinal effects:* Nausea, vomiting and diarrhea are common but usually mild. Other gastro-intestinal symptoms including constipation and abdominal pain occur occasionally.
3. *Mucocutaneous effects:* Alopecia is common; stomatitis is occasional but usually mild; skin rash is rare.
4. *Miscellaneous effects:*
   a. Fever, headache, fatigue, and weakness are common (15– 25%) but rarely severe.
   b. Microscopic hematuria is occasional.
   c. Dyspnea occurs occasionally, but it is uncommon for it to be severe.
   d. Infection as a consequence of severe leukopenia is common.

TOREMIFENE

Other name: Fareston.

Mechanism of Action

A selective estrogen receptor modulator that inhibits estrogen effects by competing with estrogen for binding on the cytosol estrogen receptor protein in cancer cells. The receptor-hormone complex ultimately controls the promoter region of genes that affect cell growth.

Primary Indication

Metastatic carcinoma of the breast in post-menopausal women with estrogen receptor—positive (or unknown) tumors.

Usual Dosage and Schedule

60 mg PO daily.

Special Precautions

1. Presently it is uncertain whether it has any carcinogenic effects on endometrium as have been observed with tamoxifen.
2. May result in increased prothrombin time in patients taking warfarin (Coumadin).
3. Cytochrome P450 3A4 enzyme inhibitors such as phenobarbital, phenytoin and carba-mazepine increase the rate of toremifene metabolism, lowering the concentration in the serum.

Toxicity

1. *Myelosuppression and other hematologic effects:* Uncommon and mild.
2. *Nausea, vomiting and other gastrointestinal effects:* Minimal nausea is common early in treatment; vomiting is occasional.
3. *Mucocutaneous effects:* Dry eyes and cataracts are rare. May cause an increase or decrease in vaginal secretions, which may result in difficult or painful intercourse.
4. *Miscellaneous effects:* These include the following:
   a. Hot flashes are common.
   b. Sweating is occasional.
   c. Vaginal bleeding and menstrual irregularity are occasional.
   d. Hypercalcemia is uncommon.
   e. Thromboembolic phenomena is rare.

131-I-TOSITUMOMAB

Other name: Bexxar.

Mechanism of Action

131-I-Tositumomab is a murine IgG2a monoclonal anti-CD20 antibody radiolabeled with 131-I, an emitter of both beta and gamma radiation. The mechanism of action includes antibody mediated cytotoxicity and cellularly targeted radiotherapy (radioimmunotherapy).

Primary Indication

Non-Hodgkin's lymphoma, chemotherapy refractory, CD20 positive, low grade or transformed low grade.

Usual Dosage and Schedule

Before dosimetric and therapeutic doses, patients are premedicated with acetaminophen 650 mg and diphenhydramine 50 mg. A saturated solution of potassium iodide, 2 to 3 drops PO three times daily, is given beginning 24 hours before the dosimetric dose and continuing for 14 days after the therapeutic dose to prevent uptake of 131-I by the thyroid.

1. *Dosimetric dose:* 450 mg of unlabeled tositumomab is given as a 1 hour infusion followed by a 20-min infusion of 5 mCi (35 mg) of 131I-tositumomab to determine the patient-specific activity (millicuries) of radiolabeled tositumomab to deliver a therapeutic dose of 65 to 75 cGy 7 to 15 days later.
2. *Therapeutic dose:* 450 mg of unlabeled tositumomab is given as a 1-h infusion followed by a 20-min infusion of patient specific (in millicuries), activity labeled to 35 mg of tositumomab (median 90 mCi, range 50 – 200 mCi).

Special Precautions

1. Use with caution in patients with over 25 percent marrow involvement with lymphoma, prior external beam radiotherapy to over 25 percent of the bone marrow, or a history of HAMAs or HACAs.
2. A saturated solution of potassium iodide, 2 to 3 drops PO three times daily, is given beginning 24 hours before the dosimetric dose and

continuing for 14 days after the therapeutic dose to prevent uptake of 131-I by the thyroid.

Toxicity

1. *Myelosuppression and other hematologic effects:* Myelosuppression is universal, with about 20 percent of patients having grade 4 thrombocytopenia or neutropenia. The nadir counts occur at a median of 5 to 6 weeks, with recovery to baseline by 10 weeks.
2. *Nausea, vomiting and other gastrointestinal effects:* Nausea is common; vomiting, abdominal pain and anorexia are occasional.
3. *Mucocutaneous effects:* Pruritus and rash are occasional.
4. *Miscellaneous effects:* These include the following:
   a. HAMAs or HACAs may develop (5–10%).
   b. Infusion-related fever, chills, dizziness, asthenia, wheezing or coughing, nasal congestion, headache, back pain, arthralgia and hypotension are occasional to common, more with dosimetric than therapeutic dose. Most commonly these are self-limited and mild to moderate in severity.
   c. Fatigue or asthenia is common.
   d. Cough and edema are occasional; dyspnea is uncommon.
   e. Thyroid suppression is uncommon when prophylaxis with potassium iodide is used.
   f. Myelodysplasia is occasionally seen 20 to 40 months after treatment.

TRASTUZUMAB

Other name: Herceptin.

Mechanism of Action

A recombinant humanized monoclonal antibody that targets the extracellular domain of the HER2 growth factor receptor.

Primary Indications

1. Carcinoma of the breast that has over-expression of HER2 (C-erb B-2).
2. Other carcinomas that exhibit overexpression of HER2.

Usual Dosage and Schedule

4 mg/kg IV loading dose over 90 min, then 2 mg/kg IV over 30 min weekly.

Special Precautions

1. During the first infusion and occasionally during later infusions, a systemic symptom complex similar to that seen with other human monoclonal antibodies is common. Severe hypersensitivity reactions and pulmonary adverse events have been reported but are uncommon to rare. These events include anaphylaxis, angioedema, bronchospasm, hypotension, hypoxia, dyspnea, pulmonary infiltrates, pleural effusions, noncardiogenic pulmonary edema, and acute respiratory distress syndrome. A more common symptom complex consists Immunosuppressants, Gene Therapy 129 of mild-to-moderate chills, fever, asthenia, pain, nausea, vomiting and

headache. These latter symptoms are generally well-managed by temporary slowing or interruption of the infusion and administration of acetaminophen, diphenhydramine and meperidine.

2. Cardiac dysfunction (cardiac symptoms or an asymptomatic decrease in ejection fraction of 10% or greater) occurs in about 7 percent of patients treated with trastuzumab alone but in 28 percent of patients treated with trastuzumab plus anthracycline and in 11 percent of patients treated with trastuzumab plus paclitaxel. In most cases, this improves with symptomatic therapy. Severe disability or death from cardiac dysfunction occurs in about 1 percent of patients. Extreme caution should be exercised in treating patients with pre-existing cardiac dysfunction.

Toxicity

1. *Myelosuppression:* Uncommon.
2. *Nausea, vomiting and other gastrointestinal effects:* Nausea and vomiting are occasional to common during first infusion. Diarrhea is also occasional to common.
3. *Mucocutaneous effects:* A rash is occasional to common and may be associated with urticaria or pruritus.
4. *Miscellaneous effects:* These include the following:
   a. Mild to moderate chills, fever, asthenia, pain and headache are common, primarily during the first infusion.
   b. Cardiac dysfunction occurs in about 7 percent of patients treated with trastuzumab alone but in 28 percent of patients treated with trastuzumab plus anthracycline and in 11 percent of patients treated with trastuzumab plus paclitaxel. In most cases, this improves with symptomatic therapy.
   c. Chest pain, back pain, dyspnea and cough are occasional to common.
   d. Peripheral edema is occasional.

VINBLASTINE

Other names: VLB, Velban, vincaleukoblastine sulfate (Fig. 2.32).

Mechanism of Action

Mitotic inhibition with reversible metaphase arrest due to action on microtubular and spindle contractile proteins.

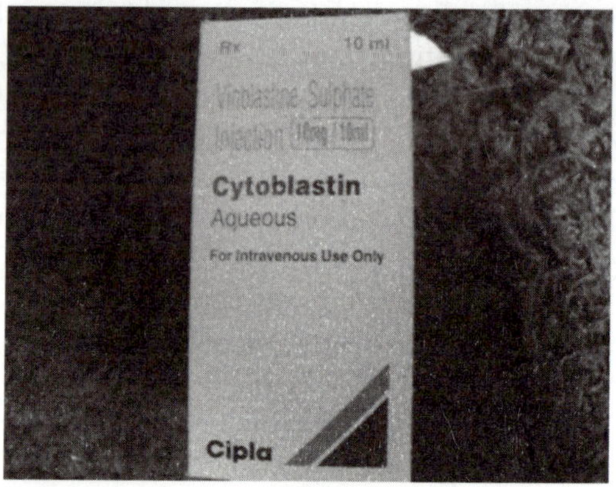

Fig. 2.32: Vinblastine injection

Primary Indications

1. Hodgkin's and non-Hodgkin's lymphomas
2. Testicular, gestational trophoblastic, kidney and breast carcinomas.

Usual Dosage and Schedule

1. 4 to 18 mg/m^2 IV weekly
2. 6 mg/m^2 IV on days 1 and 15 in combination with doxorubicin, bleomycin and decarbazine for lymphomas
3. 4.5 mg/m^2 IV on day 1 every 3 weeks in combination with doxorubicin and thiotepa for breast cancer.

Special Precaution

Administer as a slow push, taking care to avoid extravasation.

Toxicity

1. *Myelosuppression and other hematologic effects:* Dose-related leukopenia occurs with a nadir at 4 to 10 days and recovery in 7 to 10 days. Severe thrombocytopenia is uncommon.
2. *Nausea vomiting and other gastrointestinal effects:* Common but not usually severe.
3. *Mucocutaneous effects:*
   a. Extravasation may lead to severe inflammation, pain and tissue damage. Local infiltration with 1 to 6 ml of hyaluronidase (150 U/ml) may help.
   b. Mild alopecia is common.
   c. Stomatitis is occasionally severe.
4. *Miscellaneous effects:* These include the following:
   a. Neurotoxicity manifested by: (1) constipation, adynamic ileus and abdominal pain if very high doses are used; or (2) paresthesias, peripheral neuropathy and jaw pain with lower doses. Neurotoxicity is less fequent with vinblastine than with vincristine.
   b. Transient hepatitis is uncommon.
   c. Depression, headache, convulsions and orthostatic hypotension are rare.

VINCRISTINE

Other names: VCR, Oncovin and Vincasar.

Mechanism of Action

Mitotic inhibition with reversible metaphase arrest due to drug action on microtubular and spindle contractile proteins.

Primary Indications

1. Hodgkin's and non-Hodgkin's lymphomas
2. Acute lymphocytic leukemia
3. Multiple myeloma
4. Wilms' tumor, neuroblastoma, rhabdomyosarcoma and Ewing's sarcoma of childhood
5. Breast carcinoma.

Usual Dosage and Schedule

1. 1 to 2 mg/m^2 (maximum 2.0 to 2.4 mg) IV weekly

2. 0.4 mg/day as a continuous IV infusion on days 1 to 4.

Special Precautions

1. Administer as a slow IV push, taking care to avoid extravasation.
2. Because neurotoxicity is cumulative, neurologic evaluation should be done before each dose and therapy withheld if severe paresthesias, motor weakness, or other severe abnormalities occur. Underlying neurologic problems accentuate vincristine's effect.
3. Reduce dose if liver disease is significant.
4. Stool softeners or high fiber or bulk diets may avert severe constipation.

Toxicity

1. *Myelosuppression and other hematologic effects:* Mild and rarely of clinical significance.
2. *Nausea, vomiting are not seen unless paralytic ileus occurs:* Constipation is common.
3. *Mucocutaneous effects:* Severe local inflammation if extravasation occurs. Alopecia is common.
4. *Neurotoxicity:* Dose dependent and dose limiting. Mild paresthesias and decreased deep tendon reflexes are to be expected. More extensive peripheral neuropathies, severe constipation, and ileus are indications to reduce or hold therapy. Autonomic dysfunction with orthostatic hypotension or urinary retention may be seen.
5. *Miscellaneous effects:*
   a. Uric acid nephropathy due to rapid tumor cell lysis and release of uric acid is always a potential problem when therapy is first given.
   b. Syndrome of inappropriate antidiuretic hormone is rare.

VINORELBINE

Other name: Navelbine.

Mechanism of Action

Binds to tubulin; depolymerizes microtubules, causing mitotic inhibition, similar to other vinca alkaloids. Lower affinity for axonal microtubules associated with lower neurotoxicity.

Primary Indications

1. Nonsmall cell carcinoma of the lung
2. Metastatic carcinoma of the breast.

Usual Dosage and Schedule

1. 30 mg/m^2 IV as 6 to 100 min rapid infusion weekly when used with a single agent or with cisplation.
2. 20 to 25 mg/m^2 IV as a 6 to 10 min rapid infusion in various schedules, when used with other myelotoxic agents.

Special Precautions

1. Administer infusion through the sidearm of a freely flowing IV line, taking care to avoid extravasation.

2. Reduce dose by 50 percent for serum bilirubin levels of 2.1 to 3 mg/dl and by 75 percent for bilirubin levels of over 3 mg/dl.

Toxicity

1. *Myelosuppression and other hematologic effects:* Granulocytopenia is common and dose limiting, with nadir at 7 to 10 days. Thrombocytopenia is uncommon. Anemia is occasional to common.
2. *Nausea, vomiting and other gastrointestinal effects:* Nausea and vomiting are common but usually mild to moderate. Diarrhea occurs occasionally.
3. *Mucocutaneous effects:* Alopecia, mild diarrhea and stomatitis are occasional. Severe local inflammation can occur with extravasation.
4. *Miscellaneous effects:*
   a. Regarding neurotoxicity, cumulative but reversible constipation and decreased deep tendon reflexes are occasional; paresthesias are uncommon.
   b. Erythema, pain, and skin discoloration at injection site are common; phlebitis at injection site is occasional.

ZOLEDRONIC ACID

Other name: Zometa.

Mechanism of Action

A bisphosphonate that inhibits osteoclastic resorption of bone and calcium release induced by tumor cytokines.

Primary Indications

1. Hypercalcemia associated with malignancy.
2. Bone metastases from breast cancer, prostate cancer (after progression on hormonal therapy), and other solid tumors in conjucntion with standard antineoplastic therapy.
3. Osteolytic and osteoporotic bone lesions of multiple myeloma.

Usual Dosage and Schedule

1. Hypercalcemia of malignancy, 4 mg IV as a 15 min infusion. May be repeated every 1 to 8 weeks as needed.
2. Multiple myeloma or metastatic bone lesions. 4 mg IV as a 15 min infusion every 3 to 4 weeks.

Special Precaution

Do not infuse for less than 15 min. Potential for renal tubular damage, particularly if infused more rapidly, serum creatinine should be measured prior to each dose. The risk of adverse reactions, particularly renal adverse reactions, may be greater in patients with impaired renal function. Dose adjustments are not necessary so long as initial serum creatinine is under 4.5 mg/dl. Withhold if there is deterioration in renal function (creatinine increase of 0.5 mg/dl in patients with normal baseline creatinine or 1 mg/dl in patients with abnormal baseline creatinine). Use caution when administered concurrently with aminoglycosides. Serum electrolytes and renal function should be monitored closely.

Toxicity

1. *Myelosuppression and other hematologic effects:* Rare.
2. *Nausea, vomiting and other gastrointestinal effects:* Abdominal pain, anorexia constipation, nausea, and vomiting are uncommon to occasional.
3. *Mucocutaneous effects:* Infusion site reaction is occasional.
4. *Miscellaneous effects:* These include the following:
   a. Flu-like syndrome with fever, chills, skeletal aches and pains is occasional.

Chapter 3 Targeted Cancer Therapy

CANCER BIOLOGY

Cancer is thought to be a clonal disorder, because there is evidence that most cancers arise from a single cell that has suffered a disruption in its regulatory mechanisms for proliferation and self-elimination. Malignant cells differ from their normal tissue counterparts in a number of ways:

- They are often immortal, or at least have the ability to divide many more times than cells from normal somatic tissues, which tend to senesce after 50 or 60 doublings.
- They often grow more rapidly than cells of the same tissue of origin—though not necessarily faster than the normal cell can divide if given the stimulus.
- They fail to show normal cell-to-cell interactions, which results in their ability to invade, metastasize and grow in a foreign environment. The change from completely normal tissues to a frankly malignant metastasizing tumor frequently occurs in a number of discreet steps over a period of time. These "steps", which are the result of mutations, deletions, or gene changes in growth regulators, may occur spontaneously as a consequence of random errors, or they may result from exposure to agents as diverse as chemical mutagens, ionizing radiations, ultraviolet light, and viruses.

MECHANISMS OF CARCINOGENESIS

Carcinogenesis appears to be a multistep process with multiple genetic alterations occurring over an extended period of time; at least, that is how it appears. Sometimes these genetic alterations are carried in the germline, as for example in the cancer-predisposing syndromes such as retinoblastoma.

Most alterations that lead to cancer are acquired in the form of somatic mutations; chromosomal translocations, deletions, inversions, amplifications, or simply point mutations.

The control of cell proliferation is the consequence of signals affecting cell division

Gain-of-function mutation in an oncogene → Malignant transformation ← Loss-of-function mutation in a tumor suppressor gene

Malignant transformation

The process of malignant transformation may result from either a gain-of-function mutation that activates an oncogene, or a loss-of-function mutation in a tumor-suppressor gene and differentiation. These signals may be positive or negative, and the acquisition of tumorigenicity results from changes that affect these control points.

Oncogenes were first discovered from a study of retroviruses (i.e. viruses whose genomes are composed of RNA) that cause cancers in animals. The retroviruses contain modified cellular genes captured from the genomes of their vertebrate hosts. Cancer caused by a retrovirus, then, is mediated through cellular genes that have been mutated or changed. Normal versions of these genes (proto-oncogenes) are present in every mammalian cell, and many have been shown to function in regulating cell growth. Infection of cells by these viruses leads to integration of the viral oncogene into the host genome, in which it is expressed at high levels leading to overproliferation, the signature of cancer. Although a virus causes cancer by inserting an oncogene from its own genome into that of the cell, the mechanism of transformation by radiation or chemicals is to cause changes in a normal proto-oncogene indigenous to that cell, causing it to be activated. There are three principal mechanisms by which proto-oncogenes can be activated to produce a malignant cell (Figs 3.1 and 3.2).

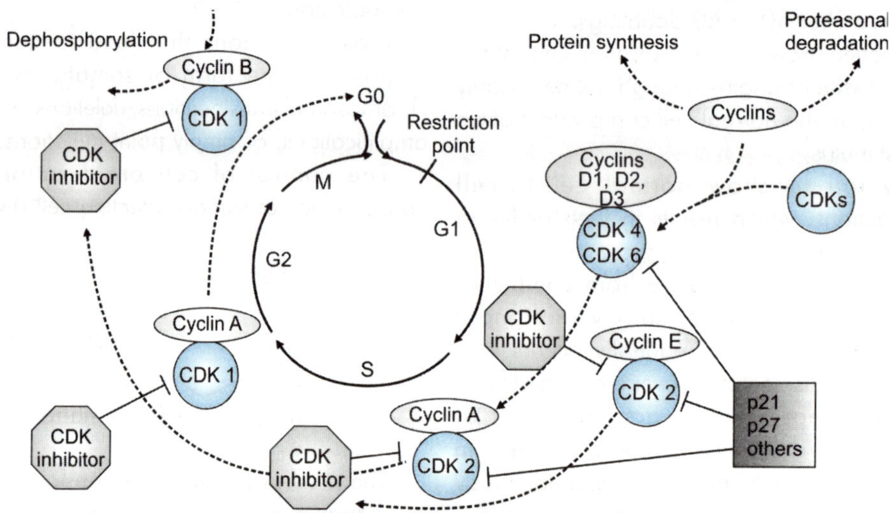

Fig. 3.1: Cell cycle regulation by cyclins and cyclin-dependent kinases (CDKs)

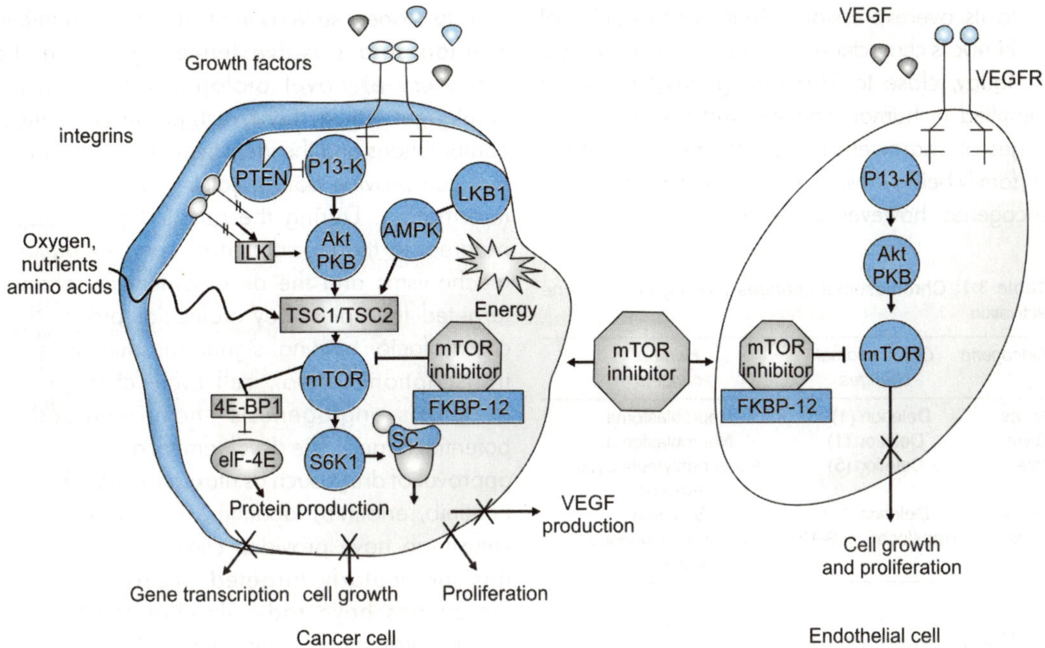

Fig. 3.2: mTOR: A central controller of tumor cell growth and angiogenesis

1. A Point mutation can occur, changing a single base pair, which subsequently produces a protein with a single amino acid change. For example, a point mutation in k-ras is found in the cancer cells of most patients suffering from colon cancer.
2. A chromosomal rearrangement or translocation can occur, often placing a proto-oncogene next to a strong promoter sequence, leading to its overexpression, or producing a new fusion gene whose product acquires a new transforming activity. Ionizing radiations are highly effective at producing DNA breaks. These chromosomal breaks may rejoin in such a way as to form a dicentric chromosome, which is almost always lethal to the cell. Translocations have been shown to be associated with several human cancers involving myc genes. For example, a translocation between chromosomes 2 and 8 is responsible for myc activation in some Burkitt's lymphomas.
3. Gene amplification, in which many new extra copies of a proto-oncogene are generated in a cell, is associated with the activation of oncogenes in several cancers. The presence of multiple copies of a proto-oncogene leads

to its overexpression. Gene amplification of N-myc is characteristic of many neuroblastomas. Today, close to 100 oncogenes have been identified in human cancers and are at various stages of characterization, with members of the ras family being most common. Presently identified oncogenes, however, are given in Table 3.1.

Table 3.1: Chromosomal changes leading to oncogene activation

Oncogene	*Chromosomal changes*	*Human cancers*
N-ras	Deletion (1)	Neuroblastoma
Blym	Deletion (1)	Neuroblastoma
fms	Deletion (5)	Acute nonlymphocytic leukemia
H-ras	Deletion (11)	Sarcoma
c-abl	Translocation (9-12)	Chronic myelogenous leukemia

The treatment of cancer is now based on an understanding of underlying biologic mechanisms and is increasingly being tailored to the molecular specificity of a tumor. Although oncology still functions within broad disease categories, the future will see an increasing shift to treatment based on the characteristic of an individual's tumor type. Interestingly, one of the first targeted therapies, all trans retinoic acid in acute promyelocytic leukemia, was first demonstrated at the bedside with a subsequent return to the bench to elucidate its underlying basis. This was a translocation resulting in disruption of the retinoic acid receptor –α gene. Since then, rigorous translational approach has led to other success stories, such as imatinib and dasatinib in Philadelphia positive leukemias. With the discovery of novel biologic agents, future challenges lie in the investigation of optimal combinations and the identification of biomarkers that can provide both predictive and prognostic information. During the past 20 years, rapid progress in the elucidation of complex biologic mechanisms and the development of rational, targeted therapies. Key molecular processes—growth factor binding, signal transduction, gene transcription control, cell cycle checkpoints, apoptosis angiogenesis—have emerged as potential targets. The development and regulatory approval of drugs such as rituximab, trastuzumab, imatinib, erlotinib, lapatinib, bevacizumab, and cetuximab have provided clinical validation for this molecularly targeted approach. These discoveries have radically changed the way cancer treatment is conceptualized.

Targeted therapy is exponential growth in the field of translational medicine, it is helpful to contextualize this progress within a larger historical perspective. In the past, cancer treatments evolved from empiric observation and, not infrequently, chance observation. In 1942, the sinking of a US battleship led to the recognition that mustard gas causes profound lymphoid and myeloid suppressions. Following this accidental discovery, mustine (the prototype nitrogen mustard) was used to treat non-Hodgkin's lymphoma (l). Since then, a majority of the more than 200 currently available cancer drugs were identified serendipitously from plants or fungi.

Human genome project, has led to drug discovery. In revealing a vast amount of information about normal and malignant cells, the human genome project has provided a gateway to the current era of molecular medicine. The development of rational drug therapy is now based on an understanding of the molecular genotypes and phenotypes of disease.

The histories behind the development of all-trans retinoic acid (ATRA), imatinib (Gleeves; Novartis, Cambridge, MA, USA), and decitabine (Dacogen; MGI Pharma/SuperGen, Minneapolis, MN, USA) are different versions of the bench to bedside and back paradigm.

In recent years, arsenic compounds, particularly arsenic trioxide (AS_2O_3), have shown success in the treatment to both primary cases and in relapsed and ATRA-resistant patients. During the 1990s, investigators in China reported that arsenic trioxide could induce a CR in patients with APL. Functioning by a mechanism different from that of ATRA, arsenic can induce a CR rate of more than 80 percent in relapsed patients after treatment with ATRA. Trials in the United States showed molecular remission in more than 80 percent of relapsed APL patients, as measured by RT-PCR of marrow specimens for PML-RAR α transcript. Currently, arsenic is considered a first-line therapy for relapsed APL patients. Because arsenic does not completely eradicate leukemic cell, the optimal postremission therapy remains undefined. Outcomes of autologous stem cell transplantation in patients with a second molecular remission after arsenic therapy have demonstrated a good success rate.

The theme of "kinase-dependent" cancers explains cancers whose growth is driven by a specific set of kinases (Fig. 3.3). The distinct molecular abnormality underlying Philadelphia positive leukemia is activation of ABL tyrosine kinase Action of TKI by a chromosome translocation (Figs 3.4A and B). Imatinib, a small-molecule tyrosine kinase inhibitor, is a direct inhibitor of BCR-ABL, KIT, and the platelet-derived growth factor receptor (PDGFR) alpha and beta. Imatinib binds competitively with ATP to BCR-ABL, blocking abnormal signaling and selectively inhibiting proliferation of BCR-ABL-positive cells.

The observation that imatinib other kinases, notably the oncoprotein c-Kit, led to another successful clinical translation of the drug for the treatment of GISTs.

The molecular hallmark of CML is the Philadelphia (Ph) chromosome, a reciprocal 9;22. Translocation that generates the fusion oncogene BCR-ABL. Since its identification in 1960, the Ph chromosome is now known to be present in more than 90 percent of CML cases. The presence of the Ph chromosome in a hematopoietic stem cell leads to cytokine-independent cell growth and survival.

Mathematical Modeling

Understanding of cancer biology require devising a mathematical framework that can describe fundamental principles underlying tumor initation and progression. Tumorigenesis is governed by principles that explain evolution—mutation and selection. An example of the application of

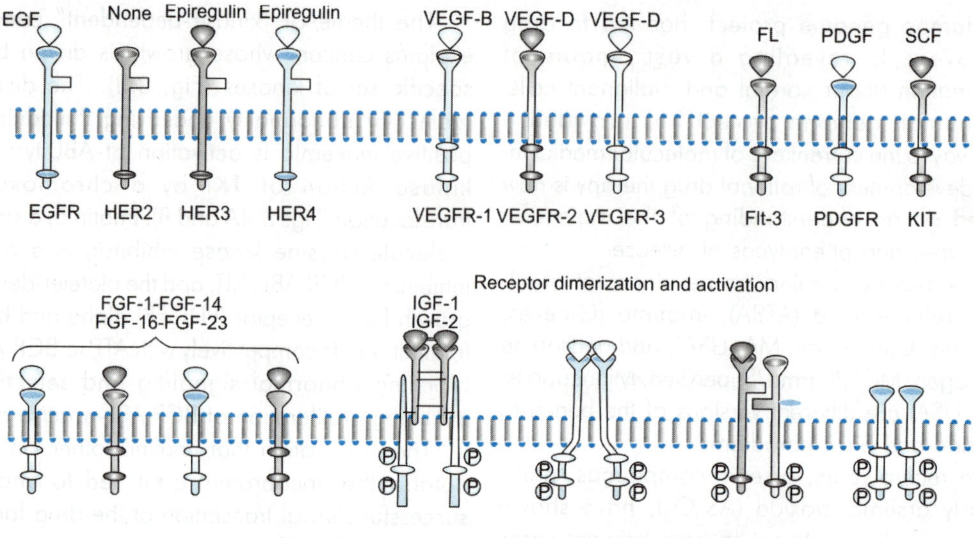

Fig. 3.3: Receptor tyrosine kinase (RTK) families and their activation

mathematical modeling to help streamline the acquisition of knowledge about molecular mechanisms is one developed for evaluating resistant populations in leukemia. A formula has been derived to calculate the probability of resistance by considering an exponentially growing leukemic stem cell population that produces resistant leukemic cells. These calculations might be helpful for determining when imatinib therapy ought to be combined with other therapies, provide an accurate prognosis for the disease, and direct is likely to take.

GISTs were rarely diagnosed until around the year 2000, when they became a focus of research. Prefiguring this increased interest was the finding the late 1990s that gain-of-function mutations of the receptor tyrosine kinase KIT play a major role in the pathogenesis of GISTs. Previously classified as leiomyomas, leiomyosarcomas, and leiomyoblastomas, GIST was first used in 1983 to describe gastrointestinal nonepithelial neoplasms that lacked the characteristics of smooth muscle cells. Historically, GISTs have been associated with a poor prognosis. The rates of recurrence after

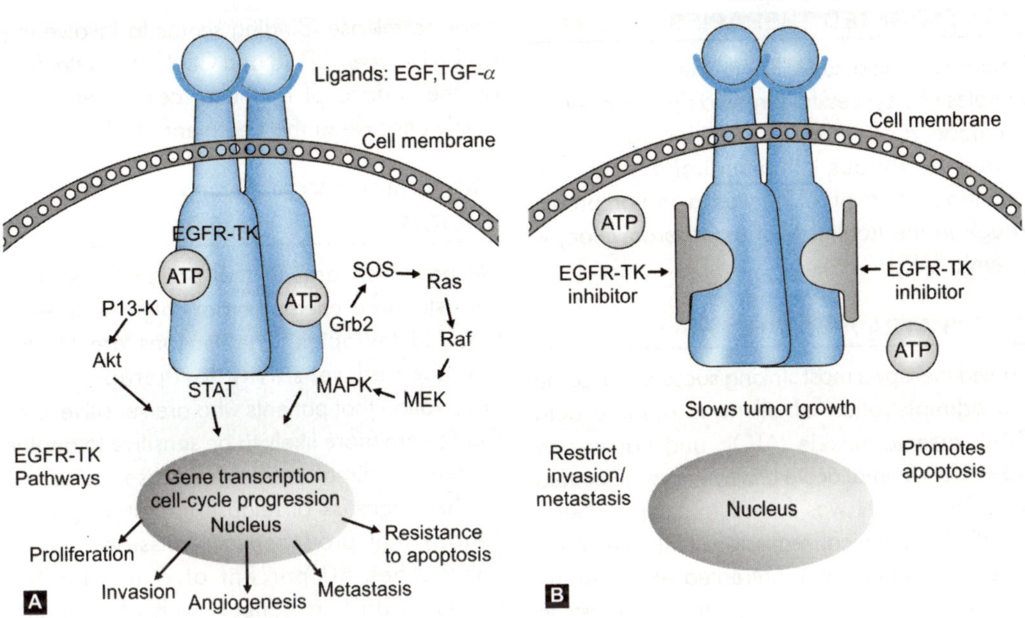

Figs 3.4A and B: Receptor tyrosine kinase induce tumor cell growth

surgical resection of GISTs are highly radiation-resistant and chemoresistant. RRs to singl-agent or combination chemotherapy have ranged from none to 9 percent in the presence of metastatic desease. A combination trial using mesna, doxorubicin, ifosfamide, and dacarbazine reported an objective RR of 22 percent, but these results have been questioned.

Preclinical evidence showed that most GISTs demonstrated gain-of-function mutations in the KIT (c-kit) proto-oncogene. Constitutive activation of KIT in GISTs leads to uncontrolled cell proliferation and resistance to apoptosis. GISTs also commonly demonstrate mutations of PDGFR α kinase. Imatinib's known mechanism of the tyrosine kinases KIT and PDGFR α provided a rationale for its clinical evaluation in GIST.

Immediate milestone is to transform cancer into a manageable disease. The language of translational medicine has enabled open communication and understanding between basic scientists researchers that will further refine targeted therapies to support a chronic disease model.

FIRST TARGETED THERAPIES

All-trans retinoic acid (ATRA) is one of the earliest examples of a successful targeted drug and serves as a model for developing novel biologic agents tailored to various other malignant tumors. The introduction of ATRA was a major breakthrough in the treatment of acute promyelocytic leukemia (APL).

WHAT IS ATRA AND ATO?

Targeted therapy's most striking success has come from administration of all-trans retinoic acid (ATRA), arsenic trioxide (ATO), and particularly ATO+ ATRA to treat acute promyelocytic leukemia (APL). This ability was found to be paralleled clinically by a clinical remission (CR) rate of 80 percent to 90 percent in untreated APL, with the CR (<5% abnormal promyelocytes and blasts in the marrow, platelet and neutrophil counts >100,000 and 1000/ul, respectively) not preceded by marrow aplasia but by differentiation of promyelocytes into myelocytes/metamyelocytes and eventually neutrophils. In 20 percent of cases there is a substantial increase (e.g. to >50,000) in the number of circulating mature myeloid cells, often accompanied by fever, effusions, edema, and lung infiltrates, constituting an "APL differentiation syndrome" ATRA syndrome but now recognized to occur after ATO as well. The pathogenesis of the APLDS is thought to involve ATRA-mediated up regulation of CD38 on the surface of blood cells and subsequent binding of these cells to epithelial cells with consequent cytokine release. Binding seems to involve interaction between CD38 and CD31, the letter found on the surface of epithelial cells. Steroids are highly effective in the treatment of APLDS.

CANDIDATES FOR TARGETED THERAPIES

We previously argued that patient in remission after standard chemotherapy might well-receive targeted therapies. The reasons are (1) their documented sensitivity to therapy; (2) the observation that patients who are sensitive to one therapy are more likely to be sensitive to another; (3) their minimal residual disease status; and (4) their high-risk of relapse if continued on the therapy that produced a remission. This risk approaches 50 percent at 6 months from remission date in patients with abnormalities involving more than three chromosomes, thus providing a counterargument to the belief that such patients have "no active disease to follow".

There is increasing use of targeted therapies in untreated, especially older, patients rather than patients in relapse.

Trastuzumab (Herceptin) is ant humanized monoclonal antibody against the extracellular domain of HER2. Trastuzumab inhibits cancer cell proliferation, induces apoptosis and reduces tumor- induced angiogenesis in preclinical breast cancer models.

The exact mechanism of trastuzumab activity remains however, preclinical date suggest that the drug induces antibody-mediated cytotoxicity as well as sequesters HER2 and prevents interactions with other members of the HER family.

Trastuzumab has demonstrated activity as a single agent (PR=24% –35%) in patients with metastatic breast cancer whose tumors overexpress HER2 64.

Dosing schedule (8 mg/kg loading followed by 6 mg/kg every 3 weeks) 3-week dosing schedule was similar in efficacy and toxicity compared to weekly dosing, but offered increased easy of administration and fewer patient visits for therapy.

Trastuzumab also augments the effects of chemotherapy. Disease response rate, median duration of response, and overall survival were all improved in patients who received chemotherapy with trastuzumab. Although earlier phase trials did not demonstrate significant cardiac toxicity with single a higher rate of congestive heart failure (CHF) was noted in patient treated with trastuzumab. When compared to the antracycline/ trastuzumab arm, the incidence of CHF was less in patient receiving antracycline/trastuzumab.

Chemotherapy Drugs Commonly Combined Trastuzumab

Drug (s)	Response rate
Paclitaxel	36-77%
Docetaxel	58-79%
Gemcitabine	36-44%
Capecitabine	60-76%

To date, the optimal duration of trastuzumab administration (1 year versus 2 years) remains undefined.

The Breast Cancer International Research (BCIR) group trial alternatively questioned the role for anthracyclines in the adjuvant setting for patients with HER2- overexpressing breast cancer. Patients enrolled in the control arm received doxorubicin- cyclophosphamide (AC) followed by docetaxel. Patients treated in the trastuzumab-containing arms received either AC followed by docetaxel with trastuzumab or docetaxel and platinum (carboplatin or cisplatin) with trastuzumab. This study demonstrated that one year of trastuzumab improved the DFS compared to adjuvant chemotherapy alone, however, longer follow-up is needed to determine if anthracyclines are necessary for the treatment of HER2- positive breast cancer.

Bevacizumab (Avastin) is a recombinant, humanized antibody against VEGF. The drug has demonstrated single—agent response rate of 6.7 percent to 17.0 percent in breast cancer patients with previously treated metastatic disease. When given in combination with capecitabine as a second-to third-line therapy for metastatic breast cancer, bevacizumb did not significantly improve DFS.

Targeted Therapy in Chronic Lymphocytic Leukemia

Chronic lymphocytic leukemia (CLL) is characterized by a monoclonal population of mature, activated B lymphocytes. It is a heterogeneous disorder with a variable clinical course. Although in recent years the introduction of chemo-immunotherapeutic combinations such as fludarabine, cyclophosphamide, and rituximab (FCR) has induced response rates of 95 percent in previously untreated patients and increased the rates of failure-free survival, CLL remains incurable for many patients. However, a better understanding of the molecular basis of CLL has led to the development of several novel therapeutic strategies that target molecular pathways. These targeted therapies inhibit signaling pathways involved in growth and proliferation in CLL cells. Among the targeted therapies being investigated in CLL are the following: monoclonal antibodies against CD52 (alemtuzumab), CD20 (rituximab, ofatumumab), and CD40 (HCD122); agent that target molecular pathways, such as cyclin-dependent kinase inhibitors (flavopirido); peptidase inhibitors (talabostat;) Bcl-2- targeting agents (antisense oligonucleotide, oblimersen; small molecule inducing apoptosis, gossypol); heat shock protein 90 inhibitors that target 7-kDa zeta-associated protein(17-AAG, CNF2024); immunomodulating agents (lenalidomide; immunostimulatory oligonucleotides CpG); hypomethylating agents (decitabine; valproic acid); antiangiogenic agents (bevacizumab); and gene therapis. This chapter reviews the use of targeted therapies as single agents and in combination with chemotherapy for CLL.

ALEMTUZUMAB

Alemtuzumab (Campath-1H), an anti-CD52 humanized monoclonal antibody, has been extensive investigated in CLL. It has significant antileukemic activety, which is high in the blood, bone marrow and spleen and low in lymph node. The Food and Drug Administration (FDA) has approved alemtuzumab for patients with B-cell CLL who have been treated with alkylating agents and for whom fludarabine therapy has failed.

As a first-line therapy, alemtuzumab administered subcutaneously three times weekly for 18 weeks induced a response rate of 87 percent and clearance of CLL cells from the blood and CR or nodular PR rates in the bone marrow of 95 percent and 65 percent, respectively. The response rate in lymph nodes was 87 percent (CR 29%). The most noteworthy adverse events were transient injection site reactions (90% of patients) and cytomegalovirus reactivation (10%), which responded to ganciclovir therapy. Alemtuzumab has mainly been investigated in relapsed or refractory CLL.

Rituximab (IDEC-C2B8) is a chimeric antibody that binds to the B-cell surface antigen CD20. Although highly effective in follicular lymphoma, with an overall response rate of 60 percent, single-agent rituximab has inferior clinical activity in small lymphocytic lymphomas (overall response rate 13%). Rituximab has clinical activity in B-cell CLL; but compared with its activity in follicular lymphoma, it is less effective in clearing disease from the bone marrow and the response duration is short. Single-agent rituximab induces response in 23 percent to 45 percent of previously treated patients rituximab was administered 375 mg/m^2 weekly for 4 consecutive weeks as a first-line therapy in CLL and was repeated at 6-month intervals. Rituximab has been used in combination with granulocyte-macrophage colony-stimulating factor (GM-CSF) on the basis of *in vitro* and clinical data in indolent lymphoma showing increased antitumor activity when combined with GM-CSF. This regimen resulted in a 79 percent response rate (CR 36%) in patients with indolent lymphoma.

Ofatumumab (HuMax CD20), a monoclonal antibody, which targets a different epitope of CD20 than that targeted by rituximab, is thought to kill rituximab-resistant cells.

Two most important drugs given below (FDA has approved):

1. ***Soranib:*** Available as 200 mg tablets it blocks the all tumor cells proliferations as well as tumor angiogenesis by help of various factors like VEGF, EGF, TKI very effective in metastatic renal cell carcinoma[progression free survival from 12 weeks conventional treatment to 24 weeks, also use full inhepatocellular carcinoma, side effects are cardiotoxicity, hypertension hand and foot syndrome dose-400 mg bd, dose may be decreased during side effects to 200 mg od.
2. ***Bortezomib:*** {ps341, proteosome inhibitor}—It is tripeptide in structure proteosome action is cell cycle progression as well as inhibit apoptosis, dose 1.3 mg/meter squre as BSA on d1.d4, d8, d11, three weekly cycle recommended drug side effects are peripheral neuropathy most comman in 30 percent cases, myelosuppresion, activation of herpes zoster infection.

Chapter 4 New Hope with Gene Therapy

CYCLOSPORINE

It markedly and selectively inhibits T lymphocyte proliferation, IL-2 and other cytokine production and response of inducer Tells to IL-1 without any effect on suppressor T cells.

IMMUNOSUPPRESSANT ANTIBODIES

Muromonab CD3: It is murine monoclonal antibody against the CD3 glycoprotein located near to the T cell receptor on helper T cells. Binding of muromonab CD3 to the CD3 antigen obstructs the binding of MHC II- antigen to the T cell receptor—participation of T cells in the immune response is prevented and T cells rapidly disappear from circulation leading to an immune blocked state. Gene therapy refers to introduction of functional genetic material into target cells to replace or supplement defective genes. In contrast to all other drugs this kind of therapy can impart new functions to a cell. Conceived in the 1960s and started in the1980s, gene therapy is still in its infancy but holds great promise for curing a number of diseases which at present can at best be only palliated or controlled. Gene defects result in failure to synthesize a functional protein or in the synthesis of dysfunctional protein. Equipping the cell (specially the one which physiologically expresses it) with a normal copy of the defective gene would overcome the deficiency at the site where it is needed on a long-term (may be permanent) basis. The major thrust area of gene therapy are a number of acquired diseases such as malignancies, immunological disorders including AIDS, cardiovascular, neurological and infective diseases, in many of which even short-term expression of the introduced gene could be therapeutic.

APPROACHES IN GENE THERAPY

Gene therapy endeavors to either modify or transfer genes.

Gene Modification

This involves correction of the defective portion of a genomic sequence or removal of the whole defective gene and its replacement by the normal copy or alteration of the sequences controlling its expression. These are technically quite difficult in the *in vivo* setting.

Gene Transfer

This involves introduction of one or more genomic expression cassettes without removing or altering the existing ones. Significant progress has been made in this approach. Gene transfer is carried out by using various physical, chemical or biological delivery methods (vectors).

Physical Methods

These include microinjection in a single cell, introduction of DNA complexed with gold particles/dextran/lipids, use of microprojectiles or direct parenteral injection of uncomplexed DNA. However, efficiency of gene transfer is low and duration of expression is short.

Chemical Methods

These use liposomes or other specific cellular legends. The liposomes can carry genes to the intracellular location in large amounts, are nonimmunogenic and technically simpler, but the level of gene transfer achieved is lower than by use of viral vectors. Liposomal delivery has been used in certain human gene therapy trials.

Biological Methods

These methods includes fusion of recipient cell with bacterial spheroblasts, erythrocyte membrane vesicles, whole cell fusion, etc. but the most efficient and widely used are viral vectors. Adenoviruses, Vaccinia virus, Herpes simplex virus have been utilized but retroviruses are the most popular vectors. For using viral vector its 'gag'; 'pol' and 'env' genes which carry out viral replication are removed and replaced by the genes to be transferred using recombinant DNA technology.

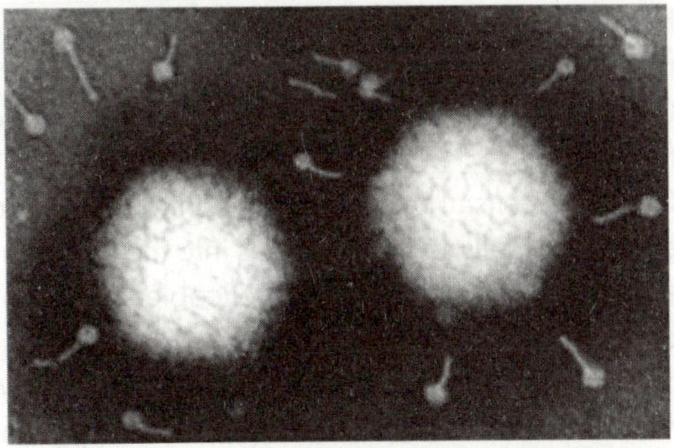

Fig. 4.1: Adenoviruses use for gene transfer

Adenoviruses (Fig 4.1) may be used for gene transfer. These viral particles are then introduced into cell line previously equipped with the gag, pol and env genes which then produce multiple viral particles carrying the desired gene. The retroviral vector is then allowed to infect host cells so that the desired DNA is inserted into a random site in the host genome which subsequently expresses the transferred gene (Fig. 4.2).

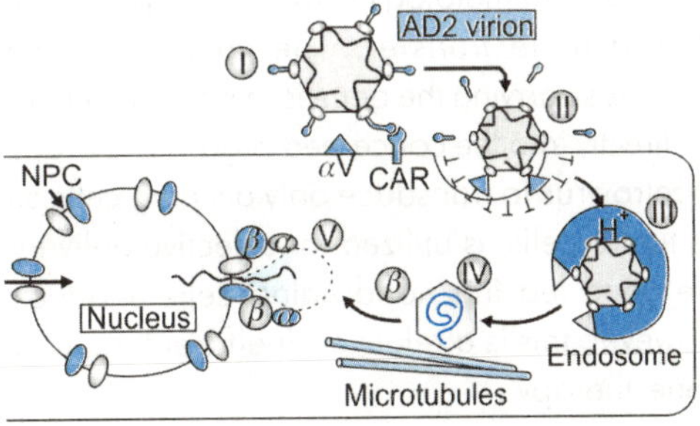

Fig. 4.2: Adenoviruses entry into cell

However, the duration of expression of the transferred gene is variable.

Gene transfer could be carried out into the following:

Germline cells: The new gene is introduced into embryonal cells so that it passes into the next generation. This is ethically not applicable to humans at present.

Somatic cells: Certain somatic cells like the bone marrow stem cells, fibroblasts, hepatocytes or myocytes of the recipient receive the new gene. This is being extensively persued.

Specific organ directed delivery of genes: To the tissues that actually require it is being tried. Success has been achieved in transferring genes into liver cells, vascular smooth muscle and endothelial cells, pulmonary cells, etc. *The techniques of gene therapy* may utilize either *ex vivo* or *in vivo* gene transfer.

Ex vivo gene transfer: These are then transfected with the vector carrying the relevant gene and injected back into the patient and are been widely utilized in the treatment of single gene defects, metabolic, hematological and immune disorders.

In vivo gene transfer: The vector, usually a retrovirus carrying the gene is injected systemically or directly into the concerned organ. The property of retrovirus to transduce only dividing cells,such as tumor cells, is utilized for selective delivery of the gene leaving nondividing cells unaffected. However, this is a relatively inefficient method of gene therapy.

APPLICATIONS OF GENE THERAPY

There are diverse applications of gene therapy, the prominent ones are:

- *Cystic fibrosis:* By introducing cystic fibrosis transport regulator (CFTR) gene into respiratory epithelial cells. This gene regulates expression of an apical chloride channel which is dysfunctional in cystic fibrosis.
- *Severe combind immunodeficiency disease (SCID):* By introducing gene for adenosine deaminase which is deficient.
- *Growth hormone deficiency:* By implanting cultured myoblasts transfected with GH gene.
- *Familial hypercholesterolemia:* By introducing LDL receptor gene into hepatocytes.
- *Lesch-Nyhan syndrome:* By introducing hypoxanthine phosphoribosyl transferase gene to correct deficiency of this enzyme in the CNS which causes severe neuropsychiatric disorder.
- *Parkinsonism:* By introducing the gene for tyrosine hydroxylase to augment dopamine production in basal ganglia.
- *Alzheimer's disease, Huntington's chorea, familial amylotropiclateral sclerosis, Gaucher's disease:* By supplementing the defective genes.
- *Stroke, head injury, multiple sclerosis:* By delivering nerve growth factor gene.
- *Duchenne muscular dystrophy:* By administering muscle dystropin gene.
- ***Cancer:***
  i. By genetic introduction of an enzyme (viral thymidinekinase) into tumor cells followed

by a prodrug that is converted to the toxic metabolite—tumor cells are selectively killed.

ii. By inserting TNF, IL-2 and other cytokine genes into tumor cells to increase their immune recognition and destruction by tumor infiltrating lymphocytes.

iii. By introducting promoter antisense gene or suppressor gene which negatively regulate tumor growth.

iv. By introducing multidrug resistance gene into bone marrow cells and rendering them less susceptible to destruction by myelosuppressant drugs. Thus a limiting toxicity of many anticancer drugs can be overcome. As yet gene therapy is only a research modality. A number of technological, toxicological and ethical problems have to be solved before it could be available for mass application.

Chapter 5 Side Effects of Chemotherapy

WHAT CAUSES SIDE EFFECTS WITH CHEMOTHERAPY?

Cancer cells tend to grow fast and chemo drugs kill fast-growing cells. But because these drugs travel throughout the body, they can affect normal, healthy cells that are fast-growing too. Damage to healthy tissue causes side effects. Although side effects are not always as bad as you might expect, many people worry about this part of their cancer treatment.

DURING CHEMOTHERAPY REMEMBER THESE LINES

The normal cells most likely to be damaged by chemo are blood-forming cells in the bone marrow; hair follicles; and cells in the mouth, digestive tract, and reproductive system. Some chemo drugs can damage cells in the heart, kidneys, bladder, lungs and nervous system. In some cases, medicines can be given with the chemo to protect the body's normal cells.

- ♦ Ensure full patient participation in treatment decisions
- ♦ Tailor treatment based on side effect and risk profile
- ♦ Identify and address patient's needs before treatment begins
- ♦ Increase home nurse visits, if needed
- ♦ Monitor patient's bone density and evaluate treatments to attenuate bone loss
- ♦ Instruct patient on symptoms of thromboembolism

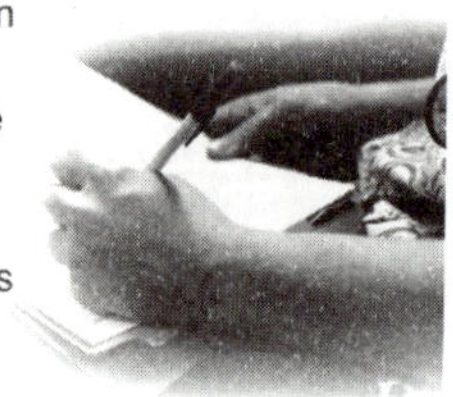

What are common side effects?

You are not alone if you have questions about side effects. Before chemo starts, most people worry about whether they will have side effects and, if so, what they will be like. The most common side effects of chemo are listed here. They are discussed in more detail toward the end of this section.

- Anemia (low red blood cell count)
- Fatigue (extreme tiredness)
- Hair loss
- Increased chance of bruising, bleeding and infection
- Nausea and vomiting.

Chemo may affect parts of your body in the following ways:

- Intestinal and stomach problems
- Appetite and weight changes
- Sore mouth, gums and throat
- Nerve and muscle problems
- Dry and/or discolored skin

- Kidney and bladder irritation
- Sexual and fertility issues because of effects on reproductive organs.

What should I remember about side effects?

Every person does not get every side effect and some people get few, if any. The severity of side effects varies greatly from person-to-person. Be sure to talk to your doctor and nurse about which side effects are most likely with your chemo, how long they might last, how bad they might be and when you should call the doctor's office about them? Your doctor may give you medicines to prevent some side effects before they happen.

CHEMO AGENTS AND ITS TOXICITY

Many people have no long-term problems from chemo. And although side effects can be unpleasant, they must be measured against the need to kill the cancer cells.

How Long do Side Effects Last?

Most side effects slowly go away after treatment ends because the healthy cells recover overtime. The time it takes to get over some side effects and regain energy varies from person-to-person and depends on many factors, including your overall health and the drugs you were given.

Many side effects go away fairly quickly, but some may take months or years to completely go away. Sometimes the side effects can last a lifetime, such as when chemo causes long-term damage to the heart, lungs, kidneys or reproductive organs. Certain types of chemo sometimes cause delayed effects, such as a second cancer that may show up many years later.

Patients often become discouraged about how long their treatment lasts or the side effects they have. If you feel this way, talk to your doctor. You may be able to change your medicine or treatment schedule. If needed, your doctor should be able to suggest ways to reduce any pain and discomfort you have.

COMMON SIDE EFFECTS

Anemia

What is anemia?

When you have too few red blood cells, your body tissues do not get enough oxygen to do their work. This condition is called *anemia*. You may have these symptoms:

Tiredness (fatigue)

Tendency to feel breath weakness called "Fatigue" if your anemia is making you feel very tired. Let your doctor or nurse know, if you have any of the symptoms listed above. Your doctor will check your blood cell count (also called a complete blood count or CBC) often during your treatment. If your red blood cell count falls too low, you may need a blood transfusion. Some people can be treated with a *growth factor* to boost the number of red blood cells the bone marrow makes.

What is fatigue?

Fatigue is one of the most common side effects of cancer treatment. It can range from mild lethargy to feeling completely wiped out. It is different from feeling tired after a long day and does not get better with rest or sleep. Fatigue tends to be the worst at the beginning and at the end of a treatment cycle. Like most other side effects, it usually goes away once chemo is complete. Things that may help you with fatigue: get plenty of rest and allow time during the day for rest periods. Talk with your doctor or nurse about a regular exercise program. Eat a well-balanced diet and drink plenty of liquids. Limit your activities. Do only the things that are most important to you. Get help when you need it. Ask family, friends and neighbors to pitch in with activities, such as child care, shopping, house-work or driving. For example, you might ask neighbors to pick up some items for you at the grocery store while doing their own shopping. Get up slowly to help prevent dizziness after sitting or lying down. Let your doctor know if you are having a hard time sleeping at night.

How do I deal with losing my hair?

Hair loss (*alopecia*) can be devastating. But not all chemo drugs will make you lose your hair. Some people have mild thinning that only they notice. Your doctor will be able to tell you if your medicines are likely to make you lose your hair. If you do lose your hair, it will almost always grow back after the treatments are over. But it might be a different color or texture. You can lose your hair on all parts of your body, not just your scalp. Eyelashes and eyebrows, arm and leg hair, underarm hair and pubic hair all may be affected. It usually does not happen right away. More often, hair loss begins after a few treatments. At that point, your hair may fall out slowly or in clumps. Any hair that remains may become dull and dry.

Things that may help you with hair loss:

- Use mild shampoos
- Use soft-bristle hair brushes
- Use low heat if you must use a hair dryer
- Do not use brush rollers to set your hair
- Do not dye your hair or get a perm
- Have your hair cut short.

A shorter style will make your hair look thicker and fuller. It also will make hair loss easier to deal with if it does happen. Use a sunscreen, hat, scarf, or wig to protect your scalp from the sun. Use a satin pillowcase. Sometimes, either during the regrowth of your hair or when you are bald, your scalp may feel extra tender, dry and itchy. It may help to keep your scalp clean by using a moisturizing shampoo and conditioner. Also use gentle creams or lotions on your scalp as needed. Even a gentle scalp massage may make your scalp feel better.

After chemo, your hair's texture and fullness may change. Hair dyes contain chemicals like peroxide that can damage hair. Although there is no research that supports hair dye doing more damage to hair after chemo, most doctors recommend patients do not use hair dyes until hair returns to normal. This may be as long as 6 months after treatment.

Should I cover my head if I lose my hair?

Some people who lose all or most of their hair choose to wear turbans, scarves, caps, wigs, or hairpieces. Others leave their heads uncovered. Still others switch back and forth, depending on whether they are in public or at home with family and friends. Here are tips to follow if you choose to cover your head with a wig or hairpiece: Shop for your wig or hairpiece before you lose a lot of hair so you can match your natural color, texture, and style. You may be able to buy a wig or hairpiece at a specialty shop just for cancer patients. A sales person may be able to come to your home to help you.

AFTER EFFECT OF CHEMOTHERAPY

If you need a hairpiece because of cancer treatment, it is a tax-deductible expense. It may also be at least partly covered by your health insurance. Be sure to check your policy and ask your doctor to write a prescription for a "hair prosthesis." Increased chance of bruising, bleeding and infection. How will chemo affect my blood cell counts? The bone marrow produces three important parts of your blood: *red blood cells*, which carry oxygen to cells throughout the body. *White blood cells*, which fight infection *Platelets*, which help blood to clot and stop bleeding chemo destroys some of the bone marrow cells, so fewer blood cells are produced. A drop in the levels of any one of these cells leads to specific side effects. Your doctor will check your *blood cell count* by doing a test called a complete blood count or CBC. This will be done often during your treatment. Bleeding or clotting problems Chemo can affect the bone marrow's ability to make platelets. These are the blood cells that help stop bleeding by plugging up damaged blood vessels and helping your blood to clot. If you do not have enough platelets, you may bleed or bruise more easily than usual, even from a minor injury. A shortage of platelets is called thrombocytopenia. Report these signs of thrombocytopenia to your doctor: Unexpected bruising small red spots under your skin red or pink urine black or bloody bowel movements. Any bleeding from your gums or nose, bad headaches Dizziness an increase in weakness. Pain in joints and muscles your doctor will check your platelet count often during your treatment. If it falls too low, you may need a platelet transfusion. Things that may help you avoid problems if your platelet count is low: Do not take any medicine without first checking with your doctor or nurse. This includes aspirin and aspirin-free pain relievers, like acetaminophen (Tylenol®), ibuprofen, and any other medicines you can buy without a prescription. Some of these medicines can weaken the platelets and make bleeding problems worse. Do not drink any alcohol (beer, wine, or liquor) unless your doctor says it's all right. Use an extra-soft bristle toothbrush to clean your teeth and talk to your doctor before using dental floss. If you have a runny nose, blow gently into a soft tissue. Take care not to cut or nick yourself when using scissors, needles, knives, or tools. Be careful not to burn yourself when ironing or cooking. Use a padded glove rather than a potholder when you reach into the oven. Avoid contact sports and other activities that might cause an injury. Drink plenty of fluids and eat enough fiber to reduce the chances you will get constipated. Use an electric shaver instead of a razor. When bending over, keep your head above your heart. Infection having a low white blood cell count decreases your body's ability to fight infections. One type of white blood cell, the neutrophil, is especially important in fighting infections. A shortage of neutrophils is called *neutropenia*. Infections can begin in almost any part of your body and most often start in your mouth as oral candidiasis (Fig. 5.1) skin, lungs, urinary tract and rectum. If your white blood cell count drops too much, your doctor may hold treatment, give you a lower dose of chemo, or give you a growth factor shot that makes your bone marrow put out more white blood cells. Things that may help you prevent infections: Wash your hands often during the day, especially before you eat and after you use the bathroom. Stay away from crowds. Stay away from people who have diseases you can catch, such as colds, flu, measles, or chicken pox. Do not get any immunization shots (vaccines) without first checking with your oncologist (cancer doctor). Stay away from people who have recently had an immunization, such as a vaccine for chicken pox or small pox. Check with your doctor about which vaccines are important and how long you should stay away from people who have had them. Clean your rectal area very well but gently after each bowel movement. Ask your doctor or nurse for advice if the area becomes sore or if you have hemorrhoids. Also, check with your doctor before using enemas or suppositories. Do not cut, bite, or tear the cuticles of your nails. Be careful not to cut or nick yourself when using scissors, needles, or knives. Use an electric shaver instead of a razor to prevent breaks or cuts in your skin. Use an extra-soft bristle toothbrush that will not hurt your gums and talk to your doctor before using dental floss. Do not squeeze or scratch pimples. Take a warm (not hot) bath, shower, or sponge bath every day. Pat your skin dry using a light touch. Do not rub. Use lotion or oil to soften and heal your skin if it becomes dry and cracked. Clean cuts and scrapes right away with warm water and soap. Use an antibiotic ointment and cover with a bandage. Wear waterproof gloves when gardening or cleaning up after animals and others, especially small children. Wash your hands afterward, since gloves can get holes that are too small to see. Even if you are extra careful, your

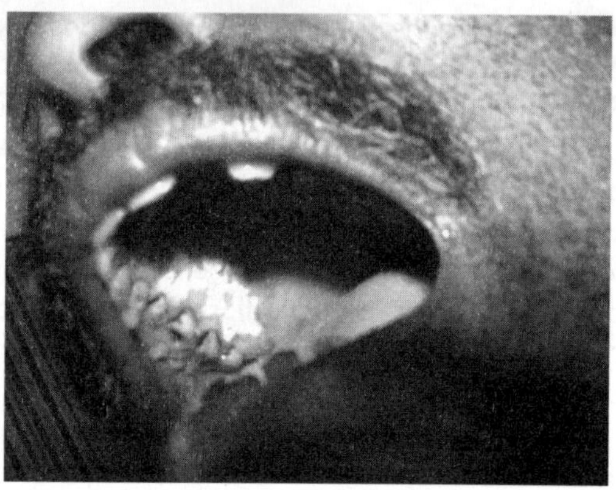

Fig. 5.1: Oral candidiasis

body may not be able to fight infections when your white blood cell count is low. Look out for and check your body regularly for signs and symptoms that you might have an infection. Pay special attention to your eyes, nose, mouth and genital and rectal areas. The symptoms of infection could be: Fever of 100.5°F or greater when your temperature is taken by mouth chills sweating loose stools (This can also be a side effect of chemo). A burning feeling when you urinate a bad cough or sore throat unusual vaginal discharge or itching redness, swelling, or tenderness, especially around a wound, sore, pimple, IV site, or central venous catheter. Abdominal (belly) pain report any signs of infection to your doctor right away. If you have a fever, do not use aspirin, acetaminophen (Tylenol®), or any other medicine to bring your temperature down without first checking with your doctor.

Nausea and Vomiting

What can I do about nausea and vomiting?

Nausea and vomiting are two of the most common and most dreaded side effects of chemo. How often you feel these side effects and how bad they are depend on the drugs you are getting and how they affect you. Nausea and vomiting may start during treatment and last a few hours. Sometimes, but less often, severe nausea and vomiting can last for a few days. Be sure to tell your doctor or nurse if you are very nauseated, if you have been vomiting for more than a day, or if your nausea is so bad that you cannot keep liquids down. The good news is that nausea and vomiting can almost always be lessened by a change in the way you eat and with drugs that help relieve both symptoms (these drugs are called *antiemetics*). Different antiemetics work for different people. You may need to try more than one before you get relief. Do not give up! Keep working with your doctor and nurse to find the antiemetics that work best for you. About half of the people getting chemo feel queasy even before treatment begins. This is called anticipatory nausea and it is very real. The best way to handle anticipatory nausea is by taking effective antiemetics to prevent vomiting and by using relaxation techniques.

Things that may help you with nausea and vomiting: Avoid big meals so your stomach will not feel too full. Eat frequent, small meals throughout the day instead of 1, 2, or 3 large meals. Drink liquids at least an hour before or after mealtime instead of with your meals. Eat and drink slowly. Stay away from sweet, fried, or fatty foods. Eat foods cold or at room temperature so you would not be bothered by strong smells. Chew your food well for better digestion. If nausea is a problem in the morning, try eating dry foods, such as cereal, toast, or crackers, before getting up. (Do not try this if your mouth is too dry, or if you have sores in your mouth or throat). Drink cool, clear liquids, such as apple juice, tea, or ginger ale that has lost its fizz. Suck on ice cubes, mints, or tart candies. (Do not eat tart candies if you have mouth or throat sores). Try to avoid odors that bother you, such as cooking smells, smoke, or perfume.Rest in a chair after eating, but do not lie flat for at least 2 hours after you have finished your meal. Wear loose-fitting clothes. Breathe deeply and slowly when you feel nauseated. Distract yourself by talking with friends or family members, listening to music, or watching a movie or TV show. Use relaxation techniques. Other chemo side effects and tips to manage them Appetite changes. There may be days when you just can not eat because of things like nausea or mouth and throat problems. You also can lose your appetite if you feel depressed or tired. When you have a poor appetite, try these tips: Eat small meals or snacks whenever you want. You don't have to eat three regular meals each day. Vary your diet, and try new foods and recipes. Take a walk before meals whenever you can. This may make you feel hungrier. Change your mealtime routine. For example, eat by candlelight or in a different place. Eat with friends or family members. When eating alone, listen to the radio or watch TV. If you live alone, you might want to arrange for meals on wheels or a program like this to bring food to you. Ask your doctor, nurse, or local American Cancer Society office about services in your area. Constipation some people become constipated from chemo. Others may become constipated because they are less active, eat less than usual, have diet changes, or because they are taking certain pain medicines. Tell your doctor if you have not had a bowel movement in two or more days. You may need to take a laxative or stool softener, but do not use these unless you have checked with your doctor, especially if your white blood cell count or platelet count is low. Things that may help you deal with constipation: Drink plenty of fluids to help keep your stool soft. Warm and hot fluids work especially well. Eat a lot of high-fiber foods. High-fiber foods include bran, whole-wheat breads and cereals, raw or cooked vegetables, fresh and dried fruit, nuts, and popcorn. Get some exercise. Just getting out for a walk can help, as can a planned exercise program. Be sure to check with your doctor before increasing your physical activity. *Diarrhea When* chemo affects the cells lining the intestine, it can cause diarrhea. Diarrhea is most often defined as two or more loose stools in 4 hours. If you have diarrhea that lasts for more than 24 hours, or if you have pain and cramping along with it, call your doctor. In severe cases, the doctor may have you take an antidiarrheal medicine, but do not take any over-the-counter antidiarrheal medicines without asking your doctor first. Things that may help you control diarrhea: Eat smaller amounts of food, but eat more often. Avoid coffee, tea, alcohol, and sweets. Avoid high-fiber foods, which can lead to diarrhea and cramping. High-fiber foods include whole-grain breads and cereals, raw vegetables, beans, nuts, seeds, popcorn, and fresh and dried fruit. Low-fiber foods, such as white bread, white rice or noodles, creamed cereals, ripe bananas, canned or cooked fruit without skins, cottage cheese, yogurt, eggs, mashed or baked potatoes without the skin, pureed vegetables, chicken or turkey without the skin and fish. Stay away from fried, greasy, or spicy foods. Avoid milk and milk products if they make your diarrhea worse. Eat more potassium-rich foods, such as bananas, oranges, potatoes and peach and apricot nectars, unless your doctor has told you otherwise. Drink plenty of fluids to replace those you have lost through diarrhea. Mild, clear liquids, such as apple juice, water, weak tea, clear broth, or ginger ale are best. Make sure they are at room temperature and drink them slowly. Let carbonated drinks lose their fizz before you drink them. If your diarrhea is severe (meaning that you have had 7 or 8 loose movements in 24 hours), tell your doctor right away. Ask if you should try a clear-liquid diet to give your bowels time to rest. As you feel better, slowly add the low-fiber foods. A clear-liquid diet does not have all the nutrients you need, so do not follow it for more than 3 or 4 days. If your diarrhea does not get better, you may need to get IV fluids to replace the water and nutrients you have lost. Mouth, gum, and throat problems good mouth care is important during cancer treatment. Chemo can cause sores in the mouth and throat. It can make these areas dry and irritated or cause them to bleed. Mouth sores are not only painful, but they can also become infected by the many germs that normally live in your mouth. Infections can be hard to fight during chemo and can lead to serious problems. It's important to take every possible step to prevent them. Ways to keep your mouth, gums and throat healthy: Have your teeth cleaned and take care of any cavities, abscesses, gum disease, or poorly fitting dentures before you start chemo. Ask your dentist to show you the best ways to brush and floss your teeth during chemo. Ask about a daily fluoride rinse or gel to help prevent decay because chemo can make you more likely to get cavities. Brush your teeth and gums after every meal. Use an extra-soft bristle toothbrush and a gentle touch; brushing too hard can damage soft mouth tissues. Ask your dentist to suggest a special type of toothbrush, floss or dental ribbon, and toothpaste if your gums are very sensitive. Rinse your toothbrush well after each use, and store it in a dry place. Avoid commercial mouthwashes. They often contain irritants such as alcohol. Instead, ask your doctor or nurse about a mild mouthwash or a mouthwash with antibiotics to help prevent mouth infections. If you develop sores in your mouth (this is called (*stomatitis*), tell your doctor or nurse right away because you may need treatment. If the sores are painful or keep you from eating, try these tips: Ask your doctor if there is anything you can put right on the sores to treat them and if there is medicine you can take to ease the pain. Eat foods cold or at room temperature. Hot and warm foods can irritate a tender mouth and throat. Choose soft, soothing foods, such as ice cream, milk shakes, baby food, soft fruits (like bananas and applesauce), mashed potatoes, cooked cereals, soft-boiled or scrambled eggs, cottage cheese, macaroni and cheese, custards, puddings, and gelatin. You also can puree cooked foods in the blender to make them smoother and easier to eat. Avoid irritating, acidic foods, such as tomatoes, citrus fruit and citrus fruit juice (orange, grapefruit and lemon); spicy or salty foods; and rough, coarse, or dry foods like raw vegetables, pretzels, granola and toast. If your mouth is dry and it bothers you or makes it hard for you to eat, try these tips: ask your doctor if you should use an artificial saliva product to moisten your mouth. Drink plenty of liquids. Suck on ice chips, popsicles, or sugarless hard candy. Chew sugarless gum. Moisten dry foods with butter, margarine, gravy, sauces, or broth. Dunk crisp, dry foods in mild liquids. Eat soft and pureed foods. Use lip balm if your lips become dry.

Nerve Problems—Certain Chemo Drugs can Cause Peripheral Neuropathy

A nerve problem that causes tingling, pins and needles, burning sensations, weakness, and/or numbness in your hands and feet. You may feel any of these nerve-related symptoms: loss of balance clumsiness trouble picking up objects and buttoning, clothing problems, walking Jaw pain, hearing loss vision changes, stomach pain. Constipation along with affecting the nerves, certain chemo drugs can affect the muscles and make them weak, tired, or sore. Nerve and muscle effects are frustrating, yet in most cases they are not serious if caught early. They are usually short term and will get better after treatment is done. Still, it is important to tell your doctor about any nerve or muscle symptoms right away. They can get worse and become quite painful if left untreated. Your doctor might want to stop the chemo for awhile or offer you treatment to ease these symptoms. Caution and common sense can help you deal with nerve and muscle problems. Follow these tips: if your fingers become numb, e.g. be very careful when handling objects that are sharp, hot, or otherwise dangerous. If your sense of balance is affected, move carefully, use handrails on stairs, and use a bath mat in the tub or shower. Skin and nail changes you may have minor skin problems during treatment, including color changes, redness, itching, peeling, dryness, rashes, and acne. You can take care of most of these problems yourself using these tips: if you develop acne, try to keep your face clean and dry. For itching, try cornstarch. To help avoid dryness, take quick, warm showers rather than long, hot baths. Apply creams or lotions after bathing, while your skin is still moist. Do not use perfume, cologne, or after shave lotion. These products often contain alcohol, which can make your skin dry. When given through an IV, certain chemo drugs, may darken your skin along the vein. This discoloration will usually fade over time after treatment ends. Most skin problems are not serious, but a few need to be taken care of right away. For example, certain drugs given through an IV can cause serious, long-term tissue damage if they leak out of the vein. Tell your doctor or nurse right away if you notice swelling or feel any burning or pain near your IV site when you are getting IV drugs. These symptoms do not always mean there's a problem, but they should always be checked out right away. Let your doctor or nurse know right away if you develop sudden or severe itching, if your skin breaks out in a rash or hives, or if you start wheezing or have any other trouble breathing. These symptoms may mean you are having an allergic reaction that needs attention right away. Some chemo drugs may make your skin more sensitive to the sun. Check with your doctor or nurse about using sunscreen. You may need to completely avoid direct sunlight. Wear long-sleeved cotton shirts, hats and pants to block the sun. Your nails may become darkened, brittle, or cracked, or they may develop vertical lines or bands. Protect your nails by wearing gloves when washing dishes, gardening, or doing other work around the house. Some over-the-counter products might strengthen your nails, but these products may also cause irritation. Get advice from your doctor if any skin and nail problems do not respond to your efforts. Be sure to let your doctor know if you have redness, pain, or changes around your cuticles or any other skin problems that you are worried about. Urine changes and bladder and kidney problems. Some chemo drugs can irritate your bladder or cause short- or long-term kidney damage. They may also cause your urine to change color (orange, red, or yellow) or take on a strong or medicine-like odor. For a short-time, the color and odor of semen may be changed too. Ask your doctor if your chemo may have these effects. And let your doctor know if you have any symptoms that might be a sign of a problem. Watch for these signs and symptoms: pain or burning when you urinate, urinating, a lot a feeling that you must urinate right away reddish or bloody urine.

(Some chemo drugs will change the color of your urine. Tell your doctor or nurse if this happens).

Drink plenty of fluids to ensure good urine flow and help prevent problems. Water, juice, coffee, tea, soup, soft drinks, broth, ice cream, popsicles and gelatin count as fluids. Weight gain, some people usually women, put on weight during chemo. We are not sure why this happens, but it may have to do with intense food cravings that develop despite the nausea. The average weight gain for women is about 7 pounds. Whether you gain weight or not, good nutrition is very important during treatment. People who eat well cope with side effects better and are better able to fight infection. Their bodies can also rebuild healthy tissues faster. Eating well- during chemo means choosing a balanced diet that contains all the nutrients your body needs. You should include foods from each of the following food groups: Fruits and vegetables; poultry, fish and meat; cereals and breads; and dairy products. You also should take in enough calories to keep your weight up and most importantly, enough protein to build and repair skin, hair, muscles and organs. You also may need to drink extra fluid to protect your bladder and kidneys during your treatment.

Chapter 6 Hormone Treatment in Cancer

The first person was Scottish surgeon Mr George Beatson who remove ovary of breast cancer patient in1896 and found that tumor regressed but recurrence soon occurred resulted into disuse of procedure, however, thirty-year later again in 1922 estrogen hormone was isolated. People again thought of ovarian irradiation or surgical oopherectomy in breast cancer patients. In 1944, Huggins Usa reported favorable outcome in prostatic cancer while removing testis. Since then lots of work on hormone treatment of breast cancer, ovarian cancer, prostatic cancer as well as in thyroid and endometrial cancer patients has been done so far directly. Breast function and development depends on estrogen and progesteron, prolactin hormone, indirectly on corticosteroids,growth hormone, thyroid hormone. Estrogen responsible for ductal growth progesterone responsible for alveolar growth.

ANTERIOR PITUITARY HORMONE (FIG. 6.1)

Role of Hormone

Receptor status: There are specific cytological receptors known as estrogen and progesterone receptors present in breast tissue. These hormones stimulate cell growth by binding hormone receptor. This hormone receptor ligand complex goes into nucleus attached to specific site of DNA and stimulate gene responsible for production of several growth factors named as, fibroblastic transforming growth factors as well as insulin like growth factor, epidermal growth factor. Estrogen and progesteron receptors are cytosol protein that can be identified on primary tumor or metastastic tissues by commonly used technique like, immuno-chemistry, fish (fluorescent *in situ* hybridization) methods. ER, PR, positive status in premenopausal women found in 45 percent cases ER and RR positive status in postmenopausal women found in 65 percent cases thus hormone treatment in breast cancer in postmenopausal women is more effective. Now we know biopsy required to study receptor status. ER and PR, considered positive when, ER is more than 10 fammol/mg, PR is more than 5 fammol/mg of tissue. Study for ER, PR status must be done, prior to chemotherapy or radio-therapy, because, adjuvant treatment might change the receptor status due to inheritant tumor biology, as well as precaution must be taken during surgery by avoiding cauterization because hormone receptor are heat labile. On study cases negative for both ER, as well as PR receptor, also have response to hormone treatment although response rate is as low as 10 percent only because ER, PR, study is a quantitative assessment.

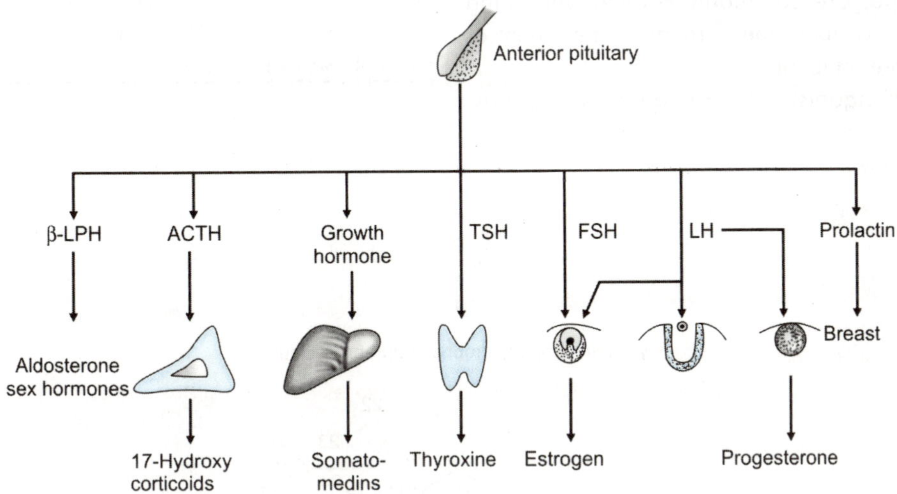

Fig. 6.1: Role of anterior pituitary in production and secretion of various hormones

Tamoxifin: It is an antiestrogenic drug but with a week agonist action on endometrium its block the estrogen hormone action on estrogen receptor thus it block production of several growth factors responsible for tumor growth it also arrest the cell division at g1 phase ues as 10 mg bd or 20 mg od, it also useful in very old age lady not suitable for surgery, or radio therapy, side effects of tamoxifin are several as hotflushes most common in 40 percent cases, vaginal dryness, fluid retention, irregular menstruation thromboembolism 2 percent, 1 percent risk of endometrial cancer due to endometrial hyperplagia, some patients do not response to tamoxifin treatment why we know tamoxifin has antiestrogenic as well as week estrogenic effect some breast cancer cells shows cellular hypersinsatization to week estrogenic effect of tamoxifin known as tamoxifin resistance.

Aromatase inhibitor: We know in postmenopausal women major source of estrogen is from adrenal gland it produces androestradian which gets converted into estrogen at peripheral adipose tissues by the help of aromatase enzyme thus aromatase inhibitor can be use as antiestrogenic drugs in breast cancer patients like letrazole 2.5 mg, anstrazole as 1mg daily as od doses indications are, postmenopoausal women, women having history of tamoxifin resestance, women having history of deep vain thrombosis, women with her neu positive status, ***side effects of aromatase inhibitor*** are, hot flushes, vaginal dryness, musculoskeletal pain, osteoporosis, headache, are commonly known, only thing uncertain is about the duration of treatment or aromatase inhibitor.

LHRH agonist in breast cancer is in use as, goserelin 3.6 mg SC monthly, leuprolide 3.7 mg SC monthly

HORMONE PRODUCTION—HOW ANDROGEN AND ESTROGEN PRODUCED (FIG. 6.2)?

Progesterone-medroxyproges tren acetate (provera) 400 mg PO daily or in injection 500 mg weekly

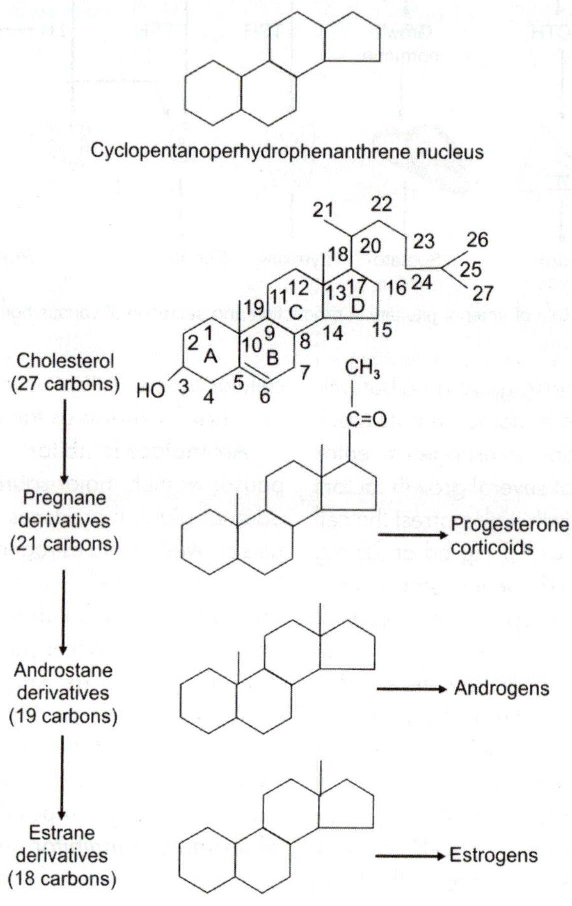

Fig. 6.2: Estrogen and androgen production

use in breast cancer patients less commonly, pure antiestrogen (fulvestrant) 250 mg IM monthly recommended in breast cancer patients.

HORMONE TREATMENT IN CANCER PATIENTS

Hormone treatment can be given in ***prostatic cancer*** in form of adjuvant treatment.

Androgen Block

Before or after surgery or radiotherapy in order to increase survival as well as to decrease size of tumor for better surgical approach, only treatment with hormone is insufficient combine treatment with orchidectomy is highly recommended.

Without hormone treatment, in localized disease failure rate is 10 percent, in extracapsular involvement failure rate is 25 percent, in seminal vesical involvement, failure rate is as high as 75 percent, thus hormone treatment is corner stone in the management or prostetic cancer. Estrogen act by suppresing LHRG and LH release thus taking away stimulus for testerion production but major side effect is cardiovascular toxicity by doing orchidectomy, we rapidly brings down serum testerion level up to 1/10 to the pretreatment level. LHRH agonist also in use, LHRH naturally secreted by hypothalamus but when large dose of LHRH agonist build up then pituitary become refectory to LHRH stimulus thus stop secreting LH hormone result in decrese production of testerion (Fig. 6.3) and (Table 6.1). However, due to initial surge of testisterion production due to LHRH agonist treatment might increase the symptoms called as *flare phenomena*. It can be avoided by initialy at start of LHRH agonist treatment combined with antiandrogenic drugs like flutamide 250 mg tds daily for few days (Fig. 6.4).

Table 6.1: Secretory products of the adrenal glands

Adrenal cortex	*Adrenal Medulla*
Glucocorticoids	Epinephrine
Cortisol	Norepinephrine
Corticosterone	Dopamine
Mineralocorticoid	
Aldosterone	
Deoxycorticosterone	
Sex hormones	
Dehydroepiandrosterone	
Androstenedione	

NONSTEROIDAL ANTIESTROGENIC DRUGS

Flutamide/bicalutamide they are androgen receptor antagonist. They act by inhibiting action of testerion and dihydrotesterion to androgen receptor in target tissue, recommended doses are like flutamide 250 mg tds daily or bicalutamide 50 mg OD daily up to 2 years. Side effects are gynecomastia dyspepsia, derange liver function test, but its advantages are no cardiotoxicity and preservation of sexual potency, treatment with flutamide and orchidectomy can lead significant survival in metastastic prostatic cancer.

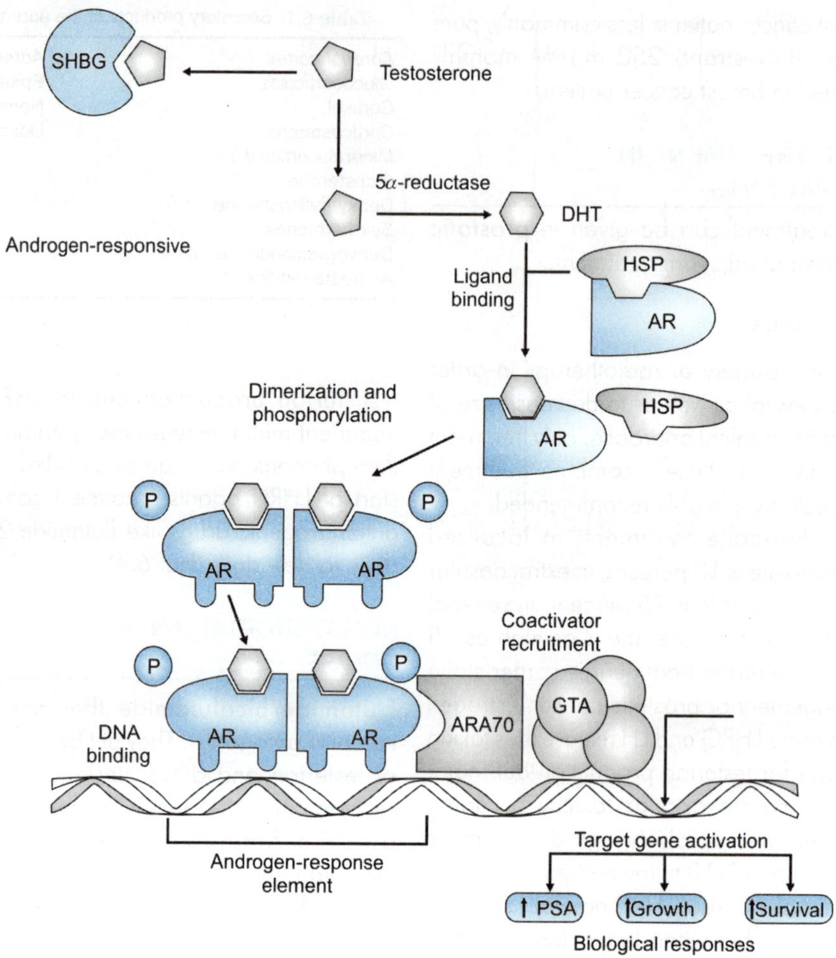

Fig. 6.3: How androgen leads to certain tumor cell growth in human?

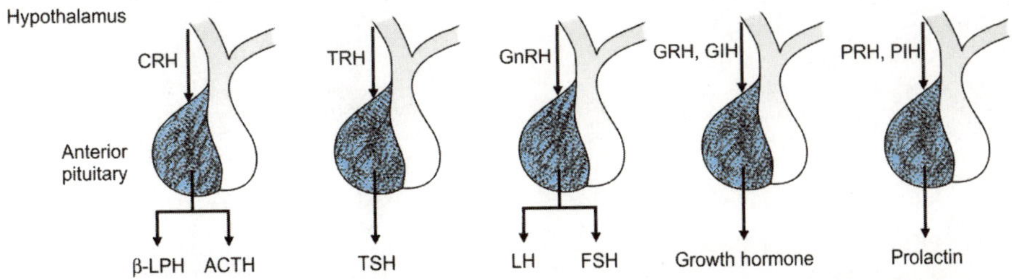

Fig. 6.4: Effects of hypophysiotropic hormones on the secretion of anterior pituitary hormones

HORMONE TREATMENT IN THYROID CANCER

Differenciated thyroid cancer patient after surgery and radioiodine treatment patient developed hypothyroidism, thus after radioiodine treatment, patients of thyroid cancer should be given lifelong thyroxin treatment with two main objective first. After surgery to avoid difieciency of T3, T4, hormone second is because after surgery left over cancer cells might repopulate underinfluence of TSH hormone thus to decrease TSH level done by external thyroxin replacement treatment.

Section-B

General Management in Oncology

Chapter

7 Management of Cancer Pain

Pain is associated symptom in advanced malignancies. More than 50 percent of all cancer patients suffer from unrelieved pain.
cancer breast 52 percent, cancer lung 45 percent, Bone tumor 85 percent, Head and neck 85 percent, Genitourinary 75 percent, Lymphoma 20 percent.

TYPES OF NEUROGENIC CANCER PAIN

1. Pheripheral neuropathy
2. Plexopathy
   a. Brachial
   b. Lumbar
   c. Sacral
3. Leptomeningeal metastasis
4. Spinal cord
   a. Epidural spinal cord compression
   b. Intramedullary metastasis.

Chemotherapy Induced Neurogenic Pain Occurs

1. Vincristine
2. Vinblastine
3. Docetaxel
4. Paclitaxel
5. Cisplatin
6. Oxaliplatin
7. Capecitabine.

Neurogenic Pain due to Direct Tumor Involvement

1. More than 50 percent cases of neurogenic cancer pain due to direct tumor involvement.
2. In head and neck cancer refferd to forehead and ear.
3. Scan figure from snell.
4. Locally advanced Ca cervix/urinary bladder/ prostate/rectum.
5. Tumor cells infiltrate into sacral plexus leading to pelvic pain radiating up to thigh.
6. LABC large axillary lymphnode involve bracial plexus causing severe shoulder pain radiating up to hand and fingers.

Types of Pain

1. Pain is always a subjective phenomena.
2. History of surgery/RT/chemo must be taken may be cause of pain.
3. Pain acute type/chronic type
4. **Intensity of pain may be:**
   a. Mild
   b. Moderate
   c. Severe
5. **Pain may be:**
   a. Somatic

   b. Visceral
   c. Neuropathic
6. Breakthrough pain: When patient having acute and chronic pain but, during 24 hours period he or she experience severe pain.

Commonly Used Drug for Neurogenic Pain

1. Carbamazepine 100 mg to 300 mg tds
2. Gabapentin 300 mg tds
3. Tricyclic antidepressants
   a. Amitryptyline
   b. Imiparamine
4. Steroids dexamethasone 16 mg 96 mg tds.
5. Phenytoin 300 mg tds or 100 mg IV tds.

Dose Titration for Gabapentin

D_1	1 capsule at bed time
D_2 D_4	1 capsule bd
D_5 D_7	1 capsule tds
D_8 D_{10}	2 capsule tds
D_{11} D_{14}	3 capsule tds

PHENYTOIN DRUG

It is Less Commonly used because:

1. Its a barbiturates analog but has a poor sedative property.
2. Most commonly use drug during seizure and to prevent seizure.
3. It has a stabilizing influence on neuronal membrane.
4. Prevent repetitive detonation of normal brain cells during depolarization shift that occurs in epileptic patients.
5. Because this drug inhibit high frequency discharge this confirms it's role in management of severe neurogenic cancer pain.

Nerve block procedure can also be used to relieve cancer pain but major limitation for nerve block procedure limited number of practitoners are expert in their use.

Chronic Pain

- Outlasts the initial injury
- Subjective exceeds the objective findings
- Poor response to conventional therapy
- Serves no beneficial purpose
- Poor response from family and care givers
- Cost ineffective therapy
- Accompanied by major psychosocial co-morbidity
- High incidence of substance abuse
- Persistent pain.

Neuropathic Pain

Pain secondary to biochemical and structural changes within the central and peripheral nervous system.

Pain transduction
↓
Pain conduction
↓
↓ Pain processing ↓ Pain perception
↓ Pain expression ↓ Pain assessment

Patient suffering depression loss of function drug abuse financial loss domestic disruption (Fig. 7.1).

THE PAIN HISTORY

The pain itself characterized by intensity/radiation, type of relieving and exacerbating factors, should be asked by oncologist during history taking of pain, pain starts slowly and then it increases in its intensity then required initially low-dose and only non opiods treatment the nopiods treatment on WHO ladder puller given in (Fig. 7.2).

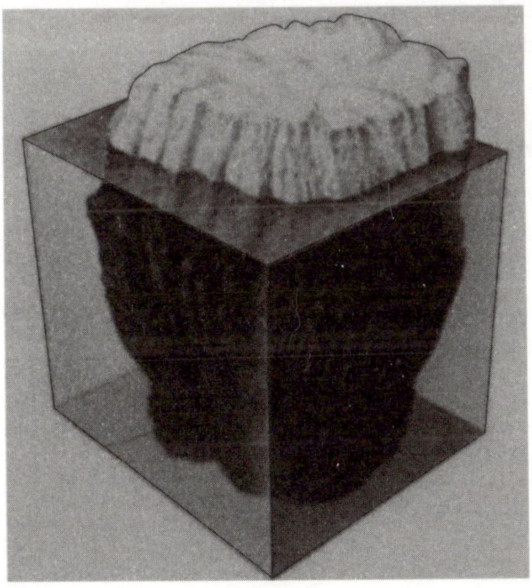

Fig. 7.1: Only upper tip felt by most of the oncologists for cancer pain

Pain Assessment

- Characterize the pain
- Characterize the disease, relationship between pain and disease and potentially treatable etiologies
- Clarify syndromes and infer pathophysiology
- Determine need for urgent therapy
- Identify other needs
- Develop a therapeutic strategy.

PAIN INTENSITY RATING SCALES

Visual analog scale (VAS)

No pain .... Worst pain

Numerical Rating Scale

0 10

No pain imaginable Worst pain

Categorical Scale

Worst pain imaginable

None (0) Mild (1–4) Moderate (5–6) Severe (7–10).

Approach to the Pain Therapy

Drug use are expression, inhibition can be anxiolytics inhibition amitryptyline venlafaxine, clonidine decrease and prevent inflammatory conduction centralization gabapentin, cox 2, opioids, NSAIDS, carbamazepine, Ketamine, opioid agonists steroids.

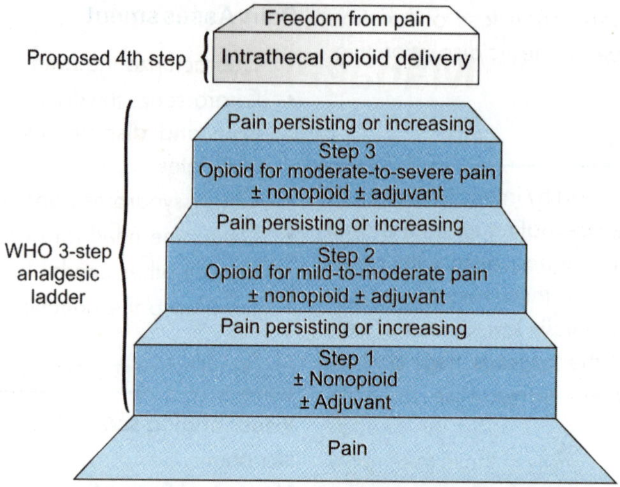

Fig. 7.2: WHO cancer pain ladder treatment with drugs

Principles of Breakthrough Pain Therapy should not exceed 25 percent of the daily dose should stay within the therapeutic window, should have minimal side effects should not be randomly escalated. If needed more than 4 hourly. Increase ATC. Assess for abuse vs. tolerance.

Precaution with Antidepressants Therapy

With the antidepressants: Start at lowest dose available escalate slowly every 10 to 14 days. Slow weaning, over a week beware of drug interactions. ***Check for*** Glaucoma, prostatic obstruction, heart block.

Chapter

8 Management of Anemia

Anemia is a common side effect of cancer and cancer therapy. Its prevalence varies with tumor type, stage and therapy used. The negative impact of anemia symptoms, such as fatigue, on patient quality of life (QoL) is substantial (Fig. 8.1). In addition, anemia may compromise patients' tolerance of treatments, resulting in the need to reduce the duration or intensity of those treatments. Prior to 1993, when recombinant human erythropoietin (rHuEPO) was approved by the US Food and Drug Administration (FDA), RBC transfusion was the sole option for the treatment of anemia in cancer. The availability of a therapeutic option with an apparently superior risk-benefit ratio has changed clinical practice and resulted in increased understanding of the impact of anemia treatment on the lives of cancer patients. During radiotherapy or cancer chemotherapy anemia as well as due to myelo suppression dead's to low white blood cells as well, which turn cases severely threatening injection. It can be manage by human granulocyte colony stimulating factor GCSF available as 300 μg to be used subcutaneously (Fig. 8.2).

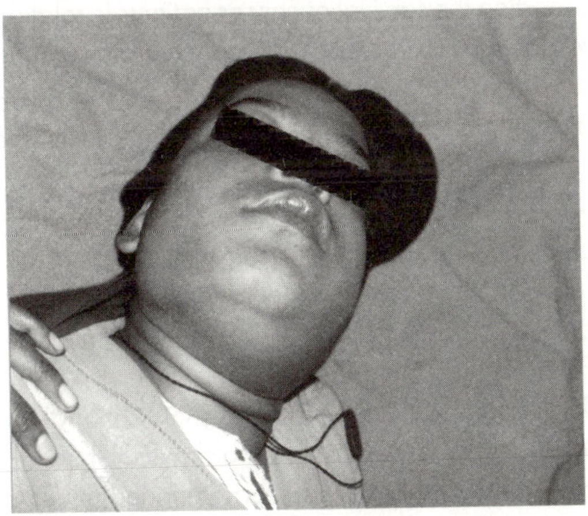

Fig. 8.1: Severe anemia in cancer patient

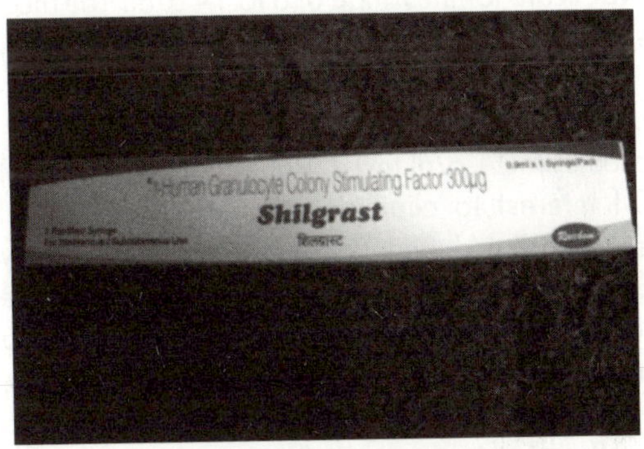

Fig. 8.2: GCSF injection

ERYTHROPOIETINE

rHuEPO was initially studied in anemic cancer patients receiving chemotherapy based on the observation that endogenous EPO concentrations were inadequate to account for the observed degree of anemia. Accordingly, the FDA limited the approval of rHuEPO to patients with nonmyeloid malignancies whose anemia was caused by the effects of chemotherapy.

CHANGES IN HEALTH-RELATED QOL PARAMETERS

In recent years, improvements in cancer care have allowed oncologists and patients to focus on QoL as a central issue. The relationship between hemoglobin level and QoL parameters in cancer chemotherapy patients trials documented significant improvements in energy, activity and overall QoL, associated with a significant increase in hemoglobin level. An increase in hemoglobin consequent to treatment was associated with an improvement in QoL score for the range of 8 to 14 g/dl. The most substantial improvements in QoL scores, for every 1 g/dl increment in the level of hemoglobin, occurred when the hemoglobin concentration increased from 11 g/dl to 12 g/dl (range, 11–13 g/dl) Of interest to clinicians, a hemoglobin level between 7 g/dl and 10 g/dl correlated with only a slight improvement in QoL. This was the range for management of patients' anemia receiving transfusions before the advent of rHuEPO therapy. Since, hemoglobin level was seldom improved to >10 g/dl, it is not surprising that physicians and patients did not note significant differences in QoL. In contrast, with an incremental improvement in hemoglobin level between 11 g/dl and 13 g/dl, substantial changes were noted in the overall QoL assessment. However, given the methodological limitations inherent in community-based studies, these findings should be interpreted only as an additional support to the results of randomized clinical trials, which are the gold standard of evidence-based medicine. In this regard, benefits to health-related QoL following treatment of cancer-related anemia with rHuEPO have been demonstrated more convincingly in recent reports.

CANCER THERAPY OUTCOMES

Anemia has been reported as an independent prognostic factor in a variety of cancer types and treatments. A systematic review of 60 articles reporting the survival of cancer patients in relation to anemia and hemoglobin concentration found a 65 percent higher relative risk of death for anemic patients than for nonanemic patients.

DOSING REGIMENS

Despite uncertainties regarding the optimal regimen, the doses of rHuEPO taken forward into phase III studies became the current standard. Following the meta-analysis report, the American Society of Clinical Oncology (ASCO) and the American Society of Hematology (ASH) jointly published guidelines that recommended rHuEPO as a treatment option for patients having chemotherapy-associated anemia (hemoglobin level <10 g/dl), advising subcutaneous (Sc) administration at a starting dose of 150 IU/kg three times weekly. If an adequate hematologic response is not seen at week 4, the dose may be doubled. An alternative weekly dosing regimen (40,000 IU/week; 60,000 IU/week in non-responders), also cited in the guidelines of the National Comprehensive Cancer Network (NCCN).

Comparisons between Erythropoietic Agents

To date, just one large, head-to-head trial of erythropoietic agents in cancer-related anemia has been published. Schwartzberg et al. recently reported the results of a randomized comparison of darbepoetin alfa (200 μg Sc every 2 weeks) and epoetin alfa (40,000 U Sc once a week) in 312 patients with breast cancer, nonsmall cell lung cancer, or gynecological cancer receiving concurrent chemotherapy. Three identical but separate protocols were used, one for each tumor type, with a combined analysis of all data from each trial prespecified in each protocol. Doses were increased to 300 μg every 2 weeks for darbepoetin alfa or 60,000 U weekly for epoetin alfa if, after 4 weeks of treatment, hemoglobin levels did not increase by 1 g/dl from baseline. Furthermore, doses for either drug were withheld if hemoglobin levels were >13 g/dl and were restarted at the previous dose once hemoglobin levels were 13 g/dl. The results were analyzed based upon the achievement and maintenance of a target hemoglobin threshold (11 g/dl) and range (11–13 g/dl).

More than 80 percent of patients in both arms of the study achieved target hemoglobin levels. Transfusions were similar in the two treatment groups, at 16 percent for the darbepoetin alfa group and 17 percent for the epoetin alfa group. After achievement of a hemoglobin level >11 g/dl, the mean hemoglobin level was maintained at approximately 12 g/dl for the remainder of the trials in both treatment groups. Eighty-one percent of patients in the darbepoetin alfa group remained in the target range, versus 75 percent in the epoetin alfa group. No differences in the percentages of patients who had to increase the dose, the median times to achieve the target hemoglobin level, or the incidences of adverse events were observed.

These results should be interpreted cautiously because efficacy and safety of the two agents were secondary objectives of the trials and the sample size was not formally powered to test noninferiority. In fact, the study's primary end point was validation of the Patient Satisfaction Questionnaire for Anemia Treatment (PSQ-An), which assessed the impact of receiving anemia treatment. More definitive evidence should be provided by the results of a National Cancer Institute—sponsored randomized trial, including approximately 1,200 patients and specifically designed to compare the efficacy and safety of darbepoetin alpha and epoetin alpha.

Iron Supplementation and Response to Erythropoietic Agents

The pathogenesis of cancer-related anemia is complex and multifactorial but is known to involve absolute or functional iron deficiency, with access to iron stores inadequate to support the increased demand associated with erythropoiesis-stimulating therapy. The most accurate method for detecting functional iron deficiency in cancer patients is the measurement of the percentage of hypochromic RBCs or reticulocyte hemoglobin content). Such measurements, however, require specialized instrumentation that is not widely available. An alternative method for evaluating available iron stores is transferrin saturation. A transferrin saturation of 20 to 30 percent is thought to indicate sufficient iron stores to support erythropoiesis in rHuEPO-treated patients, whereas lower levels may reflect functional iron deficiency. A randomized trial of iron supplementation was conducted recently in patients with chemotherapy-related anemia (hemoglobin 105 g/l, serum ferritin 450 pmol/l or 675 pmol/l with transferrin saturation 19%) receiving epoetin alfa. The results suggest that the erythropoietic response is greater when parenteral iron is given in addition to rHuEPO than when patients receive oral iron or no iron support. Although additional trials are needed, intravenous (IV) iron supplementation is reasonable in anemic patients with iron deficiency, whether or not they are receiving an erythropoietic agent.

SAFETY AND TOLERABILITY

Early comparative studies reported similar adverse-event profiles for rHuEPO and placebo except for shortness of breath, which was twice as frequent in patients receiving placebo. Five percent of rHuEPO-treated patients experienced hypertension, compared with 3.5 percent of placebo-treated patients. Although the difference was not significant, it is recognized that erythropoietin-treated patients may occasionally experience hypertension. In patients with solid tumors, the adverse event profiles were similar in the rHuEPO and placebo groups, though a few more cases of deep vein thrombosis occurred in the rHuEPO group. In six trials in patients with anemia due to an underlying hematologic malignancy, there was a statistically significant higher rate of hypertension (10% versus 1%; $p = .011$) and a nonsignificantly higher rate of thromboembolic events (3% versus 0%; $p = .55$) among rHuEPO-treated patients. The incidences of adverse events were similar in three community-based, open-label trials and generally lower than those reported in the comparative trials.

PHARMACOECONOMIC CONSIDERATIONS

Studies of rHuEPO cost-effectiveness have been challenging to conduct and analyze. The costs of some outcomes, such as QoL indicators or the impact of anemia on an individual patient's productivity, have been difficult to quantify. Also, a proper evaluation of the affordability of rHuEPO should include a comparison of both the costs of administration and the costs of the consequences of transfusion. Recent economic analyses of erythropoietin for chemotherapy-induced anemia have reported varying results depending upon the methodology used to determine costs or cost-effectiveness.

In Europe, the cost of the prophylactic use of rHuEPO for four cycles of chemotherapy at the recommended dose (150 U/kg three times a week) was estimated to be US$4,400 per patient; transfusion for the same patients was US$206 moreover, rHuEPO was effective at abolishing transfusional needs in only half the patients, and a cost-effectiveness analysis that considered all the risks and benefits of the two treatment strategies resulted in an incremental cost-effectiveness ratio of US$189,652/quality-adjusted life year In patients treated with cisplatin chemotherapy, rHuEPO added US$190,142/quality-adjusted life year. In general, this is considered to be a high figure relative to other commonly used healthcare interventions in other settings. However, it has been argued that cost per quality-adjusted life year gained may not be the most appropriate measure to use in economic evaluations when comparing two supportive care measures with no difference in survival.

Results suggest that the cost-effectiveness of rHuEPO therapy relative to transfusion is mostly dependent on the cost of the drug. Inability to predict response to rHuEPO therapy can add to its perceived expense Therefore, strategies to improve the cost-effectiveness ratio include both a better tailoring of its use in patients with a high probability of response and reducing the market cost of the drug.

Finally, it has been shown that changes in dosing and pricing overtime can have profound effects on the cost per quality-adjusted life year ratios. For example, the cost per quality-adjusted life year of rHuEPO in chronic renal failure was more than 100,000 British pounds in 1992 but has recently been estimated at 17,000 British pounds and it may well be that estimates produced by more recent cost-effectiveness studies of rHuEPO in cancer-related anemia are nearer the threshold of acceptability.

CONCLUSION

Despite the abundance of data, the role of erythropoietic agents in the treatment of anemia in cancer still presents many unresolved issues. Most patients eligible for epoetin or darbepoetin therapy on the basis of having hemoglobin levels <10 g/dl during chemotherapy do not receive treatment mainly because of financial considerations for the treatment of anemia related to cancer therapy, since they can reduce the need for transfusions and improve hemoglobin levels. Although erythropoietins are well-tolerated, they are slow to exert an effect and ineffective in a substantial proportion of patients. On the other hand, transfusion of RBCs is associated with a small risk of infection and other complications. However, no study has produced comparative results of toxicity between erythropoietins and transfusions in cancer patients, and the purported superior risk-benefit ratio of erythropoietic agents remains to be fully demonstrated. Blood transfusion is reliable, with a prompt hemoglobin increase in most patients treated. Another important consideration is that, in many patients with cancer, anemia is a feature of advanced disease. Therefore, a substantial proportion of these patients will not live long enough to experience the long-term hazards of blood transfusion. In others, anemia is a transient problem caused or aggravated by cancer therapy. These patients require few, if any, blood transfusions and their risk of incurring lasting damage is small. Indeed, treatment with erythropoietins is attractive in patients with a long-life expectancy and chronic transfusion dependency, such as patients with low-risk myelodysplastic syndromes. Unfortunately and ironically, only a minority of these patients are likely to respond.

An issue that might tilt the balance in favor of erythropoietin therapy would be a positive impact on cancer treatment outcome. To date, a possible survival trend favoring rHuEPO has not been confirmed in recent reports, which have raised concern about thromboembolic risks and the potential stimulation of tumor cell growth by the study drug. However, we underline the fact that the two recent trials with negative outcomes involved attempts to maintain hemoglobin concentrations in a range higher than those currently approved for the use of erythropoietic agents. The use of either rHuEPO or darbepoetin alfa in this setting should continue to be considered only in the context of well-designed, clinical investigations with appropriate safeguards for patients.

Cost-effectiveness issues are also of major importance and the number of patients needed to be treated with erythropoietins to avoid one transfusion. Currently, the strongest arguments to support the use of erythropoietic agents in cancer patients seem to be the effects on health-related QoL parameters. All studies that have specifically assessed QoL have produced convincing data indicating an improvement in this end point.

Chapter 9

Management of Bleeding in Cancer Patient's

Hemorrhaging occurs in approximately 6 to 10 percent of patients with advanced cancer. When visible, it can be particularly distressing to patients and their caregivers. In some patients, it may be the immediate cause of death. This article focuses on hemorrhaging that is visible, as opposed to occult bleeding. It reviews treatment options in the context of advanced cancer.

ETIOLOGY AND CLINICAL PRESENTATION

Bleeding may result from local vessel damage and invasion or from systemic processes such as disseminated intravascular coagulopathy (DIC) or abnormalities in platelet functioning and number. The underlying causes of these abnormalities are varied and include liver failure, medications such as anticoagulants, chemotherapy, radiotherapy, surgery and the cancer itself. Occasionally, concurrent diseases, such as idiopathic thrombocytopenia, may be responsible.

PHYSIOLOGY OF HEMOSTASIS

Hemorrhaging may manifest in a variety of ways, including hematemesis, hematochezia, melena, hemoptysis, hematuria, epistaxis, vaginal bleeding, or ulcerated skin lesions. It may also present as echymoses, petechiae, or bruising. Hemorrhage may occur as an acute catastrophic event, (Fig. 9.1) episodic major bleeds, or ongoing low-volume oozing. These characteristics provide clues as to the underlying cause and guide management.

MANAGEMENT: GENERAL MEASURES

The red cell and white cell formation occur in bone marrow mainly after the certain life span WBC

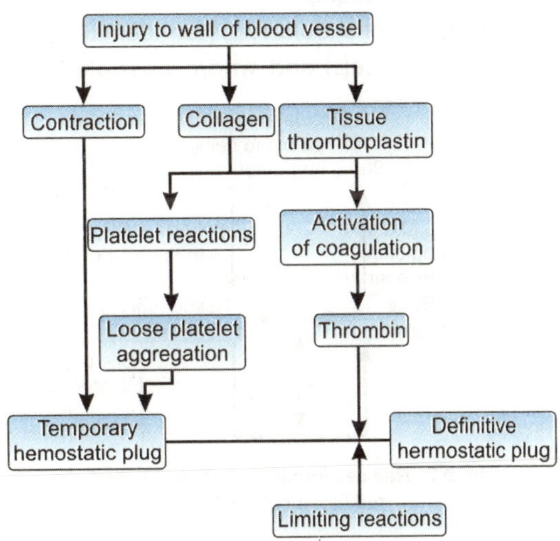

Fig. 9.1: Physiology of hemostasis

and RBC these distruction starts (Fig. 9.2). Treatment needs to be individualized and depends on several factors, including the underlying cause(s), the likelihood of reversing or controlling the underlying etiology, and the burden-to-benefit ratio of the treatment, all in the context of the patient's overall disease burden, life expectancy and goals of care. If the patient's life expectancy and overall quality of life warrants it, then management of an acute bleeding episode consists of general resuscitative measures, such as volume and fluid replacement and specific measures to stop the bleeding. On the other hand, if the patient's goals of care are palliative, then management may include measures to stop the bleeding without full resuscitative measures. Comfort measures only may be most appropriate for end-stage patients.

Management should focus on identifying the underlying cause(s) and where possible, controlling the bleeding. A comprehensive history and examination is self-evident. A review of concurrent medications and other illnesses may be helpful in identifying the etiology or contributing factors, such as the concurrent use of nonsteroidal anti-inflammatory drugs, which may exacerbate or precipitate bleeding through their actions on the gastrointestinal tract and platelet functioning. The burdens and risks of prophylactic anticoagulation may outweigh the benefits in patients with very advanced disease. Even when treated with appropriate therapeutic doses of anticoagulants, the incidence of bleeding complications remains higher in patients with advanced cancer than in those with earlier-stage disease. Investigations may be helpful. Full blood counts and clotting profiles may reveal systemic problems, while angiography or endoscopic studies may identify the site of bleeding. Goals of care should be explored. General measures may include applying pressure over the wound, and protecting the bleeding area from trauma and from the remaining infected granulation tissue.

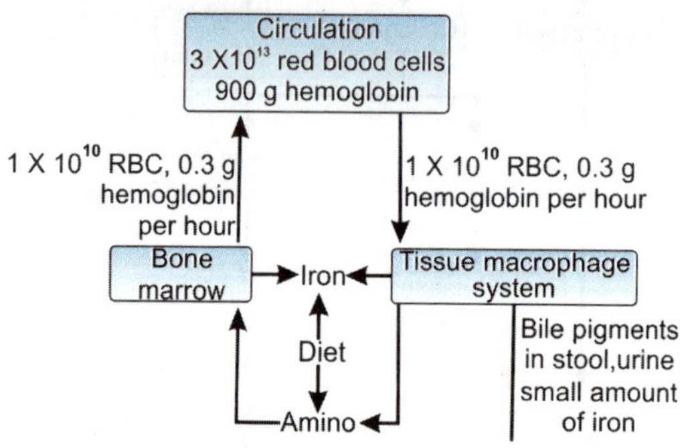

Fig. 9.2: Red cell formation and destruction of red blood cells (RBCs)

Patients at high-risk for bleeding should be identified and preventative measures should be taken before a crisis occurs. Episodic, low-volume bleeding (e.g. hemoptysis) may herald larger, catastrophic hemorrhages. Caregivers of patients at risk for major bleeds ought to be informed and prepared for such an event. However, this should be done sensitively so as not to invoke too much fear.

MANAGEMENT: LOCAL INTERVENTIONS

Packing, Hemostatic Agents and Dressings

Packing can be used with or without pressure to achieve hemostasis when bleeding originates in the nose, vagina or rectum. Surgical swabs of varying sizes may be used. These can be coated with chemicals that facilitate hemostasis; for example, acetone in vaginal packing and cocaine in nasal packing. If possible, the frequency of dressing changes should be reduced and nonadherent dressings should be used. Specially designed catheters with inflatable balloons may be used to control severe epistaxis. Foley catheters have also been used for this purpose. Such measures are temporary, since prolonged pressure may cause local ischemia.

A variety of agents and dressings, mostly designed for surgical procedures, has been reported to be of benefit for exterior, topical use in patients with advanced cancer. The evidence to support this, however, is largely based on case reports. The high costs of some of these products may also be prohibitively expensive for regular usage. Thromboplastin, a natural blood-clotting agent obtained from bovine plasma, is available as a powder for topical application. Systemic injection or absorption can lead to serious clotting. Absorbable gelatin is available as a sterile sponge-like dressing or sterile powder. It can be applied dry or saturated with sterile sodium solution and is absorbed within 4 to 6 weeks. When applied, fibrin is deposited in the interstices of the foam, resulting in swelling of the sponge, thereby forming a large synthetic clot. When applied to nasal, rectal, or vaginal mucosa, it liquifies within 2 to 5 days. Other bioabsorbable topical hemostatic agents include fibrin sealants and oxidized cellulose. Fibrin sealants are derived from human plasma and reproduce the final steps in the coagulation pathway to form a clot. They are used in a broad range of surgical procedures to assist hemostasis, including cardiovascular, hepatic and splenic surgery. Some are impregnated with clotting factor XIII and a solution of thrombin and calcium chloride. Collagen is another agent with inherent hemostatic activity. When applied as a bovine-derived mesh it comes into contact with blood, provokes the clotting cascade and forms a clot. Alternatively, oxidized cellulose compounds and highly absorbent alginate dressings, derived from seaweed, are available for topical use.

Vasoconstricting or cauterizing agents provide an alternative modality to managing localized, capillary-based bleeding. Epinephrine may be used, but its liberal use is discouraged. Prostaglandins E2 and F2 have been used to control intractable hemorrhagic cystitis. Bladder spasms, however, may limit their utility. Silver nitrate, an inorganic silver salt, induces a chemical cauterization and has been used to control bladder hemorrhages and epistaxis. Formalin, 2 percent or 4 percent, acts as a chemical cautery and has been used to control intractable rectal and bladder hemorrhaging. In one case series, topical formalin controlled bleeding in 49 of 55 patients (89%) with radiation-induced rectal bleeding. Aluminum astringents, such as 1 percent alum, can be delivered by continuous bladder irrigation. Bladder spasms are controllable with antispasmodic medications. Sucralfate has shown some benefit in controlling cancer-related gastrointestinal bleeding and cutaneous oozing. In the latter, a gel is prepared by dispersing one 1 g tablet of sucralfate in 5 ml of water soluble gel (e.g. K-Y® Jelly; McNeil-PPC, Inc.; Skillman, NJ) and is applied once or twice daily.

Radiotherapy

External-beam radiotherapy has been shown to decrease hemoptysis caused by lung cancer, with control occurring in up to 80 percent of patients. The optimal dose and fractionation remain controversial. Hypofractionation appears to be as effective as multiple fractions (often 10 or more daily fractions). A single fraction of 10 Gy has been shown to be as effective as multiple fractions in patients with hemoptysis due to lung cancer. Total doses of either 20 Gy (via multiple fractions) or 8 Gy (via hypofractionation) are often suggested. Radiotherapy should also be considered for bleeding from cancerous lesions of the vagina, skin rectum, and bladder. External-beam radiotherapy may be successful in controlling bleeding in up to 85 percent of cases of rectal bleeding and 60 percent of cases of hematuria from bladder cancer. One study found that a hypofractionated regimen (17 Gy in two fractions over 3 days) for patients with symptoms from advanced bladder cancer was as well tolerated as and less distressing to patients than a regimen of 12 fractions given over 26 days (45 Gy). Upper gastrointestinal hemorrhaging from malignant processes is less amenable to radiotherapy. While radiotherapy can be useful in controlling bleeding from head and neck cancers, many of these patients have already received maximal doses of radiotherapy when they present with bleeding, thereby excluding further radiation. Single or reduced fraction regimens appear to be as effective as multiple fractions in controlling bleeding.

Endoscopy

Endoscopy-based treatments have, for a long-time, been used in managing bleeding from upper gastrointestinal varices, particularly after systemic therapies such as vasopressin or somatostatin analogs have failed. This treatment method has been reported to be superior to balloon tamponade. It involves the injection of sclerosing agents into the varices or ligation of the vessels. Endoscopic interventions have also been proven to be useful for managing cancer-related hemorrhaging of the upper gastrointestinal tract, lungs and bladder. Ethanol hyperosmotic saline epinephrine, gelatin solutions and sodium tetradecyl sulfate are injected into the site of bleeding. Alternatively, the vessels may be cauterized by heat or by polar or laser coagulation *Akhtar* and colleagues reported on a series of 48 consecutive patients with esophagogastric cancer who underwent endoscopic argon-beam plasma coagulation for symptom and disease control. Bleeding was well controlled in three of the five patients treated for bleeding. Hemostasis was achieved in approximately 70 to 90 percent of cases treated for upper gastrointestinal bleeds. Complications occurred in 5 to 15 percent of cases and included worsening of the bleeding and perforation of the tract. Cystoscopic-assisted cautery by either heat or laser probes has been used in the treatment of hematuria in patients with bladder cancer. Its role is mainly for patients in whom continuous bladder irrigation and lavage have failed. Under direct vision, the urologist can inspect the bladder, identify the source of bleeding, and fulgurate the bleeding vessel or tumor. In the case of hemoptysis, bronchoscopy allows for ice-cold saline lavages and/or the use of balloon tamponade laser phototherapy or topical application of thrombin or fibrinogen at the site of bleeding. Endoscopic procedures have been used to control bleeds from the lower gastrointestinal tract, although these may be more challenging. Colonoscopic techniques vary and include bipolar electrocoagulation, heater probe, argon and Nd:YAG lasers.

Interventional Radiology

Transcutaneous arterial embolization (TAE) may be useful in well-selected patients. The procedure is often performed via a femoral or axillary approach under local anesthetic and is generally well-tolerated, requiring only mild sedation. The blood vessel supplying the affected site is first identified by arteriography. This is followed by the insertion of a hemostatic agent, usually in the form of a coil. Limiting factors include the presence of a bleeding disorder and the availability of the appropriate expertise. Embolization is restricted to areas where the blood vessels are accessible by the catheter and where embolization of the blood vessel does not result in ischemia of key organs. Benefits have been reported in patients with cancers involving the head and neck pelvis lung, liver and gastrointestinal tract. As with other treatment options in this setting, the majority of the evidence supporting this modality relies on case reports.

TAE has been used to manage carotid artery rupture in cancer patients. *Bates* and *Shamsham* reported on a patient whose episodes of profuse (but self-limited) carotid hemorrhage were successfully controlled by an endovascular technique that combined placement of a flexible self-expanding stent-graft to protect the common and internal carotid artery with selective coil embolization of the affected external carotid artery branches. *Sakakibara* and colleagues used an endoluminal balloon to control bleeding in three patients prior to undergoing surgical ligation of the arteries.

Transhepatic arterioembolization was used to control bleeding in five patients with inoperable hepatocellular cancer who presented with gastrointestinal bleeding from a variety of sources (esophageal varices or direct invasion of the duodenum, transverse colon, or stomach). *Recordare* and colleagues described four patients who underwent TAE to control spontaneous rupture of hepatocellular carcinoma. Patients lived for 3 to 62 months following the procedure. A quality-of-life analysis was not reported. *Wu* and colleagues suggested that acute upper gastrointestinal bleeding is a potential complication following TAE in patients with hepatocellular cancer. Thirty-one of 208 patients who underwent TAE in their service experienced upper gastrointestinal bleeding after the procedure. However, given that gastric or duodenal ulcers were found in 21 of these cases. Mallory-Weiss syndrome was found in three cases and esophageal varices were found in two cases, the bleeding was likely the result of comorbidities and complications of the cancer rather than the treatment itself. Not withstanding, the importance of meticulous case selection needs to be underscored.

Surgery

Surgery may be appropriate for a small group of well-selected patients who have failed conservative measures and who are deemed fit for surgery. Surgery usually consists of ligation of larger vessels or the removal of bleeding tissue. Two surgical approaches have been described for the management of carotid artery rupture—resection with reconstruction and ligation of the artery. *Witz et al* reported on three patients with head and neck cancers who presented with acute or imminent carotid artery rupture. Those patients successfully underwent ligation of the artery with no neurological sequelae. *Yegappan* and colleagues reported on prospectively collected data from 55 women who presented with bleeding from radiation proctitis. Bleeding in six patients who did not respond to topical formalin application was controlled with surgery.

MANAGEMENT

Systemic Interventions

Vitamin K (Phytonadione, Menadiol) Vitamin K is necessary for the hepatic production of a number of clotting factors, including factors II, VII, IX and X. Liver disease, insufficient intake of leafy green vegetables (a source of vitamin K), small bowel disease or resection, as well as intrahepatic and extrahepatic biliary obstruction can lead to deficiencies in the clotting factors. Coagulation screening studies reveal a prolonged prothrombin time or international normalized ratio (INR) and partial thromboplastin time with normal thrombin time, fibrinogen and serum fibrin-fibrinogen degradation products.

Vitamin K treatment may be helpful if either a derangement of these factors or excessive warfarin therapy is implicated in bleeding in a patient with advanced cancer. Doses of 2.5 to 10 mg are recommended, depending on the severity of the situation. The jury is not out on which roule of administration is best. *Whitling* et al. evaluated four different routes of vitamin K administration for reversing excessive anticoagulation: high-dose intravenous (1–10 mg), low-dose intravenous (0.5 mg), subcutaneous (1–10 mg) and oral (2.5–5 mg). Anticoagulation was achieved in all four groups. Although the high-dose intravenous method was the most effective at lowering INR levels to <5, overcorrection occurred more frequently with that method. *Byrd* and colleagues reported the effective and safe reversal of excess warfarin anticoagulation using subcutaneous phytonadione at doses of 1 mg for INR levels >8 but <14 (group 1) and 2 mg for levels >14 (group 2). The mean INR reductions in group 1 and group 2 after 24 hours were 49 percent and 67 percent, respectively. By 48 hours, INR levels were below 4.5 in both groups. No hemorrhagic or thrombotic complications were reported. The subcutaneous administration of phytonadione did not correct the INR as rapidly or as effectively as intravenous administration in a randomized trial. Higher doses of subcutaneous phytonadione were recommended for cases where full anticoagulation reversal is required. *Nee* et al. suggested that subcutaneous administration along with modification of the warfarin dosing is acceptable, since all patients in their study achieved safe levels of anticoagulation within 72 hours of subcutaneous administration. A recent retrospective study of 105 patients reported that only two (1.9%) patients who received intravenous phytonadione experienced adverse reactions. These anaphylactoid reactions manifest as dyspnea, chest tightness, facial flushing, nausea and in severe cases, cyanosis, loss of consciousness, hypotension and possibly death. However, review of the literature reveals that these are rare occurrences. A randomized, double-blind, placebo-controlled study comparing oral phytonadione (2.5 mg) plus the omission of further warfarin therapy with omission alone for reversing excessive warfarin anticoagulation in 30 asymptomatic patients (INR levels of 6–10) found that the addition of oral phytonadione reduced the time to achieve a normal INR by 1 day. Adverse effects did not differ between the two groups. *Fondevila* et al. on the other hand, reported no advantage of adding oral phytonadione (1 mg) to a regimen of simply discontinuing the warfarin in patients with excessive oral anticoagulation. Oral menadiol (20 mg daily for 3 days) was found to be as effective as intravenous phytonadione (1 mg daily) in normalizing INR levels in 26 patients with cholestasis. Therefore, when possible, vitamin K should be given by the subcutaneous or oral routes. When intravenous administration is considered unavoidable, the drug should be injected slowly, probably not exceeding 1 mg per minute. If, in 6 to 8 hours after parenteral administration, the INR is not satisfactorily lowered, the dose may be repeated. The role of prophylactic vitamin K administration for asymptomatic patients with elevated INR levels from liver involvement is unclear.

Vasopressin/Desmopressin

Vasopressin is a posterior pituitary hormone that causes splanchnic arteriolar constriction and reduction in portal pressure when injected intravenously or intra-arterially. This method has been extensively used in managing variceal bleeding related to portal gastropathy. Its use has also been reported in oncology. In a controlled trial, vasopressin therapy stopped bleeding in about half the patients with active upper-malignancy-related gastrointestinal bleeding. Doses range from 0.1 to 0.4 mg by continuous infusion. Vasoconstrictor effects on the myocardial, mesenteric, and cerebral circulation are the most notable potential side effects.

Somatostatin Analogs

Octreotide, an analog of somatostatin, has been used to manage upper gastrointestinal bleeds. Somatostatin reduces splanchnic flow and pressure via venous dilatation, thereby reducing portal pressure and portal venous flow. A starting dose of 50 to 100 µg twice daily is recommended. The dose may be titrated, as needed, up to 600 µg per day. An alternative regime consists of a bolus of 50 µg given intravenously or subcutaneously, followed by a continuous subcutaneous or intravenous infusion of 50 µg/hour for 48 hours. At low doses, very few side effects are reported, but at doses greater than 100 µg/hour, nausea, abdominal discomfort and diarrhea may occur. Except for preventing perioperative bleeding in pancreatic cancer resections, there are no reports related to the use of octreotide/somatostatin in controlling bleeding in cancer patients.

Antifibrinolytic Agents

Tranexamic acid (TA) and aminocaproic acid (EACA) are synthetic antifibrinolytic agents that block the binding sites of plasminogen, thereby inhibiting the conversion of plasminogen into plasmin by tissue plasminogen activator. The end result is a decreased lysis of fibrin clots. Tranexamic acid is approximately 10 times more potent than EACA *in vitro*. Fibrinolytic inhibitors have been used successfully in a variety of nononcologic settings. These include the control of bleeding following dental extractions subarachnoid hemorrhages, and gastrointestinal bleeds. Several case reports and a few studies have been published that suggest a role for these agents in the oncology setting.

TA and EACA have been administered orally and intravenously. The suggested intravenous dose of TA is 10 mg/kg three to four times a day, infused over about 1 hour. The suggested intravenous dose of EACA is 4 to 5 g in 250 ml over the first hour then 1 g/hour in 50 ml administered continuously for 8 hours, or until the bleeding is controlled. The most common adverse effects are gastrointestinal in nature (nausea, vomiting, and diarrhea) and occur in 25 percent of cases. Adverse effects appear to be dose dependent. Thromboembolism is uncommon. These antifibriolytics can also be applied topically, rectally, or by intrapleural instillation.

A systematic review of randomized trials found that hemostatic medications (TA, EACA, desmopressin and aprotinin) used for reducing surgery-related bleeding have limited or contradictory evidence of efficacy large controlled studies of these drugs are lacking in the cancer setting.

Blood Products

The frequency and severity of hemorrhages increases as platelet count declines below 20,000/µl. The risk of severe bleeding rises only when the count is below 5 to 10,000/µl. Patients with chronic autoimmune thrombocytopenia can tolerate platelet counts in the 5 to 10,000/µl range for long periods of time. Platelet transfusion in the setting of advanced cancer should be on a case-by-case basis with the aim of controlling symptoms.

A single unit of platelets should increase the platelet count in an average adult by approximately 6,000 to 10,000/μl, assuming normal splenic pooling. Four to six units are usually required to control bleeding. There is no scientific basis for the old 20,000/μl cut off. The short half-life of platelets, which decreases further as their counts drop, limits their usefulness in severely thrombocytopenic patients with end-stage disease. *Lassauniere* and colleagues have proposed criteria for platelet transfusions in patients with advanced hematologic malignancies. These criteria include continuous bleeding of the mouth or gums, epistaxis, extensive and painful hematomas, severe headaches, or disturbed vision of recent onset, as well as continuous bleeding through the gastrointestinal, gynecological or urinary systems.

The issue of whether or not to continue platelet transfusions in thrombocytopenic patients with end-stage disease poses an ethical dilemma. While ongoing transfusions may be futile, patients and families may perceive the cessation of transfusions as withdrawal of life-sustaining therapy. Sensitive and empathic discussions among patients, their families and the attending physician and health team are essential to explore their expectations, fears and concerns and to engage in advanced end-of-life planning while ensuring ongoing support and commitment to providing optimal comfort care.

Fresh frozen plasma is reserved for a very select group of patients with life expectancies greater than days to weeks. These include: (A) patients with specific deficiencies in certain coagulation factors; (B) patients in whom the effects of warfarin need to be reversed urgently; (C) patients who require urgent invasive interventions such as thoracenteses or surgery; and (D) when appropriate, the treatment of DIC. Similarly, packed red cell transfusions are indicated when anemia resulting from blood loss causes or aggravates symptoms such as fatigue and dyspnea. Guidelines for red blood transfusions in palliative patients have been published elsewhere.

The goals of care in a patient in the terminal phases of cancer should be comfort. Invasive treatments may present more burden than benefit in these patients and comfort without invasive procedures takes precedence. In some cases, it is unclear as to whether or not a local or systemic measure will be of benefit. Time-limited or therapeutic trials (e.g. whether or not a platelet transfusion or an antifibrinolytic agent will provide benefit) may be warranted in select circumstances. When a terminally ill patient is identified as being at risk for a major hemorrhage, family members and caregivers need to be sensitively informed and prepared, since these events can be extremely distressing. Using dark towels to absorb blood, applying pressure to the site of hemorrhaging and placing patients in the lateral position (in the event of hematemesis or hemoptysis) are simple empowering measures. A rapid-acting sedative should be available for sedation. Midazolam, 2.5 mg or 5 mg intravenously or subcutaneously, serves this purpose well if necessary, it can be repeated after 10 to 15 minutes. Orders for a sedative in case of such an emergency should be entered. Families/caregivers should be instructed on how to administer the medication subcutaneously. An indwelling subcutaneous butterfly facilitates administration. Families should be informed about whom to call in case of such an emergency. Anticoagulants should be reviewed, and the benefits versus burdens of continuing with these treatments should be considered. Maintaining therapeutic INR levels in terminally ill patients taking warfarin can be challenging and may require a switch to a low-molecular-weight heparin if the benefits of continuing anticoagulation outweigh the risks and burdens. The pharmacokinetics of these drugs are more predictable, their interactions with other drugs are less, they are not affected by liver dysfunction, and they require much less monitoring, negating the need for regular blood tests in these patients.

CONCLUSION

Bleeding in patients with advanced cancer can be caused by a variety of underlying processes and presents clinically in many different ways, from chronic, low-volume bleeding to acute episodes of major hemorrhaging. Identifying the underlying cause(s) is an important first step in managing it. Whether the bleeding originates from capillaries or from larger vessels will affect the treatment plan. Several local modalities are available to manage localized bleeding. These include topical hemostatic agents and dressings, radiotherapy, endoscopic procedures and TAE or balloon placement through interventional radiology. The use of interventional radiology is increasing. Systemic treatments are also available, particularly for more generalized bleeding or oozing. The majority of these treatments are supported only by case reports and series in the setting of advanced cancer. Comparative and controlled trials are lacking in this patient population. Patients at risk for major hemorrhages should be identified, and their families and caregivers should be prepared. End-of-life decision-making should be based on comfort and the optimization of quality of life.

Chapter 10 Role of Steroids in Cancer

Hearing the word steroid you may think of "roid rage" and muscle-bound gym rats with shrunken testicles. But if your doctor prescribed steroids as part of your treatment for cancer or another serious illness, do not worry. It is not "that" kind of steroid.

Your doctor is actually talking about cortisol, a form of steroid that your body produces naturally. It is different from anabolic steroids, which are the illegal muscle-building kind in human body steroids as formed by the help of cholestrol (Fig. 10.1).

HOW STEROIDS HELP?

Although the cortisol-type steroids prescribed for cancer treatment are different from anabolic steroids, you still need to take them under the close supervision of your doctor or medical specialist.

You will probably get a manmade version of the natural steroid cortisol, such as: cortisone, hydrocortisone, prednisone, methylprednisolone. These can help with your treatment in a variety of ways: reduce nausea associated with chemotherapy and radiation, kill cancer cells and shrink tumors as part of chemotherapy, decrease swelling, reduce allergic reactions (before transfusions, for example), lessen headaches caused by brain tumors. Sometimes, your doctor will recommend steroid treatments just to help you sleep, eat and feel better. Doctors can prescribe steroids for cancer treatment several ways: by injection through an intravenous (IV) drip in liquid or pill form as a cream (Table 10.1).

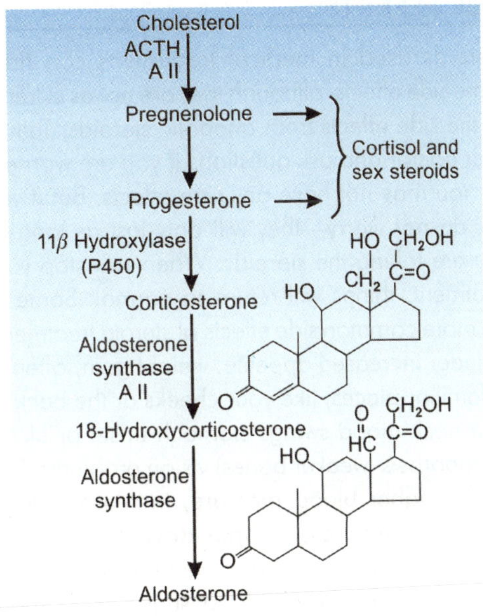

Fig. 10.1: Hormone synthesis

Table 10.1: Glucocorticoids and their relative potency

Compound	*Antli-inflammatory potency*	*Mineralocorticoid potency*	*Approximate equivalent dose (mg)*
Short-acting (<12 hours)			
Cortisol	1	2	20
Cortisone	0.8	2	25
Intermediate-acting (12 to 36 hours)			
Prednisone	4	1	5
Prednisolone	4	1	5
Methylprednisolone	5	0	4
Triamcinolone	5	0	4
Long-acting (>36 hours)			
Paramethasone	10	0	2
Betamethasone	25	0	0.75
Dexamethasone	25	0	0.75

SIDE EFFECTS

Steroids used in medical treatments can have some side effects, although they are not as extreme as the side effects from anabolic steroids. Talk to your doctor and ask questions if you are worried.

You may not have any side effects. But if you do, do not worry—they will only last as long as you are taking the steroids. When you stop your treatment, things will return to normal. Some of the more common side effects of steroid treatments include: increased appetite, weight gain, often in unfamiliar places, like your cheeks or the back of your neck mood swings stomach upset or ulcers osteoporosis (weaker bones) vision problems (Fig. 10.2). higher blood pressure, increased blood sugar. Sometimes, people develop diabetes temporarily. If you already have diabetes, you will need to monitor your blood sugar levels more closely. For girls, irregular menstruation (missed or late periods). Less common side effects include: bruising more easily, difficulty fighting infections, acne flare-ups and increased facial hair.

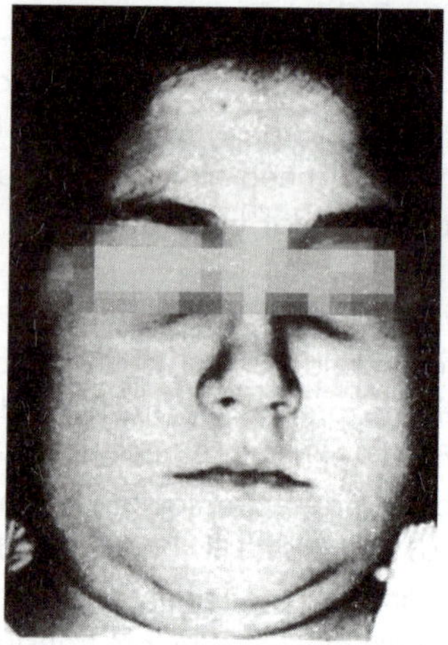

Fig. 10.2: Steroid side effects

If you develop several of these symptoms, you have a condition called Cushing syndrome. Sometimes it gets better if you make changes in the way you take the steroids. If you are having problems with these side effects, talk to your doctor.

Remember, you may not have any side effects. If you do, you will probably find that they are overshadowed by the benefits of the treatment. But check with your doctor about ways to make them easier to live with.

Tips on taking steroids for cancer treatment: Your doc will give you all the details, of course, but there are some things to remember when taking steroids for cancer treatment. Here are a few: Do not stop taking the medication without your doctor's guidance. If you notice anything strange while you are being treated with steroids, tell your parents and doctor right away. Do not stop taking the steroid, though. Your body makes less cortisol when you are having steroid treatments, so you need to ease off the medication and give your body a chance to get its own production back up to normal again. If you do not, your body could go through a potentially serious withdrawal. Weaning your body off the medication is easy to do, and your doctor will guide you through it.

Chapter

11 Role of Antacids

ACID-RELATED PATHOPHYSIOLOGY—THE STOMACH SECRETES

Stomach is consist of body function and pyloric part (Fig. 11.1). Hydrochloric acid (HCl), bicarbonates, pepsinogen, mucus, prostaglandins, stomach lining of inner mucosa having many secretory glands (Fig. 11.2).

Glands of the Stomach

- Cardiac
- Pyloric
- Gastric

The gastric glands are the largest in number (Fig. 11.2).

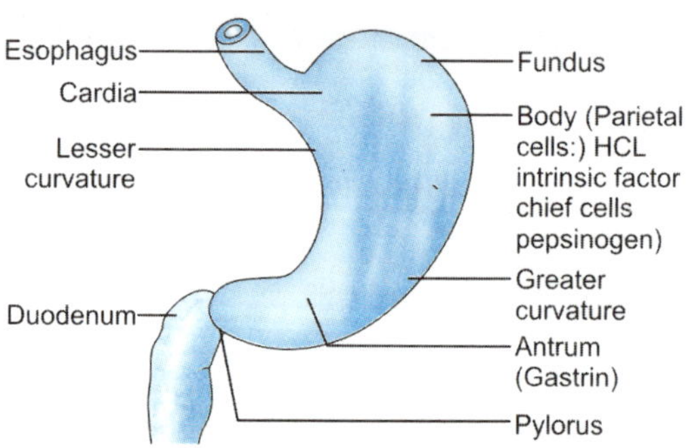

Fig. 11.1: Anatomy of stomach

Cells of the Gastric Glands

- *Parietal cells:* Produce and secrete HCl. Primary site of action for many acid-controller drugs.
- *Chief cells:* Secrete pepsinogen (pro-enzyme). Pepsinogen becomes pepsin when activated by exposure to acid. Pepsin breaks down proteins (proteolytic).

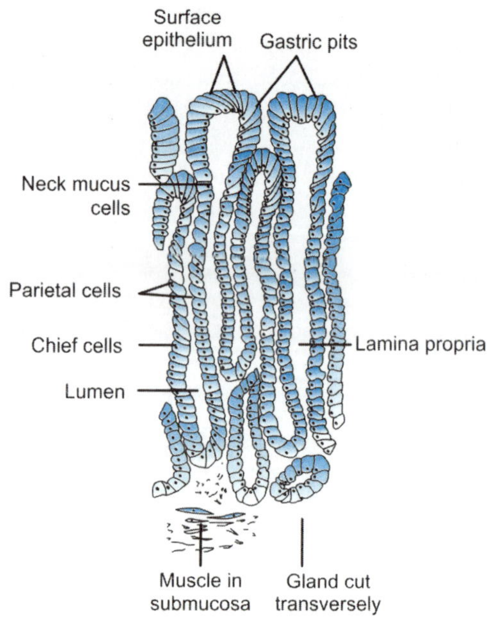

Fig. 11.2: Stomach mucosal glands

- *Mucoid cells:* Mucus-secreting cells (surface epithelial cells). Provide a protective mucous coat. Protects against self-digestion by HCl.

Secretion of HCl

HCl is secreted by the parietal cells. Maintains stomach at a pH of 1 to 4. Secretion stimulated by: large, fatty meals, excessive amounts of alcohol, emotional stress.

PARIETAL CELLS STIMULATION SECRETION

Acid-related diseases caused by imbalance of the three cells of the gastric gland and their secretions. Most common: hyperacidity. Most harmful: peptic ulcer diseases (PUD). Lay terms for overproduction of HCl by the parietal cells: indigestion. Sour stomach, Heartburn—Acid stomach.

Antacids mechanism of action promote the gastric mucosal defense mechanisms: Secretion of mucus: protective barrier against HCl. Bicarbonate: helps buffer acidic properties of HCl. Prostaglandins: prevent activation of proton pump. Antacids do not prevent the over-production of acid. Acids neutralize the acid once it's in the stomach.

Antacids Drug Effects

Reduction of pain associated with acid-related disorders. Raising gastric pH from 1.3 to 1.6 neutralizes 50 percent of gastric acid. Raising gastric pH point from 1.3 to 2.3 neutralizes 90 percent of the gastric acid. Antacids OTC formulations available as: capsules and tablets, powders, chewable tablets, suspensions, effervescent granules and tablets.

Antacids

Magnesium salts: Forms: carbonate hydroxide, oxide, trisilicate. Commonly cause a laxative effect. Usually used with the other agents to counteract this effect. Dangerous when used with renal failure-the failing kidney cannot excrete magnesium, resulting in accumulation. For example: magnesium hydroxide (MOM); combination products such as maalox, aluminum and magnesium.

Calcium salts:Forms: many but carbonate is the most common. May cause constipation. Their use may result in kidney stones. Long duration of acid action may cause increase of gastric acid secretion (hyperacidity bound). Often advertised as an extrasource of dietary calcium. For example: calcium carbonate.

Sodium bicarbonate: Highly soluble. Quick onset, but short duration. May cause metabolic alkalosis. Sodium content may cause problems in patients with hypertension or renal insufficiency.

Aluminum salts: Forms: carbonate, hydroxide, phosphate. Have constipating effects. Often used with magnesium to counteract constipation. For example: aluminum carbonate.

Antacids and Antiflatulents

Antiflatulents: Used to relieve the painful symptoms associated with gas. Several agents are used to bind or alter intestinal gas and are often added to antacid combination products. OTC Antiflatulents: activated charcoal. Simethicone: O alters elasticity of mucus-coated bubbles, causing them to break. O Used often, but there are limited data to support effectiveness.

Antacids Side Effects

Minimal and depend on the compound used: aluminum and calcium

Magnesium: Diarrhea

Calcium carbonate: Produce gas and belching; often combined with simethicone. Assess for allergies pre-existing conditions that may restrict the use of antacids, such as: fluid imbalances—Renal disease, pregnancy-GI obstruction.

Antacids Nursing Implications

Patients with hypertension should use low-sodium antacids. Use with caution with other medications due to many drug interactions. Most medications should be given 1 to 2 hours after giving antacid. Antacids may cause premature dissolving of enteric—coated medications, resulting in stomach upset. Monitor for side effects: nausea, vomiting, abdominal pain, diarrhea. With calcium-containing products: constipation, acid rebound.

HistamineType 2 (H_2) Antagonists and H_2 Antagonists

Drug effect: Suppressed acid secretion in the stomach.

Therapeutic uses: Shown to be effective for:

- Gastric ulcer
- Upper GIT bleeding
- Gastroesophageal reflux disease (GERD)
- Duodenal ulcer with or without *H.pylori*.

Can be also effective for: Stress ulcers-peptic esophagitis.

H_2 Antagonists side effects: Overall, less than 3 percent incidence of side effects. Cimetidine may induce impotence and gynecomastia.

Drug Interactions

Cimetidine: O Binds with P 450 microsomal oxidase system in the liver, resulting in inhibited oxidation of many drugs and increased drug levels. O All H_2 antagonists may inhibit the absorption of drugs that require an acidic GI environment for absorption.

H_2 Antagonists

Drugs interactions: Smoking has been shown to decrease the effectiveness of H_2 blockers. Nursing implications: Assess for allergies and impaired renal or liver function. Use with caution in patients who are confused, disoriented or elderly. Take one hour before or after antacids. Ranitidine may be given intravenously.

Proton Pump Inhibitors

The parietal cells release positive hydrogen ions (protons) during HCl production. This process is called the " Proton pump." H_2 blockers and antihistamines do not stop the action of this pump.

Mechanism of action: Irreversibly bind to H^+/K^+ ATPase enzyme. This bond prevents the movement of hydrogen ions from the parietal cell into the stomach. Result: achlorhydria "All gastric acid secretion is blocked." In order to return to normal acid secretion, the parietal cell must synthesize new H^+/K^+ ATPase. Total inhibition of gastric acid secretion:

- Lansoprazole (Zollipak)
- Omeprazole (Omepak)
- Rabeprazole
- Pantoprazole
- Esomeprazole.

Therapeutic uses: GERD maintenance therapy. Erosive esophagitis: short-term treatment of active duodenal and begin gastric ulcers. Zollinger-Ellison syndrome. Treatment of *H.pylori*-induced ulcers.

Side effects: Safe for short-term therapy. Incidence low and uncommon.

Nursing implications: Assess for allergies and history of liver disease. Pantoprazole is the only proto pump inhibitor available for parenteral administration and can be used for patients who are unable to take oral medications. May increase serum levels of diazepam, phenytoin and cause increased chance for bleeding with warfarin. Instruct the patient taking Omeprazole: it should be taken before meals. The capsule should be swallowed whole, not crushed, opened or chewed. It may be given with antacids.

Sucralfate

Cytoprotective agent: Used for stress ulcers, erosions, PUD. Attracted to and binds to the base of ulcers and erosions, forming a protective barrier over these areas. Protects these areas from pepsin, which normally breaks down proteins (making ulcers worse). Little absorption from the gut. May cause constipation, nausea and dry especially tetracycline. Binds with phosphate. Can not be administered with other medications.

Misoprostol

Synthetic prostaglandin analog: Prostaglandins have cytoprotective activity—Protect gastric mucosa from injury by enhancing local production of mucus or bicarbonate. Promote local cell regeneration. Help to maintain mucosal blood flow. Used for prevention of NSAID-induced gastric ulcers. Doses that are therapeutic enough to treat duodenal ulcers often produce abdominal cramps and diarrhea.

Section-C

Common Cancer and Its Management

Chapter 12 Management of Cervical Cancer

TREATMENT OF CIN/DYSPLASIA

1. CIN grade-I: Cause is usually inflammatory infection should be treated patient to be kept on follow-up three monthly pap smear examination.
2. CIN grade–II /grade III:
   Local destructive method:
   - Cryosurgery
   - Fulgration coagulation
   - Laser ablation

   Excision of local tissue:
   - Conization by cold knife
   - Laser conization
   - LLETZ (large loop excision of transformation zone)

   Surgery:
   - Therapeutic conization
   - Hystectomy.

Cervical cancer usually spread via parametrium an either side (Fig. 12.1).

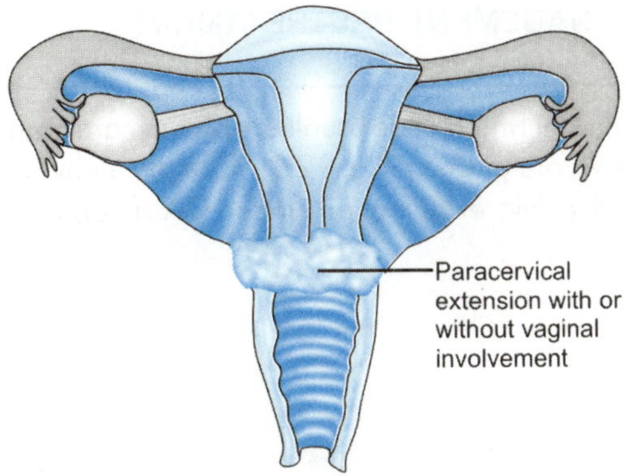

Fig. 12.1: Extension of cervical cancer

TREATMENT OF CA CERVIX

A. Preinvasive disease

Cryosurgery/Laser treatment! LEETZ, but before above treatment: One must exclude following:

a. **Entire transformation zone should be visualized colposcopically.**
b. **Endocervical curettage should be negative.**
c. **Other sites seen on colposcopic, examination are negative.**

If patients not meets above three criteria therapeutic conization should be performed.

Nowadays cryosurgery/laser treatment/ LEET has been declined why?

We prefer to long follow-up with pap smear examination for low-grade dysplasia. High-grade dysplasia warrants therapeutic conization to permit histopathological examination.

Treatment of adenocarcinoma *in situ*. Because adenocarcinoma *in situ* frequently multifocal thus cone biopsy always not reliable, thus ideal treatment of adenocarcinoma *in situ* is required type I hystectomy knowing the fact adeno-carcinoma is a radioresistant tumor.

MANAGEMENT PRETREATMENT EVALUATION

Cervical lymph node usually involve in carcinoma cervix are given in (Fig. 12.2). Complete physical and pelvic examination under GA if required. Chest X-ray IVP cystoscopy colposcopy and colposcopy directed biopsy or cone biopsy, endocervical curettage and biopsy.

Optional investigation, CT scan abdomen and pelvis for primary tumor as well as lymph node status and distant metastasis. Bone scan if required. Proctosigmoidoscopy all the patient of Ca cervix stage II B onwards para-aortic lymph node sampling must be done. I B onwards IVP is must in all cases of Cocervix. II B onwards investigation required—para-aortic LN sampling—Cystoscopy, proctosigmoidoscopy.

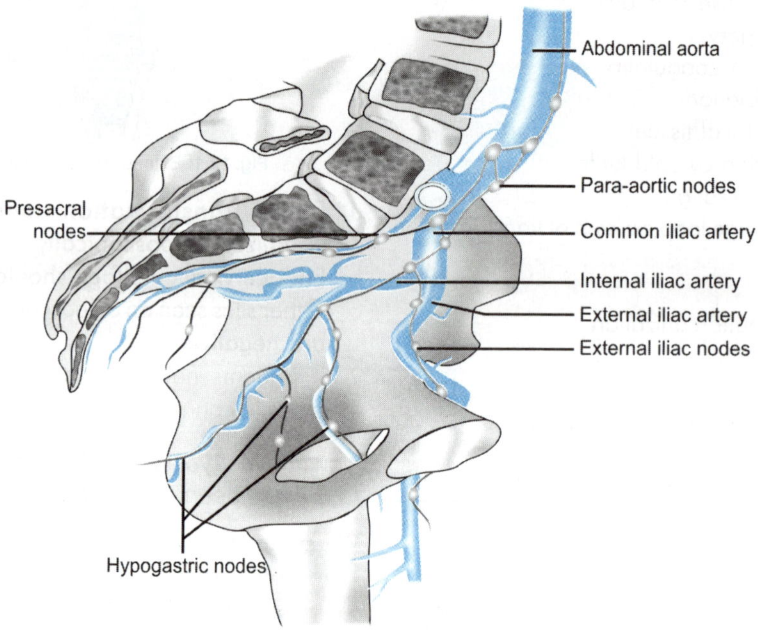

Fig. 12.2: Pelvic lymph nodes around cervix

Limitation of Biopsy and Importance of PV Examination

Since tissue obtained by punch biopsy may fail to access depth of invasion or status of pelvic wall and tumor size. Thus clinical PV examination it becomes vital to access the tumor size as well as parametric involvement. PV examination under the general anesthesia provide better inspection of upper vagina, cervix and more precise palpation of parametrium and lateral pelvic wall.

STAGE IA, TREATMENT

A1 Therapeutic conization or
Type-I hystrectomy or
ICRT 60 to 70 Gray (Gy) alone.
A2 Radical hysterectomy with pelvic LN dissection or ICRT alone 60 to 70 Gray (Gy).

STAGE IB1

EBRT + ICRT ! or radical hysterectomy with pelvic lymph node dissection. Result with surgery or radiotherapy alone 85 percent 5-year survival.

Surgery preferred young women small volume disease node negative favored candidate for surgery in order to preserve ovarian function and maintain the vaginal length.

Radiotherapy preferred old age women to avoid morbidity of surgery and here ovarian preservation is not warranted.

HOW TO TREAT EARLY B1 LESION BY RADIOTHERAPY?

We can give 60 Gy to point A, (30 Gy and 30 Gy 1 wk apart).

Now dose to the point B will be 1/3rd of the point A dose that means 20 Gy received by the parametrium. We know parametrium is to be given dose up to 50 Gy so now left over 30 Gy will be delivered by EBRT but we have to limit the dose to point A up to 75 Gy so that during 30 Gy delivery by the radiotherapy after 7 fraction we can use midline block to avoid extra dose to point A that means 1600 cGy dose can be delivered with 5 cm midline block.

USE OF MIDLINE BLOCK

Advantage

Parametrial boost can be given 10 Gy/5 fraction by EBRT.

Avoid extra dose to the rectum and bladder as well as brachytherapy dose can be increased.

Disadvantage

Overdose to the medial structure like increased dose to the point A.

Underdosing to the uterosacral ligament if disease present there.

RADIOTHERAPY

Therapeutic dose required in CA cervix 80 to 85 Gy to point A and 50 to 55 Gy to point B. Radiation given in two phases:

Phase -1 EBRT: By cobalt 60, 50 Gy in 25 fractions to whole pelvis on given in (Fig. 12.3).

Phase -2: Either by ICRT / SERVO application.

Therapeutic dose required in CACX for advance stage is 80 to 85 Gy to point A and 50

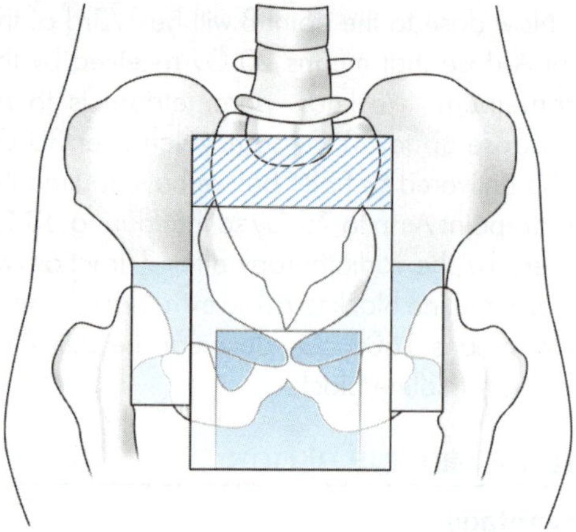

Fig. 12.3: Radiation field use in cervical cancer

to 55 Gy to point B. When given by LDR, dose pattern (Fig. 12.4) point A and B is very important in the management of carcinoma cervix via brachytherapy (Figs 12.5 and 12.6A and B).

Phase-1: EBRT Co 60 50 Gy / 25 fraction @ 200 cGy/fraction, 5 fraction/week.

Phase-2: ICRT 30 to 35 Gy to point A.

Entire treatment: EBRT+ICRT must be completed in 7 to 8 week since 5 week required for EBRT and for HDR treatment we can afford 1 week delay between EBRT and ICRT because 1 week gap required between 2 fraction of HDR.

For LDR we can afford maximum 2 week gap between EBRT and brachytherapy.

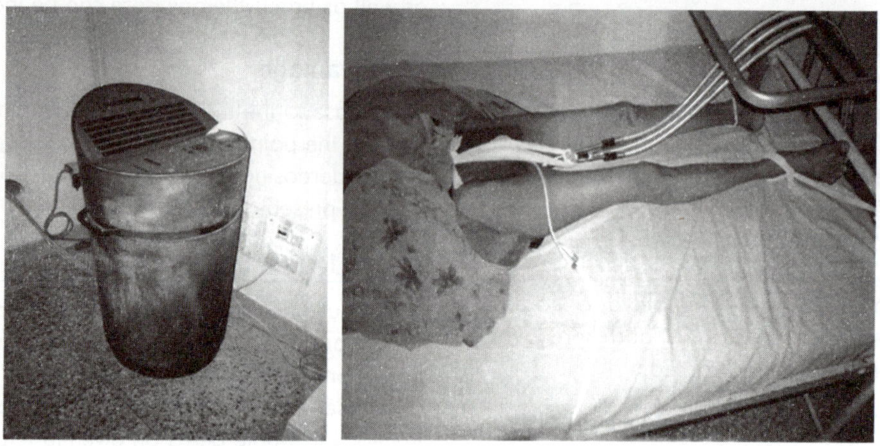

Fig. 12.4: LDR unit, patient under LDR treatment

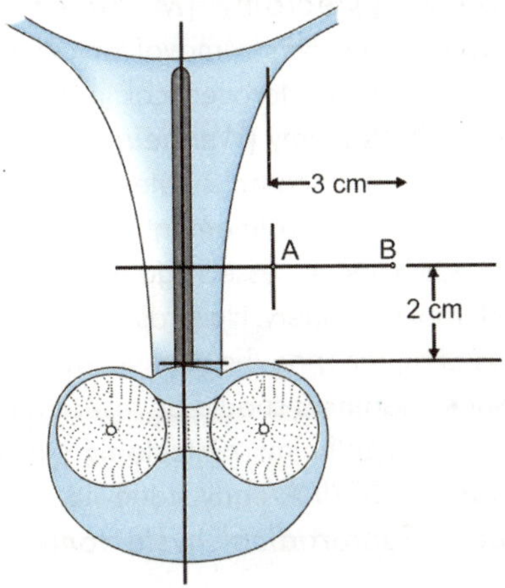

Fig. 12.5: Point A and B

STAGE IB2/ IIA TREATMENT

These lesion having high chances of pelvic lymph node recurrence thus ideal treatment surgery + postoperative radiotherapy. Postoperative radiotherapy indicated in these high-risk group

1. Pelvic lymph node
2. Positive margin
3. Residual disease
4. Lymphovascular invasion
5. High grade histology
6. Parametrial invasion.

STAGE IIB, III, IVA TREATMENT

Treatment is radical radiotherapy with concurrent chemotherapy.

EBRT preferred 15 to 18 MV photon to spare soft tissue and skin by fore field technique or by

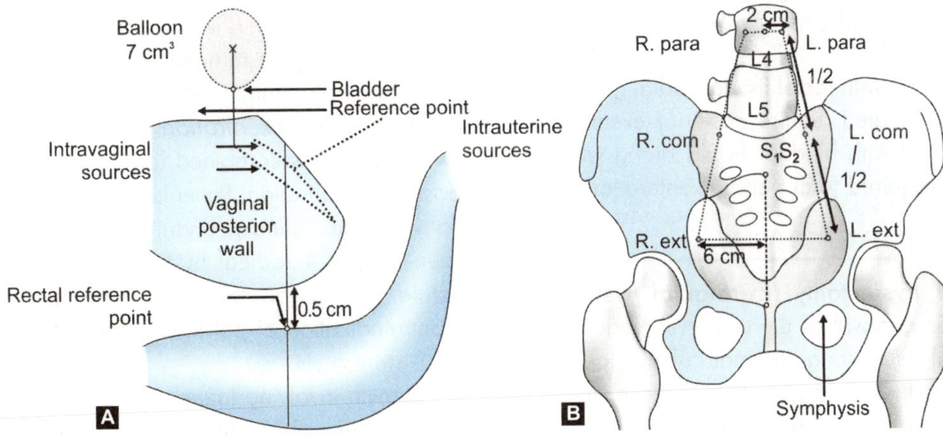

Figs 12.6A and B: Various reference point useful known for brachytherapy of cervix

two field technique but, if high energy photon is not available than 4 MV cobalt 60/linac ideally we should use 4 field technique with low energy to avoid extrareaction because beam is less penetrating. (ICRT 30-35 Gy + EBRT 50 Gy).

Concurrent cisplatin 35 mg/m^2 weekly with radiotherapy is indicated in the stage 1 B onwards only. It decreases the recurrence as much as 50 percent.

Para-aortic Lymph Node Irradiation

It is not usually taken into consideration because of high morbidity and mortality reported. However, concurrent cisplatin further decreases the importance of para-aortic lymph node irradiation.

STAGE IVA TREATMENT

Patients with bladder fistula radical radiotherapy contraindicated, surgery (Anterior exenteration) or palliative radiotherapy 30 Gy/10 fraction can be given.

Patients with rectal fistula: radial radiotherapy contraindicated require posterior exenteration.

Patient with bladder fistula along with rectal fistula required total pelvic exenteration.

TYPE OF HYSTECTOMY

Type-1 hystectomy (Extrafacial hystectomy): Involves removal of uterus cervix adjacent para-cervical tissue alongwith small cuff of upper vaginal type-I hystectomy mainly done in the microinvasive carcinoma stage- I A-1 or stage A-2.

Type-2 hystectomy (Modified radical hystectomy): Involves removal of cervix uterus paracervical tissue uterocervical ligament.

Type-3 hystectomy (Wertheims hystectomy): Involves removal of complete uterus, cervix, upper half of vagina, round ligament as well as pelvic lymph node. Uterine vessels ligated at their origin from internal iliac artery. Hazards of bladder fistula decreased by spearing the superior vesicle artery. Uterosacral ligament should be resected as much as possible. Wertheims hystectomy indicated in stage-I B-1/1 B2/II A/early stage-IIB.

Type-4 Supraradical hystectomy (involve pelvic exentration):

Anterior exentration: Include uterus cervix vagina bladder urinary conduit made ureter attached ileal segment this surgery usually done in CA cervix patient with bladder fistula.

Posterior exentration: It is done when bladder is normal but rectum is involve (RVF). Uterus cervix vagina and rectum removal is done and patient left with permanent colostomy.

Total pelvic exentration when both VVF and RVF present it is combined form of anterior and posterior exentration. Patients left with permanent colostomy and urinary conduit. High complication seen in type-4 radical hystectomy small bowel fistula/obstruction seen in 50 percent cases. Contraindication of pelvic exentration is:

a. Distent mets
b. Growth involving lateral pelvic wall
c. Poor general condition of the patient.

RECURRENCE OF CARCINOMA CERVIX

After radical surgery if pap smear becomes positive after 3 months of surgery or new mass lesion develops, treatment is radical radiotherapy. Patients with pelvic wall recurrence shows poor outcome compared to the patients those having central recurrence.

After Radical Radiotherapy Clinically One Must See

- Leg edema
- Sciatic pain
- Uretric obstruction

Above finding showed unresectable lesion at the side wall of pelvis hence, surgery is not possible but the small tumor limited to cervix can be taken care of radical hysterectomy.

AFTER TREATMENT FOLLOW-UP OF PATIENTS

Both gynecologist and radiation Oncologist should follow the patient jointly:

- Monthly up to 3 months
- 3 monthly up to 1st year
- 4 monthly up to 3rd year
- 6 monthly up to 2 to 5th year, 5 years onwards yearly follow-up lifelong nowaday current study by ICMR shown is that breast cancer is on the rise and cervical cancer on the fall shown (Fig. 12.7) celibreat.

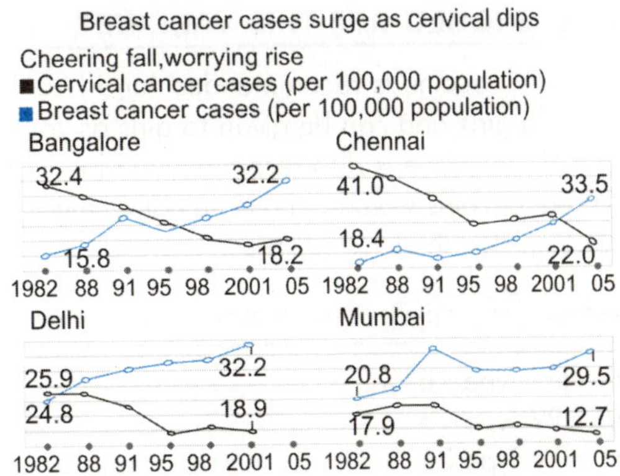

Fig. 12.7: Data showing reverse is on the way

Breakthrough in Carcinoma Cervix: Prevention and Control

In June 2006, the Advisory Committee on Immunization Practices (ACIP) voted to recommend the first vaccine developed to prevent cervical cancer and other diseases in females caused by certain types of genital human papilloma virus (HPV). The vaccine, Gardasi (r), protects against four HPV types, which together cause 70 percent of cervical cancers and 90 percent of genital warts. The Food and Drug Administration (FDA) recently licensed this vaccine for use in girls/women, ages 9 to 26 years. The vaccine is given through a series of three shots over a six-month period (0, 2 and 6 month).

WHO SHOULD GET THIS VACCINE?

The HPV vaccine is recommended for 11 to 12 year old girls and can be given to girls as young as 9. The vaccine is also recommended for 13 to 26 year old girls/women who have not yet received or completed the vaccine series.

TYPE OF STRAIN OF VIRUS

- HPV Type 16
- HPV Type 18
- HPV Type 31
- HPV Type 35
- HPV Type 45

Above said strains of human papilloma virus (HPV) known to cause carcinoma cervix (approx. 90% cases).

WHY IS THE HPV RECOMMENDED FOR SUCH YOUNG GIRLS?

Females should get the vaccine before they are sexually active. This is because the vaccine is most effective in girls/women who have not yet acquired any of the four HPV types covered by the vaccine. Girls/women who have not been infected with any of those four HPV virus types will get the full benefits of the vaccine.

WHY IS THE HPV VACCINE ONLY RECOMMENDED FOR GIRLS/WOMEN AGES 9 TO 26?

The vaccine has been widely tested in 9 to 26 years old girls/women. But research on the vaccine's safety and efficacy has only recently begun with women older than 26 years of age. The FDA will consider licensing the vaccine for these women when there is research to show that it is safe and effective for them.

SHOULD PREGNANT WOMEN GET THE VACCINE?

The vaccine is not recommended for pregnant women.

EFFICIENCY OF THE HPV VACCINE

Studies have found the vaccine to be almost 100 percent effective in preventing diseases caused by the four HPV types covered by the vaccine including precancers of the cervix, vulva and vagina and genital warts. The vaccine has mainly been studied in young women who had not been exposed to any of the four HPV types in the vaccine.

WHY DOES THE VACCINE NOT PROTECT AGAINST?

Because the vaccine does not protect against all types of HPV, it will not prevent all cases of cervical cancer or genital warts. About 30 percent of cervical cancers will not be prevented by the vaccine. So it will be important for women to continue getting screened for cervical cancer (regular Pap tests).

SAFETY OF HPV VACCINE

The FDA has licensed the HPV vaccine as safe and effective. This vaccine has been tested in over 11,000 females (ages 9–26 years) around the world. These studies have shown no serious side effects. The most common side effect is soreness at the injection site. CDC, working with the FDA, will continue to monitor the safety of the vaccine after it is in general use. Vaccine is made up of proteins from the outer coat of the virus (HPV). There is no infectious material in this vaccine.

DOSE SCHEDULE

The HPV vaccine is given through a series of three shots over a 6-month period. The second and third doses should be given 2 and 6 months (respectively) after the first dose.

Will girls/women who have been vaccinated still need cervical cancer screening?

There are three reasons why women will still need regular cervical cancer screening.

- **First**, the vaccine will not protect against all types of HPV that cause cervical cancer, so vaccinated women will still be at risk for some cancers.
- **Second**, some women may not get all required doses of the vaccine (or they may not get them at the right times), so they may not get the vaccine's full benefits.
- **Third**, women may not get the full benefit of the vaccine, if they receive it after they have already acquired one of the four HPV types.

Should girls/women be screened before getting vaccinated?

- No girls/women do not need to get an HPV test or Pap test to find out, if they should get the vaccine. An HPV test or a Pap test can tell that a woman may have HPV, but these tests cannot tell the specific HPV type(s) that a woman has.

Other Ways to Prevent Cervical Cancer and HPV

Another HPV vaccine is in the final stages of clinical testing, but it is not yet licensed. This vaccine would protect against the two types of HPV that cause most (70%) cervical cancers.

Chapter

13 Breast Cancer Management

PRETREATMENT EVALUATION

1. First to confirm diagnosis by FNAC/biopsy.
2. Chest X-ray to rule out lung metastasis (Fig. 13.1).
3. USG whole abdomen and pelvis to rule out metastasis.
4. Mammography—Opposite breast mammography also required if histology is lobular carcinoma, since bilaterality is 20 percent (Lobular vs 5% inductal carcinoma) (Fig. 13.2).
5. Routine hematological test.
6. Bone X-ray in symptomatic patients.
7. Bone scan in symptomatic patients.

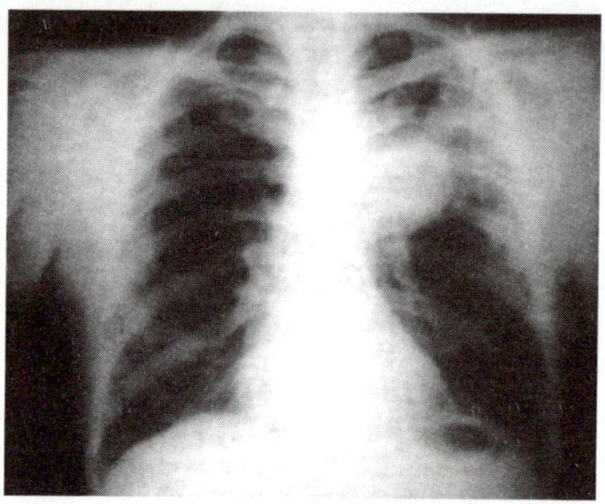

Fig. 13.1: Lung metastasis

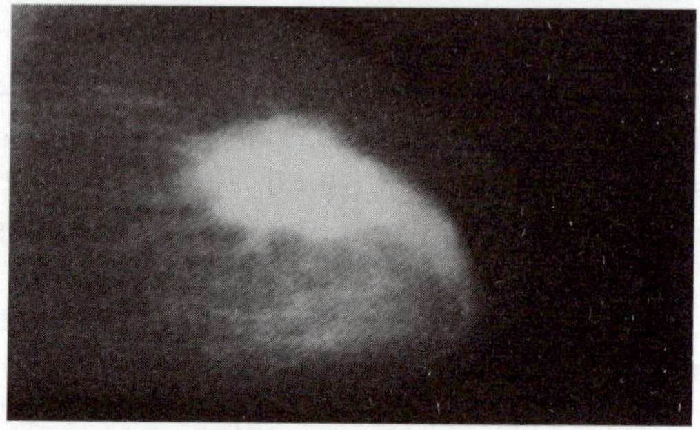

Fig. 13.2: Mammography shown breast cancer

Ductal Carcinoma *In Situ*

Lumpectomy + postoperative radiotherapy to chest wall, no axillary irradiation if tumor larger in size tumor mastectomy + chest wall irradiation require.

Lobular Carcinoma *In Situ*, Treatment

1. Bilateral total mastectomy.
2. An ipsilateral total mastectomy with mirror image biopsy from opposite breast, if found positive total mastectomy of that side also.
3. No role of postoperative radiotherapy.
4. Current recommendation is no surgical intervention, only follow-up with estrogen 20 mg

OD for 5 years. Why? : Lobular carcinoma *in situ* rarely becomes invasive carcinoma and bilateral mastectomy is too mutilating at the modern age of the treatment (Devita) (Flow chart 13.1).

Flow chart 13.1: Triple diagnosis

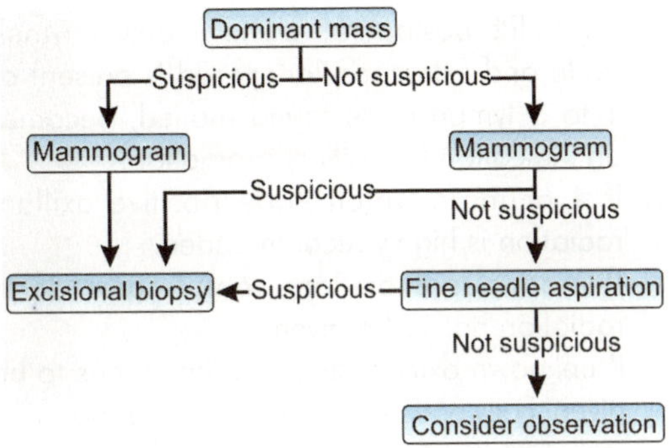

EARLY STAGE BREAST CARCINOMA

Clinical stage I and stage II

A - TO N1
- T1 N1
- T2 N0

B - T2 N1
- T3N0

Sequence of Treatment

NACT (+/–) and surgery; radiotherapy (Maintenance) and hormone treatment.

Advantages of NACT

1. According NSABP protocol B27 the purpose of chemotherapy is to decrease the tumor size up to such, extent that (Breast conservation surgery) can be performed otherwise patients has to go undermastectomy.
2. The other advantage of preoperative chemo is to assess the objective response of the type of the chemo regime patients is highly responsive.
3. Chemotherapy increased overall 5-year survival from 44 to 88 percent.
4. Why chemo is recommended in early stage breast cancer, a major trial of 552 patients with stage I to stage III not showing apparently any distant metastasis but 36 percent patients shows microscopic metastasis in bone marrow, thus, it is at present the strongest indication of NACT in early stage of breast cancer.
5. Why chemo is more effective in premenopausal women?
   - Chemo cause apart from tumor regression, ovarian ablation because of chemotoxicity thus double increase in benefit found in premenopausal age patient with chemotherapy.
   - Other cause is that, it can be a relative advantage overpostmenopausal women (more chances of chemo dose reduction has to be done in older women which is not there in premenopausal age.

a. **Surgical management**

i. Lumpectomy
ii. QUART (Milan)
iii. Simple mastectomy
iv. Radical mastectomy
v. MRM
vi. Extended radical mastectomy.

b. **Indications and contraindications of BCT**
   i. Both the points bear in the mind while performing BCT in early stage breast carcinoma.
   ii. At present treatment philosophy of axillary lymph node.

c. **By surgery**
   i. If clinically positive axillary lymph node: Treatment is axillary lymph node dissection of level 1 and level 2. Removal of level 3 does not carry any survival advantage rather increase morbidity (lymph edema brachial plexus injury).
   ii. Clinically negative axillary lymph node at present recommendation is sentinal lymph node biopsy. If found positive, axillary lymph node dissection. If found negative, no axillary dissection recommended at present.

By radiation

1. After the surgery minimum lymph node to be removed for pathological sampling should be atleast 10.
2. If all ten lymph node found negative no axillary radiation.
3. If 1 to 3 lymph node positive, axillary radiation ±, if HPE postoperative shows only 1 lymph node and extracapsular spread is present or 1 to 3 lymph node found matted, becomes an indication for axillary irradiation.
4. If 4 or more lymph node positive axillary radiation is highly recommended.
5. If inadequate axillary sampling is done radiation has to be given.
6. If unknown axillary status radiation has to be given. Fatty patient with high axillary separation radiation has to be given, tipical lymph node spread in breast cancer shown in (Fig. 13.3).

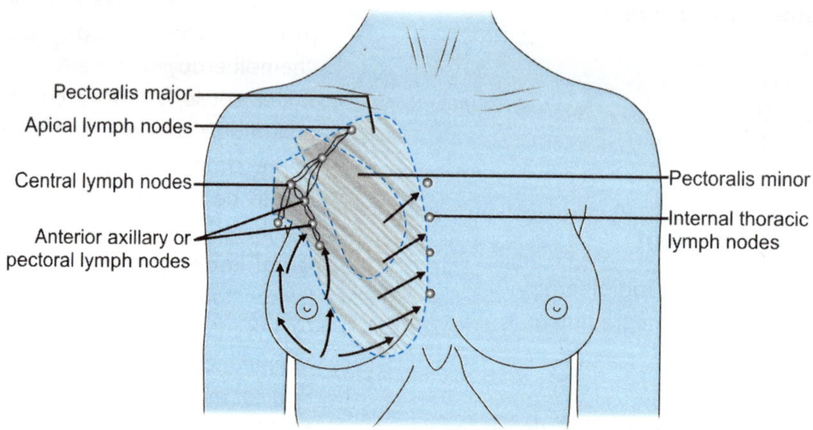

Fig. 13.3: Typical lymphatic drainage of breast

7. All the stage III A,B and C. (Excluding T3, N0, M0) radiation has to be given.

Management of Locally Advanced Breast Cancer (LABC) (Flow Chart 13.2)

1. Developing country incidence is 40 to 50 percent.
2. Developed country incidence is 2 to 5 percent.
3. The stages comprises in the LABC
   a. Operable stage LABC - T3, N0, M0
      - T3, N1, M0
   b. Inoperable stage LABC - T4, N0, M0
      - T4, N1, N2/N3

Flow chart 13.2: Treatment tree of advanced (locally) breast cancer

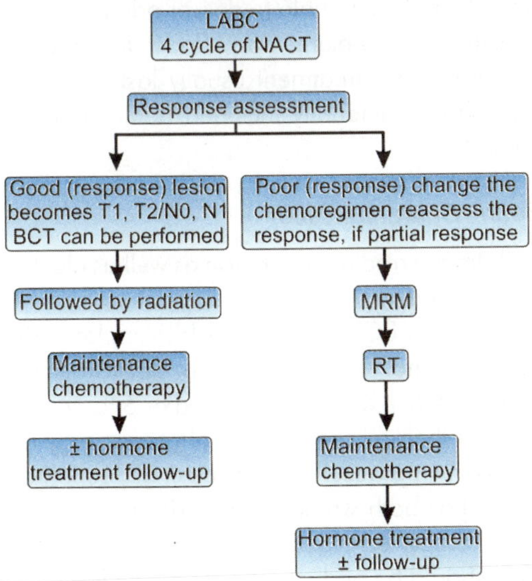

Role of Chemotherapy in LABC

1. Patients initially presenting with tumor that require mastectomy can be potentially down stage to allow BCT.
2. Response of individual can be assess *in vivo*.
3. Response to NACT is strong prognostic factor for outcome of the disease.
4. Inoperable tumor can be converted into operable.
5. Reports says after NACT if surgery is performed percentage of axillary lymph node positivity significantly decreases.

Radiotherapy Planning Technique

1. As a radiation oncologist we should know the prestaging of the tumor.
2. Postoperative HPE should be looked tumor status of excised tumor margin estrogen/ progesteron receptor status cerb+ve or –ve status, in lymph node sampling to know how many in are positive of metastasis.
3. So far as radiotherapy (EBRT) is concerned two types of planning technique we use
   a. Whole breast technique (en block)
   b. LRRT technique.

Whole Breast Technique

Here two tangantial fields are used, computerized planning is required for optimum dose delivery.

Disadvantages

Of this type planning:
- Less dose given SCF-area
- High-dose to lung tissue
- Dose involved IMC, LN

This technique is used for:
- BCT
- LABC (Locally advanced breast cancer) after induction chemotherapy.

LRRT Technique

This one is most commonly used in breast cancer Alm to treat breat/or chest wall regional lymph node (Figs 13.4 and 13.5).

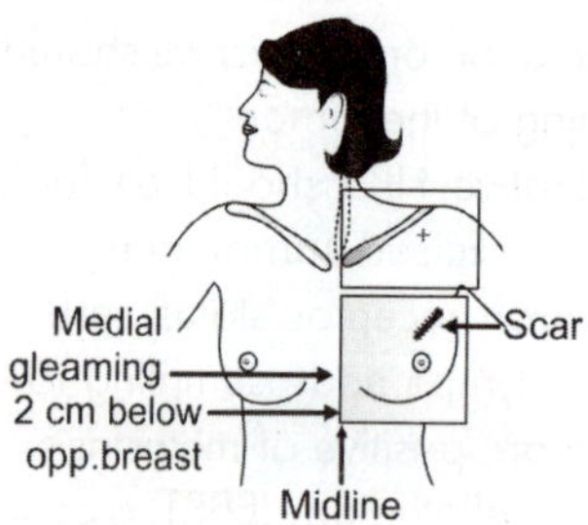

Fig. 13.4: Old field

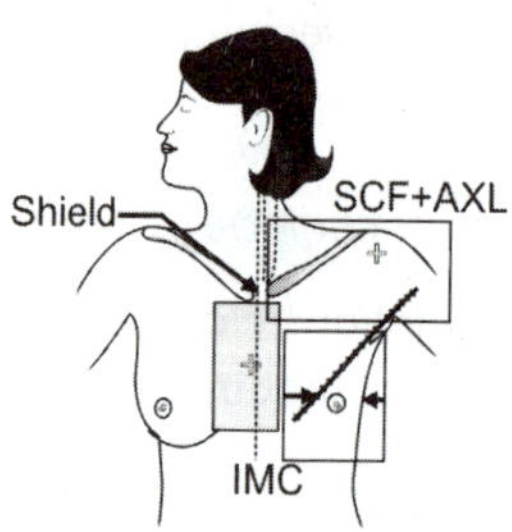

Fig. 13.5: Current breast field LRRT (locoregional radiotherapy)

Regional LN, here separate field use to irradiate.
- Chest wall
- Axilla
- SCF
- IMC

Here humoral head to be protected by circular shield because
i. Site of active hemopoiesis
ii. Joint fixity avascular necrosis of the head of humorous. Lead to joint fixity and pain in lateral life.

RECOMMENDATION FOR AXILLARY LYMPH NODE RADIATION

When axilla is heavily involved or in fatty patient when SCF dose unable to deliver adequate dose to axilla as a supplementary/ boost dose towards the end of the treatment usually last 10 to 15. IMC was traditionally included earlier but now under?

Beam Characteristics

1. Primary irradiation: Photon as well as electron are used.
2. Boost (In BCT): Electron or Ir^{192} implant EBRT occasionally use in absence of electron or Ir^{192}.

$C0^{60}$ 4 MV, 6 MV can be used or 6 to 16 MEV electron therapy can be used photon energy less than 6 MV may result in under dosing to superficial tissue. For both whole breast/LRRT (Locoreginal radiotherapy) technique patient should be in supine arms should be abducted at 90° to the ipsilateral side head turn sharply to the opposite site and shoulder tip should touche table top.

0.5 cm thick bolus used to increased dose to skin and scar but not require for T1/T2 lesion.

Role of Interstitial Implant in Breast Carcinoma

1. To give boost to the site of excision following lumpectomy.
2. After EBRT inform of scar boost treatment.
3. For small local recurrence.

Hormone Treatment

1 Women with ER/PR receptor positive status, estrogen 5 yr 20 mg OD reduce the annual risk of recurrence by 40 percent. Tamoxifen equally effective in premenopausal and postmenopausal women. *Hormone treatment is more effective in postmenopausal women, Why?* Because of following:
   a. ER/PR positive status seen in 64 percent patients in post menopausal age.
   b. ER/PR positive status seen in only 45 percent patients at premenopausal age, but l;the complication of tamoxifen is more serious in postmenopausal women.
      i. 1% risk of endometrial cancer
      ii. 2% risk of thromboembolism
      iii. Most common complication of tamoxifen is hot flashes (can be treated with a SSRI selective serotonin reuptake inhibitor Venlaflaxine)

      ER/PR positive patients response rate of tamoxifen is 78%

      ER –ve / PR +ve second best response is 45%

      ER +ve/ PR –ve third best response is 35%

      But ER –ve/ PR –ve also response to tamoxifen T/t 15% Why?

Bystander Effect?

ER –ve/ PR +ve response rate is 45%

But ER +ve/PR –ve response rate is 35%

This diversity is known as Bystander effect.

Aromatase Inhibitor

Indications

1. Used mainly in postmenopausal women who have known contraindication to tamoxifen treatment, e.g. history of thromboembolism and deep vein thrombosis, known intolerance to tamoxifen.
2. If tumor shows HER 2 neu +ve status they do not response to tamoxifen treatment but have some response to aromatase inhibitor.

Disadvantage of Aromatase Inhibitor

Compared to tamoxifen, aromatase inhibitor associated with increased rate of bone loss (Osteoporosis) thus high-risk of bone fracture is there.

Commonly Used Hormone Treatment

SERM (Selective Estrogen Receptor Modulator)

1. Tamoxifen 20 mg OD daily for 5 years
2. Toremifene 60 mg OD daily
3. Pure antiestrogen drug is fulvestant 250 mg IM monthly.

Ovarian Ablation

1. LHRH agonist
   a. Goserelin (Zoldex) 3.6 mg SC 4 weekly
   b. Leuprolide (Lupron) 3.75 mg SC 4 weekly
   c. Ovarian ablation by radiation 15 to 20 Gy/ 5 to10 fraction
   d. Progesteron (Medroxiprogesterone acetate) (Provera) 500 mg per orally daily or IM injection 500 mg weekly.
2. Aromatase inhibitors
   a. Letrazol 2.5 mg daily
   b. Anasterozole 1 mg daily

The most common dilemma in postopevative. case of CA breast, what should we do, if HPE report shows margin +ve, answer is resurgical excision of that very margin followed with postop. radiotherapy without excision of margin should not proceed for radiotherapy because local recurrence in these situations are high.

Chapter

14 Palliative Treatment in Breast Cancer

PALLIATIVE RADIOTHERAPY INDICATED IN BREAST CANCER

1. Bone pain (bone mets)
2. Preservation of fracture at critical site
3. Brain mets
4. Spinal mets
5. Choroid mets
6. Bleeding/ulceration from primary site
   Overall survival for metastatic breast cancer is 18 to 24 months.
7. Metastasis response to chemoterapy and hormone therapy as well but we practice radiotherapy for quick response. Distant metastasis can occur in breast cancer as long as 25 to 30 years after diagnosis, however, majority of the breast cancer cases. Liver metastasis see (Fig. 14.1) dose worst prognosis in compair to bone metastesis.
   Metastasis, occur within 5-year of diagnosis of primary site. If tumor size is 1 to 2.5 cm median interval of distent mets is 3½ years usually but if size more than 8 cm this period is 4 months node –ve patient this period is, 5 to 6 years node +ve patient this period is, 2½ years.

a. *Palliative radiotherapy to primary tumor:* Use for sing bleeding/discharge/ulceration/bulk of primary tumor by two parallel and opposite tangential field/electron therapy dose 30 Gy/ 10 fraction or 20 Gy/5 along with chemotherapy. But if patient is previously irradiated, radiotherapy (palliative) have invariably unsatisfactory result so, only option chemotherapy.

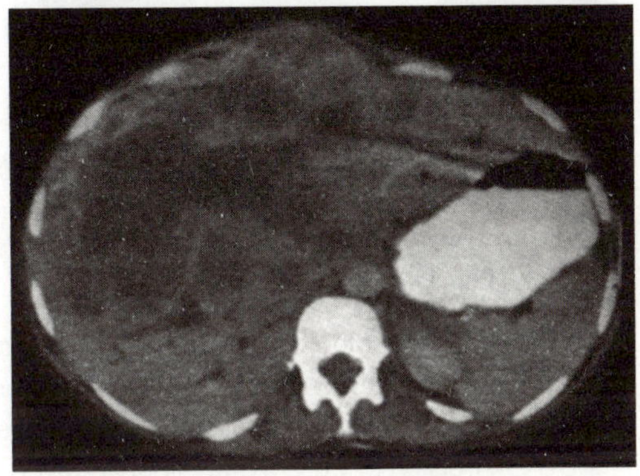

Fig. 14.1: Liver metastasis

b. *Bone mets:* Most common sites are spine/ pelvis/femur/ humerus/ since breast drain via azygous vein to Batson paravertebral veins (Fig. 14.2) thus must common spinal mets is thoracic spinal met's tumor cell destroy bone directly or produce PGE1/PGE2/IL2 which stimulate osteoclast cells leads to bone resorption, if PT

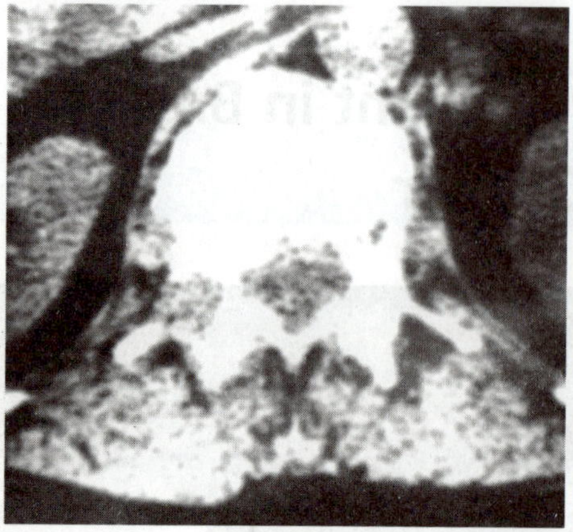

Fig. 14.2: Vertebral metastasis

comes to you in pathological fraction state then first do the bone stabilization by internal fixation or by immobilization cast then palliative RT to fracture site 8 Gy/fraction or 20 Gy/5 fraction/30 Gy/10 fraction this help in bone recalcification.

Breast chemotherapy patient with metastasis put on chemo or palliative radiotherapy response usually assessed by physical examination or imaging studies but bone metastasis is exception why? Because after palliative RT or chemotherapy healing of bone (as a blastic response) may be mistaken by radiologist as a progression of bone metastasis thus, the best response for bone metastasis after chemo or radiotherapy is improvement in the pain at metastatic site is the best guide for response assessment. In case of multiple/extensive bone mets HBI can be done, 6 Gy to upper half 8 Gy to lower half dividing line will be L4 vertebra with a gap of 4 to 6 wk to avoid myelosuppression or by use of Sr^{89}, p^{32} Radio active isotope therapy with zoledronic acid/pamidronate (Bisphosphonates)

Sr^{89} systemic radiotherapy is superior to HBI in many aspects

1. Reduces metastasis pain for long-time.
2. The recurrence or bone pain is remote dose of Sr^{89} 1.5 to 3 MBq/Kg body weight the pain relief occurs in 77 percent cases. Main side effect is bone marrow depression.

BRAIN SECONDARY

After lung, Ca breast in the most common cause of brainmets.

Brain Metastasis (Figs 14.3A and B)

Common site in brain is supratentorial cerebrum and cerebellum, brain stem is rare clinical feature headache/vomiting/higher mutar function disorder/cranial nerve palsy management-

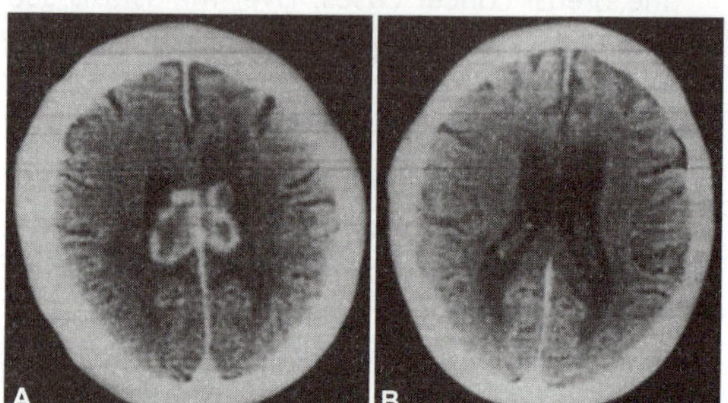

Figs 14.3A and B: Brain metastasis. (A) Performence scores of at least 80% tend to survive 5–6 months; (B) Course of 3000 cGy

steroid/radiotherapy and chemotherapy anti-convulsant/radiotherapy given by German helmet/ slanting field technique dose 20 Gy/5 fraction or 30 Gy/10 fraction median survival after D of brainmets is 3 to 6 month.

SPINAL CORD COMPRESSION

Most commonly extradural, After diagnosis of primary site of breast Ca spinal mets occur around 3 to 4 years, clinical feature pain/weakness/ sensory loss/sphincter disturbance occurs when vertebral collapse occurred RT dose 30 Gy/10 fraction or 8 Gy/fraction 2 days prior to RT high dose of IV steroid given, (60–100 mg dexamethasone). After 3 days of treatment oral steroid can be started, 60 percent patients show response in pain relief by palliative radiotherapy.

Orbital Metastasis

In women ocular mets most commonly occurs in breast Ca (Its incidence is 10–40%) mostly in eye and ocular adenexa. In 90 percent cases mets involve choroidal layer WHY? Because choroidal layer is highly vascular, thus chances of metastatic deposit becomes high (C/F diplopia, sudden blindness due to retinal detachment) in case or ocular adnexa met (C/F proptosis, periorbital swelling)

1. **Investation require:** USG eye, fundoscopy, fluoresent angiography, FNAC (US guided) to confirm diagnosis.
2. **Palliative RT dose:** 30 Gy/10 fraction by lateral and anterior field with 45° wedge to avoid other eye and brain. An average with ocular metastasis patient survive, usually up to one year.

Brachial Plexopathy

May be two types, neoplastic plexopathy, radiation induce plexopathy.

1. **RIBP (Radiation Induced Bracheal Plexopathy)** rare nowadays, why?
2. Due to restricted dose (50 Gy) its incidence is less than 1 percent RIBP cause is axillary/SCF/ field irradiation radiation causes fibrosis leads to plexopathy (radiation cause, proliferation of neurolemal sheath and obliteration of blood vessels leads to ischemia of nerve fiber treatment is exercise/pain killer/thyroxin (decrease fibrosis) RIBP usually occurs after 4 years of radiotherapy mainly upper trunk of brachial plexus involved due to RIBP clinical feature pain at shoulder girdle restricted shoulder movement.

NEOPLASTIC PLEXOPATHY

Its incidence is 3 percent mainly involved lower trunk of brachial plexus (ulnar nerve) thus C/F pain shoulder girdle/restricted movement radiating pain arm and forearm up to 4th/5th finger. This distressing pain is due to lower trunk of brachial plexus involvement C_8T_1 treatment of neoplastic plexopathy is in nonirradiated cases 50 Gy in 5 wk included field is SCF in order to cover C_8T_1 nerve root.

Lung Metastasis

In case of Bilateral multiple lung mets treatment of choice is systemic chemotherapy. In cases of repeated Pleural effusion treatment of choice is systemic chemotherapy, i.e. inter custal drainage sclerotherapy (intrapleural instillation of bleomycin) or 15 Gy/3 fraction can be given to involved chest. In sclerotherapy, agent used—Bleomycin, tetracycline, talc powder, gold Au^{198}

Indication of Radiotherapy in Pleural Effusion

1. Repeated plural effusion and drug instilation (sclerotherapy been failed),
2. When intercostal drainage is contraindicated.

Complications of Radiotherapy in Breast Cancer

1. Acute effect
2. skin changes cause by RT may present several wks to month but due to advent of megavoltage severe skin reaction no longer seen nowadays.
3. Skin reaction's like dry sequmation/most desquamation can be treated by local gention violet (antifungal, antiserum gention violet also having drying effect.
4. due to IMF irradiation esophagitis occurs towards the end of 3rd week of treatment (after 15 fraction).

Late Effects

1. Rib's fracture occurs in 3 to 5 percent case
2. Chest wall fibrosis (–5%) (now less in megavoltage era)
3. Radiation pneumonitis (1–5%)
4. Arm edema (5–20%) of irradiation to lung area radiation pneumonitis depend upon volume of radiation pneumonitis—when tangential field use along with SCF/axillary field/added without chemotherapy radiation pericarditis above 35 Gy radiation pericarditis further aggravated with the use of anthracyclines based chemo. Another late effect of radiotherapy include II malignancy due to carcinogenesis (usually malignant fibrous histiocytoma (MFH) osteogenic sarcoma occur). Then we knew that radiotherapy has a key role in managements of breast cancer and in breast conservation surgery and lung term benefits of radiotherapy outweights the radiation related morbidities.

Chapter 15 Head and Neck Cancer

The term head and neck cancer refers to a group of biologically similar cancers originating from the upper aerodigestive tract, including the lip, oral cavity (mouth), nasal cavity, paranasal sinuses, pharynx and larynx. Most head and neck cancers are squamous cell carcinomas (SCCHN), originating from the mucosal lining (epithelium) of these regions. Head and neck cancers often spread to the lymph nodes of the neck and this is often the first (and sometimes only) manifestation of the disease at the time of diagnosis. Head and neck cancer is strongly associated with certain environmental and lifestyle risk factors, including tobacco smoking, alcohol consumption, UV light and occupational exposures and certain strains of viruses, such as the sexually transmitted human papillomavirus. These cancers are frequently aggressive in their biologic behavior; patients with these types of cancer often develop a second primary tumor. Head and neck cancer is highly curable if detected early, usually with some form of surgery although chemotherapy and radiation therapy may also play an important role. The 2009, estimated number of head and neck cancer in the US is of 35,720 new cases.

Classification

Head and neck squamous cell carcinomas (HNSCC's) make-up the vast majority of head and neck cancers and arise from mucosal surfaces throughout this anatomic region. These include tumors of the nasal cavities, paranasal sinuses, oral cavity, nasopharynx, oropharynx, hypopharynx and larynx.

CANCER ORAL CAVITY

Oral Cavity

Oral cancer

Squamous cell cancers are common in the oral cavity, including the inner lip, tongue, floor of mouth, gingivae and hard palate. Cancers of the oral cavity are strongly associated with tobacco use, especially use of chewing tobacco or "dip," as well as heavy alcohol use. Cancers of this region, particularly the tongue, more frequently treated with surgery than are other head and neck cancers (Fig. 15.1). Surgeries for oral cancers include:

Maxillectomy (can be done with or without orbital exenteration).

Mandibulectomy (removal of the mandible or lower jaw or part of it).

Glossectomy (tongue removal can be total, hemi or partial).

Radical neck dissection.

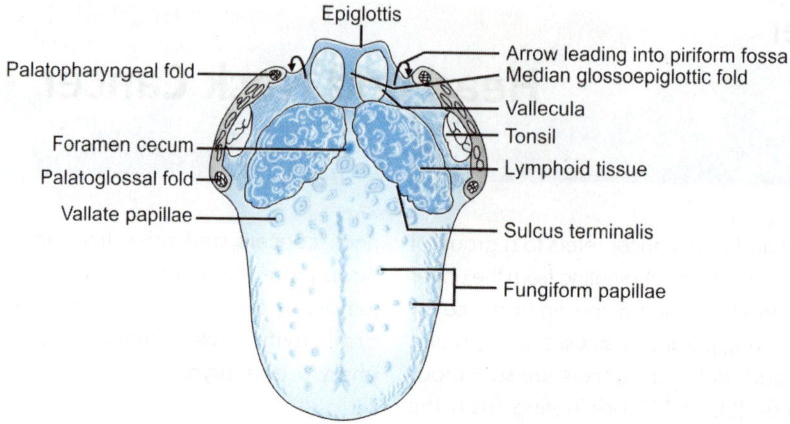

Fig. 15.1: Anatomical landmark of tongue

Moh's Procedure

Combinational, e.g. glossectomy and laryngectomy done together.

The defect is covered/improved by using another part of the body and/or skin grafts and/or wearing a prosthesis.

Nasopharynx

Nasopharyngeal cancer arises in the nasopharynx, the region in which the nasal cavities and the Eustachian tubes connect with the upper part of the throat. While some nasopharyngeal cancers are biologically similar to the common HNSCC, "poorly differentiated" nasopharyngeal carcinoma is distinct in its epidemiology, biology, clinical behavior and treatment and is treated as a separate disease by many experts.

Oropharynx

Oropharyngeal squamous cell carcinomas (OSCC) begins in the oropharynx, the middle part of the throat that includes the soft palate, the base of the tongue and the tonsils alveolar (Figs 15.2 and 15.3). Squamous cell cancers of the tonsils are more strongly associated with human papillomavirus infection than are cancers of other regions of the head and neck.

Hypopharynx

The hypopharynx includes the pyriform sinuses, the posterior pharyngeal wall and the postcricoid area. Tumors of the hypopharynx frequently have an advanced stage at diagnosis and have the most adverse prognoses of pharyngeal tumors. They tend to metastasize early due to the extensive lymphatic network around the larynx.

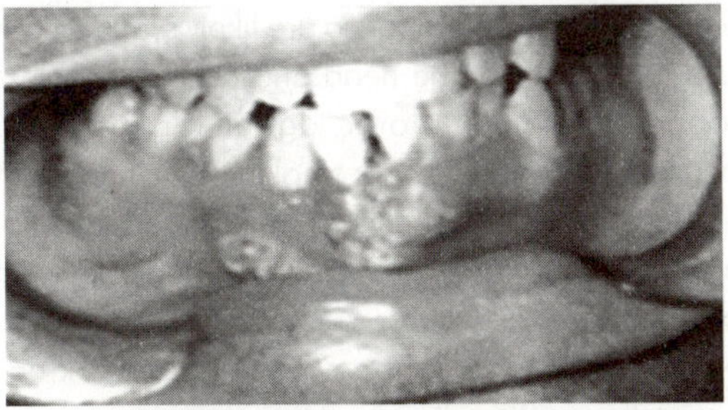

Fig. 15.2: Carcinoma-alveolar

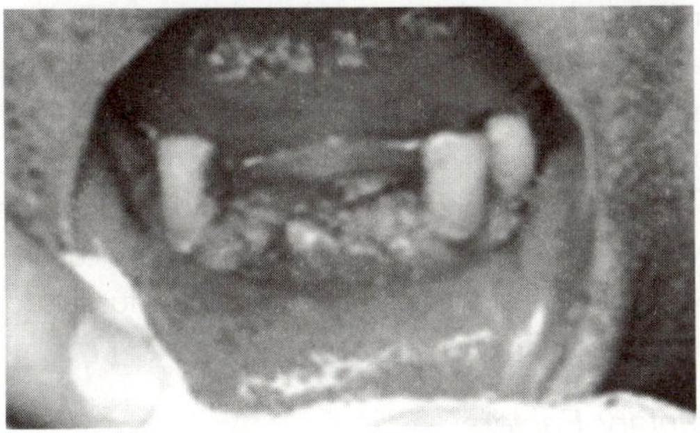

Fig. 15.3: Ca-lower alveolar

Larynx

Laryngeal cancer begins in the larynx or "voice box." Cancer may occur on the vocal folds themselves ("glottic" cancer), or on tissues above and below the true cords ("supraglottic and subglottic" cancers respectively). Laryngeal cancer is strongly associated with tobacco smoking.

Surgeries can include partial laryngectomy (removal of part of the larynx) and total laryngectomy (removal of the whole larynx). If the whole larynx has been removed the person is left with a permanent tracheostomy opening and learns to speak again in a new way with the help of intensive teaching and speech therapy and/or an electronic device.

Also anyone who has had a glossectomy (tongue removal) will be taught to speak again in a new way and have intensive speech therapy.

Trachea

Cancer of the trachea is a rare malignancy which can be biologically similar in many ways to head and neck cancer and is sometimes classified as such.

Most tumors of the salivary glands differ from the common carcinomas of the head and neck in etiology, histopathology, clinical presentation and therapy, Other uncommon tumors arising in the head and neck include teratomas, adenocarcinomas, adenoid cystic carcinomas and mucoepidermoid carcinomas. Rarer still are melanomas and lymphomas of the upper aerodigestive tract.

Signs and Symptoms

Cancer usually begins with symptoms that seem harmless enough like an enlarged lymph node on the outside of the neck, a sore throat or a hoarse sounding voice. However, in the case of throat cancer, these conditions may persist and become chronic. There may be a lump or a sore in the throat or neck that does not heal or go away. There may be difficult or painful swallowing. Speaking may become difficult. There may be a persistent earache. Other possible but less common symptoms include some numbness or paralysis of the face muscles.

Presenting symptoms include:

1. Mass in the neck
2. Neck pain
3. Bleeding from the mouth
4. Sinus congestion, especially with nasopharyngeal carcinoma
5. Bad breath
6. Sore tongue
7. Painless ulcer or sores in the mouth that do not heal
8. White, red or dark patches in the mouth that will not go away
9. Earache
10. Unusual bleeding or numbness in the mouth
11. Lump in the lip, mouth or gums
12. Enlarged lymph glands in the neck
13. Slurring of speech (if the cancer is affecting the tongue)
14. Hoarse voice which persists for more than six weeks
15. Sore throat which persists for more than six weeks
16. Difficulty swallowing food.

Change in diet or weight loss clinical streging shown in Figs 15.7A to D how, head and neck cancer spread from primary site to secondary lymphnode involvement.

Causes

Alcohol and tobacco use are the most common risk factors for head and neck cancer in the United States. Alcohol and tobacco are likely synergistic in causing cancer of the head and neck. Smokeless tobacco is an etiologic agent for oral and pharyngeal cancers. Cigar smoking is an important risk factor for oral cancers as well. Other potential environmental carcinogens include marijuana and occupational exposures such as nickel refining, exposure to textile fibers and woodworking. Cigarette smokers have a lifetime increased risk for head and neck cancers that is 5- to 25-fold increased over the general population. The ex-smoker's risk for squamous cell cancer of the head and neck begins to approach the risk in the general population twenty years after smoking cessation. The high prevalence of tobacco and alcohol use worldwide and the high association of these cancers with these substances makes them ideal targets for enhanced cancer prevention.

Dietary Factors

Dietary factors may contribute. Excessive consumption of processed meats and red meat were associated with increased rates of cancer of the head and neck in one study, while consumption of raw and cooked vegetables seemed to be protective.

Vitamin E was not found to prevent the development of leukoplakia, the white plaques that are the precursor for carcinomas of the mucosal surfaces, in adult smokers. Another study examined a combination of Vitamin E and beta carotene in smokers with early-stage cancer of the oropharynx and found a worse prognosis in the vitamin users.

Betelnut

Betelnut chewing is associated with an increased risk of squamous cell cancer of the head and neck.

Recent evidence is accumulating pointing to a viral origin for some head and neck cancers.

Human Papillomavirus

Human papillomavirus (HPV), in particular HPV16, is a causal factor for some head and neck squamous cell carcinoma (HNSCC). Approximately 15 to 25 percent of HNSCC contain genomic DNA from HPV and the association varies based on the site of the tumor, especially HPV-positive oropharyngeal cancer, with highest distribution in the tonsils, where HPV DNA is found in (45–67%) of the cases, less often in the hypopharynx (13–25%) and least often in the oral cavity (12–18%) and larynx (3–7%).

Some experts estimate that while up to 50 percent of cancers of the tonsil may be infected with HPV, only 50 percent of these are likely to be caused by HPV (as opposed to the usual tobacco and alcohol causes). The role of HPV in the remaining 25 to 30 percent is not yet clear.

Epstein-Barr Virus

Epstein-Barr virus (EBV) infection is associated with nasopharyngeal cancer. Nasopharyngeal cancer occurs endemically in some countries of the Mediterranean and Asia, where EBV antibody titers can be measured to screen high-risk populations. Nasopharyngeal cancer has also been associated with consumption of salted fish, which may contain high levels of nitrites.

There are a wide variety of factors which can put someone at a heightened risk for throat cancer. Such factors include smoking or chewing tobacco or other things, such as gutkha, marijuana or paan, heavy alcohol consumption, poor diet resulting in vitamin deficiencies (worse if this is caused by heavy alcohol intake), weakened immune system, asbestos exposure, prolonged exposure to wood dust or paint fumes, exposure to petroleum industry chemicals and being over the age of 55 years. Another risk factor includes the appearance of white patches or spots in the mouth, known as leukoplakia, in about one-third of the cases this develops into cancer.

Diagnosis

A patient usually presents to the physician complaining of one or more of the above symptoms. The patient will typically undergo a punch biopsy of this lesion and a histopathologic information is available, a multidisciplinary discussion of the optimal treatment strategy will be undertaken between the radiation oncologist, surgical oncologist and medical oncologist.

Histopathology

Throat cancers are classified according to their histology or cell structure and are commonly referred to by their location in the oral cavity and neck. This is because where the cancer appears in the throat affects the prognosis—some throat cancers are more aggressive than others depending upon their location. The stage (Fig. 15.4) at which the cancer is diagnosed is also a critical factor in the prognosis of throat cancer, most commaly histopathology in oral cancer done by punch biopsy forceps (Fig. 15.5).

Squamous Cell Carcinoma

Squamous cells are the epithelium (tissue layer) that is the surface cells of much of the body. Skin and mucous membranes are squamous cells. This is the most common form of larynx cancer, accounting for over 90 percent of throat cancer. Squamous cell carcinoma is most likely to appear in males over 40 years of age with a history of heavy alcohol use coupled with smoking.

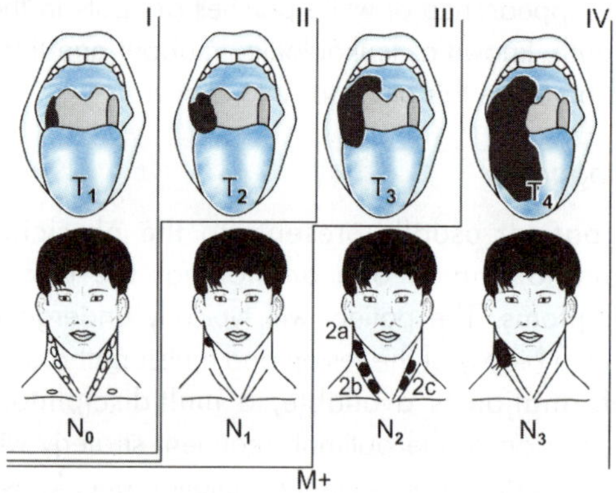

Fig. 15.4: Clinical staging of oral cavity cancer

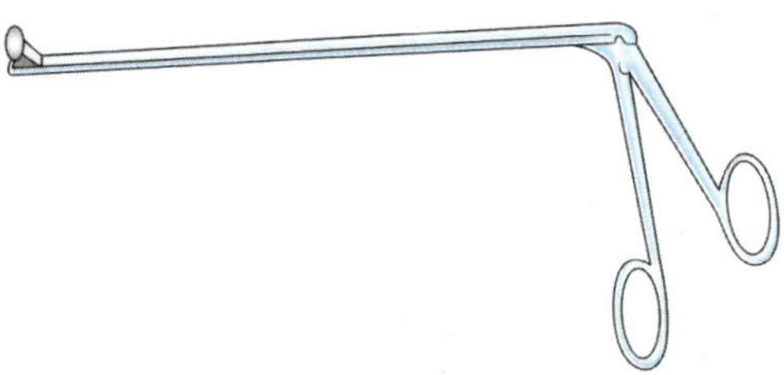

Fig. 15.5: Punch biopsy forceps

Adenocarcinoma

Adenocarcinoma is a cancer of the columnar epithelium typical of the lower esophagus. It is typical of Barrett's esophagus but may be at another location. Adenocarcinoma is thought of as a product of Barrett's oesophagus.

Prevention

Avoidance of recognized risk factors (as described above) is the single most effective form of prevention. Regular dental examinations may identify precancerous lesions in the oral cavity.

When diagnosed early, oral, head and neck cancers can be treated more easily and the chances of survival increase tremendously.

Management

Improvements in diagnosis and local management, as well as targeted therapy, have led to improvements in quality of life and survival for head and neck cancer patients since 1992, After a histologic diagnosis has been established and tumor extent determined, the selection of appropriate treatment for a specific cancer depends on a complex array of variables, including tumor site, relative morbidity of various treatment options, patient performance and nutritional status, concomitant health problems, social and logistic factors, previous primary tumors and patient preference. Treatment planning generally, requires a multidisciplinary approach involving specialist surgeons and medical and radiation oncologists.

Several generalizations are useful in therapeutic decision-making, but variations on these themes are numerous. Surgical resection and radiation therapy are the mainstays of treatment for most head and neck cancers and remain the standard of care in most cases. For small primary cancers without regional metastases (stage I or II), wide surgical excision alone or curative radiation therapy alone is used sometimes only radiotherapy informal interstitial brachytherapy is used in T1 lesion of head and neck cancer (Fig. 15.6) for brachytherapy to the early using of tongue diffrent techniques used (Figs 15.7A to D). More extensive primary

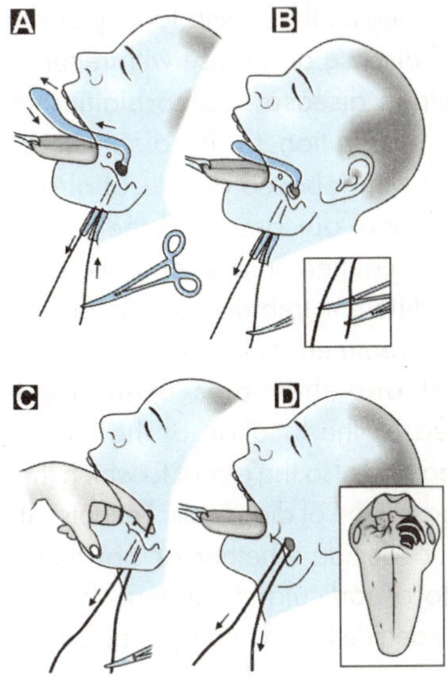

Figs 15.7A to D: Loop technique of implant

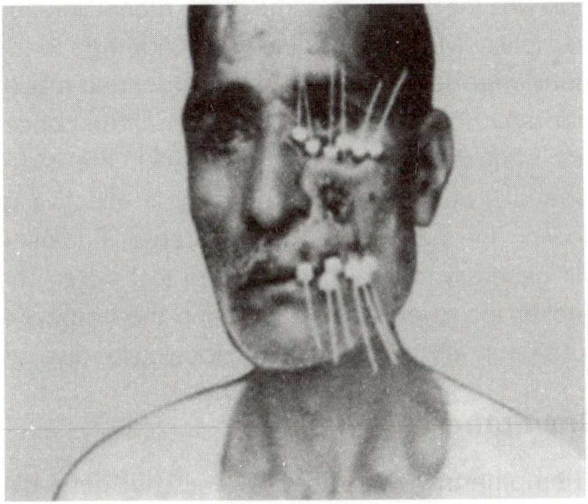

Fig. 15.6: Interstitial implant

tumors, or those with regional metastases (stage III or IV), planned combinations of pre- or postoperative radiation and complete surgical excision are generally used. Survival and recurrence risk has been roughly equivalent between surgical and radiation-based approaches, with a head-to-head comparison in only one randomized study. More recently, as historical survival and control rates are recognized as less than satisfactory, there has been an emphasis on the use of various induction or concomitant chemotherapy regimens.

Patients with head and neck cancer can be categorized into three clinical groups: those with localized disease, those with locally or regionally advanced disease and those with recurrent and/or metastatic disease. Comorbidities (medical problems in addition to the diagnosed cancer) associated with tobacco and alcohol abuse can affect treatment outcome and the tolerability of aggressive treatment in a given patient.

Many different treatments and therapies are used in the treatment of throat cancer. The type of treatment and therapies used are largely determined by the location of the cancer in the throat area and also the extent to which the cancer has spread at time of diagnosis. Patients' also have the right to decide whether or not they wish to consent to a particular treatment. For example, some may decide to not undergo radiation therapy which has serious side effects, if it means they will be extending their lives by only a few months or so. Others may feel that the extra time is worth it and wish to pursue the treatments.

Surgery

Surgery as a treatment is sometimes used in cases of throat cancer. In such cases an attempt is made to remove the cancerous cells. This can be particularly tricky, if the cancer is near the larynx and can result in the patient being unable to speak. Surgery is more commonly used to resection (remove) some of the lymph nodes to prevent further spread of the disease lymph node involvement in head and neck cancer leads to poor prognosis (Fig. 15.8) type of lymph node removal from neck and different type of incision used given in (Figs 15.9A to G).

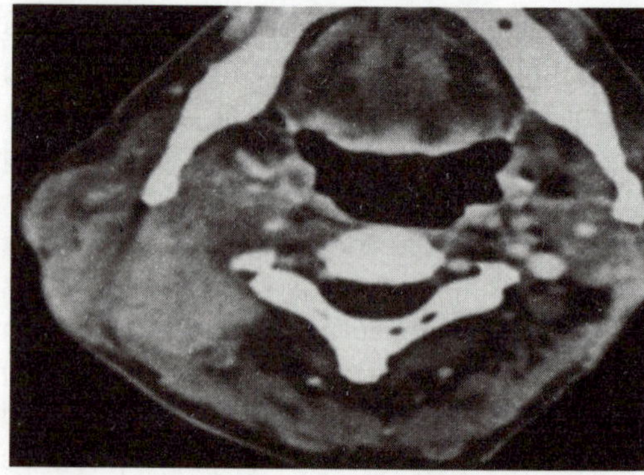

Fig. 15.8: CECT showing lymph node at rightside

Radiation therapy is the most common form of treatment.

There are different forms of radiation therapy. One of newer treatments is intensity-modulated radiotherapy or IMRT which is able to focus more precisely, so that fewer healthy cells are destroyed than was the case with some of the older radiation therapies. IMRT reduces incidental damage to the many important structures of the throat and mouth that may not be involved. However, if the cancer has metastasized or is widespread, the older form of treatment may be the most effective at slowing the progression of the disease. Radiation will generally, cause the patient to feel sicker and weaker for several weeks following the treatment, but is a very effective treatment in stopping the disease.

Chemotherapy

Chemotherapy in throat cancer is not generally used to *cure* the cancer as such. Instead, it is used

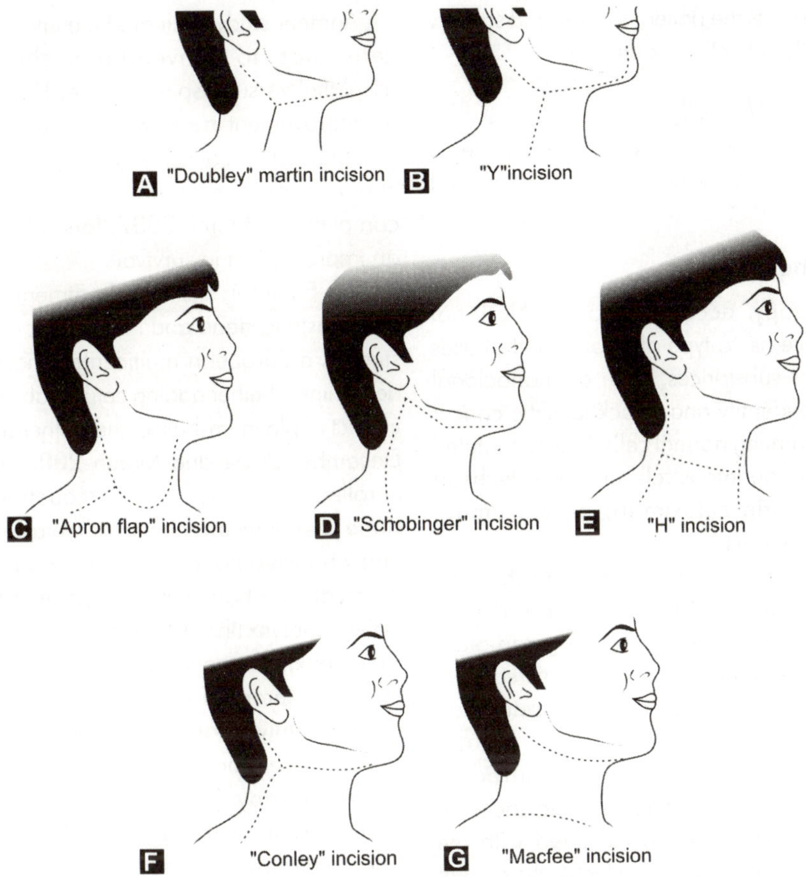

Figs 15.9A to G: Types of incision used in head and neck surgery

to provide an inhospitable environment for metastases so that they will not establish in other parts of the body. Typical chemotherapy agents are a combination of taxol and carboplatin. Erbitux is also used in the treatment of throat cancer. While not specifically a chemotherapy, Amifostine is often administered intravenously by a chemotherapy clinic prior to a patient's radiotherapy sessions.

Amifostine protects the patient's gums and salivary glands from the effects of radiation.

Photodynamic Therapy

Photodynamic therapy may have promise in treating mucosal dysplasia and small head and neck tumors.

Targeted Therapy

Targeted therapy, according to the National Cancer Institute, is "a type of treatment that uses drugs or other substances, such as monoclonal antibodies, to identify and attack specific cancer cells without harming normal cells." Some targeted therapy used in squamous cell cancers of the head and neck include cetuximab, bevacizumab, erlotinib and reovirus.

The best quality data are available for cetuximab since the 2006, publication of a randomized clinical trial comparing radiation treatment plus cetuximab versus radiation treatment alone. This study found that concurrent cetuximab and radiotherapy improves survival and locoregional disease control compared to radiotherapy alone, without a substantial increase in side effects, as would be expected with the concurrent chemoradiotherapy, which is the current gold standard treatment for advanced head and neck cancer. Whilst this study is of pivotal significance, interpretation is difficult since cetuximab—radiotherapy was not directly compared to chemoradiotherapy. The results of ongoing studies to clarify the role of cetuximab in this disease are awaited with interest.

Another study evaluated the impact of adding cetuximab to conventional chemotherapy (cisplatin) versus cisplatin alone. This study found no improvement in survival or disease-free survival with the addition of cetuximab to the conventional chemotherapy. However, another study which completed in March 2007, found that there was an improvement in survival.

The Erbitux in First-Line Treatment of Recurrent or Metastatic Head and Neck Cancer (EXTREME) study is a European multicenter phase III trial to determine whether adding cetuximab improves the impact of platinum-based chemotherapy. Between December 2004 and March 2007, researchers enrolled 442 patients in 17 countries who had stage III or IV recurrent and/or metastatic SCCHN and who were not candidates for further surgery or radiation. About half of the patients had cancer in their pharynx (throat) and a quarter in their larynx (voice box), but none in the nasopharynx (upper part of the throat). The patients averaged 57 years of age. Only about 10 percent were women. Patients were randomly assigned to receive either chemotherapy (222 patients) or the same chemotherapy with cetuximab (220 patients). Chemotherapy consisted of 5-fluorouracil plus either carboplatin or cisplatin. The trial was led by Jan Vermorken, MD, PhD, of the University of Antwerp in Belgium. Vermmorken as well as other researchers involved in the trial have various relationships with Merck KGaA, Amgen, Oxygene and sanofi-aventis. Merck KGaA provided funding for the study. (See the protocol summary.)

Results patients treated with cetuximab reduced their risk of dying by 20 percent, surviving a median of 10.1 months compared to 7.4 months for those receiving chemotherapy alone.

Head and neck cancer clinical trials employing bevacizumab, an inhibitor of the angiogenesis receptor VEGF, are recruiting patients as of March 2007. No published clinical trial information is available as of that date. Erlotinib is an oral EGFR inhibitor and was found in one Phase II clinical trial to retard disease progression. Scientific evidence for the effectiveness of erlotinib is otherwise lacking to this point. A clinical trial evaluating the use of erlotinib in metastatic head and neck cancer is recruiting patients as of March 2007.

Reovirus is an oncolytic virus that targets RAS activated cancer cells. Trial update on November 2008, showed stable disease or better in the first eight of nine patients with refractory head and neck cancer. Phase II trials are ongoing in England and the USA with phase III trials planned.

Prognosis

Although early-stage head and neck cancers (especially laryngeal and oral cavity) have high cure rates, up to 50 percent of head and neck cancer patients present with advanced disease. Cure rates decrease in locally advanced cases, whose probability of cure is inversely related to tumor size and even more, so to the extent of regional node involvement. Consensus panels in America (AJCC) and Europe (UICC) have established staging systems for head and neck squamous cancers. These staging systems attempt to standardize clinical trial criteria for research studies and attempt to define prognostic categories of disease. Squamous cell cancers of the head and neck are staged according to the TNM classification system, where T is the size and configuration of the tumor, N is the presence or absence of lymph node metastases and M is the presence or absence of distant metastases. The T, N and M characteristics are combined to produce a "stage" of the cancer, from I to IVB.

Residual Deficits

Even after successful definitive therapy, head and neck cancer patients face tremendous impacts on quality of life. Despite marked advances in reconstructive surgery and rehabilitation, intensity-modulated radiotherapy (IMRT) and conservation approaches to certain malignancies, some patients continue to have significant functional deficits.

Problem of Second Primaries

Survival advantages provided by new treatment modalities have been undermined by the significant percentage of patients cured of head and neck squamous cell carcinoma (HNSCC) who subsequently develop second primary tumors. The incidence of second primary tumors ranges in studies from 9.1 to 23 percent at 20 years. Second primary tumors are the major threat to long-term survival after successful therapy of early-stage HNSCC. Their high incidence results from the same carcinogenic exposure responsible for the initial primary process, called field cancerization.

Head and Neck Cancer has Numerous Negative Effects on the Body Systems

Digestive System

As it can impair a person's ability to swallow and eat, throat cancer affects the digestive system. The difficulty in swallowing can lead to a person to choke on their food in the early stages of digestion and interfere with the food's smooth travels down into the esophagus and beyond.

The treatments for throat cancer can also be harmful to the digestive system as well as other body systems. Radiation therapy can lead to nausea and vomiting, which can deprive a body of vital fluids (although these may be obtained through intravenous fluids if necessary). Frequent vomiting can lead to an electrolyte imbalance which has serious consequences for the proper functioning of the heart. Frequent vomiting can also upset the balance of stomach acids which has a negative impact on the digestive system, especially the lining of the stomach and esophagus.

Respiratory System

In the cases of some throat cancers, the air passages in the mouth and behind the nose may become blocked from lumps or the swelling from the open sores. If the throat cancer is near the bottom of the throat it has a high likelihood of spreading to the lungs and interfering with the person's ability to breathe; this is even more likely if the patient is a smoker, because they are highly susceptible to lung cancer. If the respiratory system is unable to bring oxygen into the body, the oxygen deprivation will cause the body's cells to wither and die causing one to become weaker and sicker.

Others

Like any cancer, metastasization affects many areas of the body, as the cancer spreads from cell-to-cell and organ-to-organ. For example, if it spreads to the bone marrow, it will prevent the body from producing enough red blood cells and affects the proper functioning of the white blood cells and the body's immune system; spreading to the circulatory system will prevent oxygen from being transported to all the cells of the body; and throat cancer can throw the nervous system into chaos, making it unable to properly regulate and control the body.

Symptoms and Side Effects

Patients with head and neck cancer may experience the following symptoms and treatment side effects:

1. Eating problems
2. Pain associated with lesions
3. Mucositis
4. Nephrotoxicity and ototoxicity
5. Xerostomia
6. Gastroesophageal reflux
7. Radiation induced osteonecrosis of the jaw.

Chapter

16 Ovarian Cancer

"Gynecological malignancies" 80 percent, cervix, 10 percent, ovary 5 percent, uterine Ca, 5 percent, rest other.

INTRODUCTION

Ovarian Ca case fatality is very high they are:

1. Difficulty in early diagnosis more than 60 percent of cases present in locally advanced stage.
2. No anatomical barriers exist to curtail the spread of growth and their distribution throughout the peritoneal cavity since whole intra-abdominal and pelvic organ and lymph node are at the risk of metastatic involvement.

INCIDENCE

Leading cause of mortality amongst all cancer of female genital tract in compare to Western countries incidence is quit lower in developing countries. Incidence rate in India is 4.7 to 8.7/ 100,000 women per year.

Usually present 4 to 6th decades of life.

ANATOMY

Ovaries are solid pink gray bodies situated in the ovarian fossa of pelvis. Its size in premenopausal stage is 3.5 × 2.5 × 1.5 cm and postmenopausal ovary get atrophied with size 2 × 1.5 × 1 cm in size. Adult ovaries lay on either side of uterus behind and below the fallopian tubes anterior margin of the ovary attached to the posterior surface of the broad ligament of uterine by mesovarium upper pole of ovary supported by infundibulopelvic ligament (Fig. 16.1).

Nulliparous ladies ovaries lies in peritoneal fossa on the lateral pelvic a wall known as fossa ovaries of Waldeyer this fossa lies below the bifurcation of common iliac artery (on X-ray point just below the sacroiliac joint on either side).

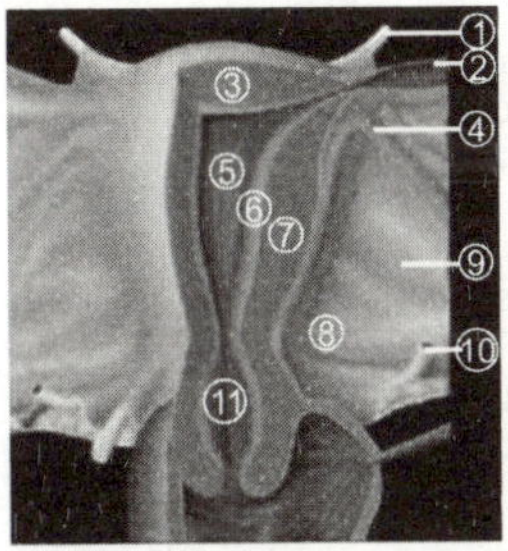

Fig. 16.1: Hysteroscopic anatomy. 1. Round ligament; 2. Uterine tube; 3. Fundus of uterus; 4. Proper ovarian ligament; 5. Uterine cavity; 6. Endometrium; 7. Myometrium; 8. Mesometrium of broad ligament; 9. Uterine artery; 10. Ureter; 11. Cervical canal

Blood Supply of Ovaries

Direct branch of aorta given immediately below the renal arteris veins draining right side to inferior vena cava (IVC) left side drain into left renal vein.

Lymphatic Drainage

We know ovary development arises near para-aortic area just below the renal hilum. Thus, para-aortic lymphadenopathy at the level of renal hilum occurs, in ovarian Ca pelvic lympha-denopathy occurs, once pelvic peritoneum involvement occurs, inguinal lymphadenopathy occurs due to blockadge of pelvic lymph node by metastatic deposit leading to retrograde lymphatic flow (Figs 16.2 and 16.3).

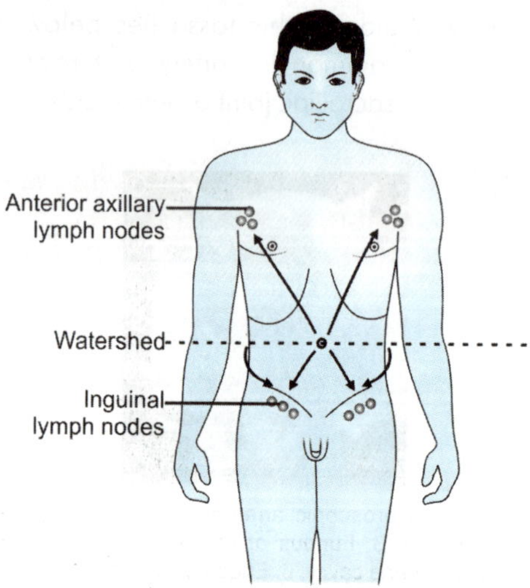

Fig. 16.2: Lymphatic drainage of skin of thorax and abdomen

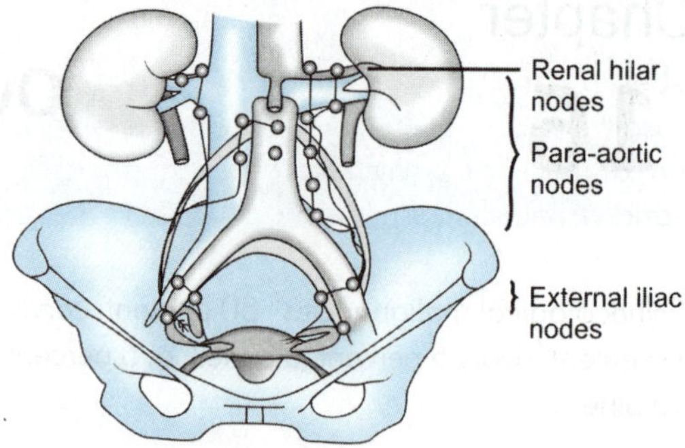

Fig. 16.3: Lymphatic drainage of ovarian cancer

LYMPH NODE METASTASIS

Etiology of ovarian cancer remains unknown. But possible causes are reproductive, endocrine, environmental, dietary, viral.

Reproductive Causes

Common in while race and developed countries and highest among the affluent class people (Diet rich in animal fat).

Ovulation has direct influence on ovaries. Thus, oral contraceptive pill using women will have an-ovulatory cycle and lesser trauma to ovaries. Thus, decrease incidence of ovarian Ca.

Increase in the level of estrogen, hyper-stimulation of ovary using clomiphene citrate or gonadotropin result in increase estrogen concentration causing multiple follicular enlargement leading and increase risk of ovarian carcinoma.

Environmental Factors

Asbestos and talc powder are regarded as causative factors. Dietary: Increase intake of meat and animal fat is also increase chances of ovarian cancer.

Viral

Mumps viral infection might offer some protection against ovarian cancer.

Hereditary

3.6 percent higher chances seen in Ist order of relative of ovarian Ca, vague complaint's are, abdominal pain, abdominal lump, dyspepsia, urinary frequency, constipation, weightloss, anorexia, pelvic discomfort lowbackache.

a. Women beyond 4th decade of her life.
b. On examination pelvic mass/abdominal mass. Benign tumor's are cystic/smooth/unitral and mobil but malignant tumor in more then 50 percent case are bilateral and immobile, size usually in more then 5 cm solid in consistency usually associated with ascites but, benign tumor solid in consistency are fibroma of ovary causing meigs syndrome present ascites right side plural effusion, krukenberg tumor malignant in nature but mobile. Functional and inflammatory enlargement of ovaries usually occurs at child bearing stage.

CLASSIFICATION OF OVARIAN CA

Benign tumor become malignant like mucinus cyst become malignant in 5 percent cases. Papillary cyst adenoma becomes malignant in 50 percent cases.

1. Common epithelial tumor of ovary
   a. Papillary cyst adenoma Ca in 50 percent
   b. Undiffrentiated tumor 17 percent
   c. Mucinous tumor in 12 percent
   d. Endometrioid tumor 10 percent
   e. Clear cell Ca 6 percent
   f. Brenner tumor 1 percent.
2. Sex cord tumor
   a. Granulosa cell tumors
   b. Androblastoma tumor (Sertoli-Leydig cell tumors)
   c. Gynandroblastoma tumor.
3. Lipid cell (lipoid cell tumor).
4. Germ cell tumor (15% of all ovarian cancers), (Fig. 16.4). Typical germ cell tumor are:

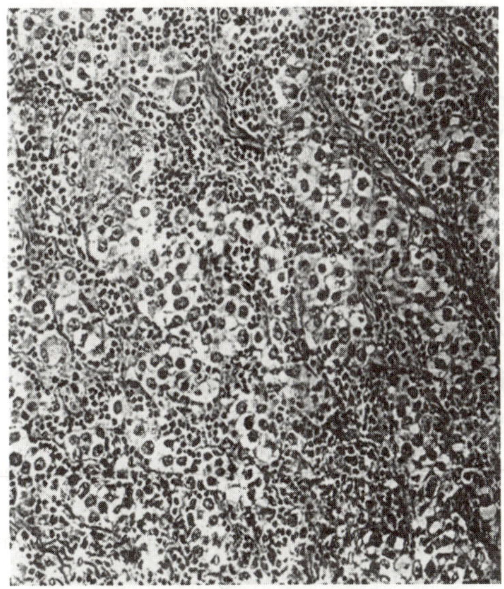

Fig. 16.4: Histological picture of germ cell tumor

a. Dysgerminona
b. Endodermal sinus tumor (yolk sac)
c. Embryonal Ca
d. Coriocarcinoma.
e. Teratoma
   i. Immature
   ii. Mature
   iii. Solid
   iv. Cystic demoid cyst

5. Secondary tumor (Metastatic tumor)
   Primary lies in pyloric antrum 70 percent
   Large bowel 12 percent
   Breast Ca 6 percent
   Rest of other (thyroid Ca/GB/ pancreas)
   Features of krukenberg tumor
   a. Invariably B/L
   b. Solid in consistency
   c. Freely mobile
   d. Capsule intact
   e. Histological presence of signet ring cells.

Importance of Histological Grade in Ovarian Carcinoma

Grading described on the basic of mitotic count per high power field under microscope nuclear cytoplasmic ratio (N/C), Proportion of solid area and neurotic areas. Stage I grade 1 to 5-year serial 90 percent, Stage I grade III 5-year serial 54 percent.

Differences Between Borderline and Malignant Tumor of Ovary

1. When atypical cells (Dysplastic cells) exceed > 4 layer's of ovarian epithelium or when stromal invasion is present than borderline stage converts into malignant stage.

Spread Pattern

Spread direct extension exfoliation of malignant cells lymphatic spread to adjacent lymph nodes. Distant spread by vascular channels is extremely uncommon. First disease involve capsule then mesovarian there after adjacent organ. Once disease involved the external surface, malignant cells may exfoliate in peritoneal cavity. Subsequently, the (transcoelomic spread in 70% cases) and then metastatic implantation occurs on peritoneal surface bowel surface (Leading bowel obstruction) ascitis occurs because of extensive peritonial implantation causing lymphatic and venus obstruction causing ascitis. Malignant cell may reach under surface of diaphragm and superior surface of liver. (Cause Right-sided hypochondrial pain) omentum implant's (Called an omentum cake) hematogenous spread to liver/ lunge/ brain/bone occurs very late stage of disease.

Complete Physical and Pelvic Examination Should be Done with Empty Bladder and Rectum Under Ga

1. On PV examination, pouch of Douglas should be palpated usually via posterior fornix one might get heard nodular ovarian tumor.
2. Simple X-ray abdomen and pelvic large soft tissue opacity. Since firm bone/teeth center seen in wall of dermoid cyst.
3. Chat X-ray to rule out lung metastasis.
4. IVP to exclude hydronephrosis due to large para-aortic in may compress renal hilum.
5. Barium meal performed to rule out primary stomach or large bowel.

6. Breast examination.
7. Transvaginal sonography (TVS) is best given you more detail.

ON TVS

Benign cyst are thin walled usually unilocular it at all loculated septal thickness would be <5 mm malignant tumor usually solid. It loculated septal thickness more than 5 mm usually bilateral

1. Laparoscopy: Very useful for staging as well as employed as a tool for IInd look surgery after successful chemotherapy.
2. Ca-125: Most sensitive tumor marker for epethilial ovarian but also increase in: endometrial Ca, abdominal tuberculosis, endometriosis. Rise of Ca-125 continued up to 6 to 8 weeks after successful surgery decline and comes down to normal less then 35 unit/ml this is a very successful tool as response to chemotherapy as well as recusant of ovarian Ca.

Other Ovarian Tumor Markers

Other ovarian tumor markers are:
C.Ea/Ca 19.9/LDH/α-FP/β-hCG) germ cell tumor marker.

Cytological examination of ascitis fluid false-negative report as high as 60 percent.

TREATMENT OPTIONS ARE SURGERY AND CHEMOTHERAPY

Radiotherapy obsolete nowadays. The biggest challenge is to diagnose an early case. Mostly we found cases in locally advance stage.

Due to better surgical technique as well as advent of paclitaxel/cisplatin based chemotherapy out look of ovarian Ca drastically improved in last two decades.

Surgery—has diagnostic as well as therapeutic role maximum possible ovarian cytoreduction. If ascitis is present fluid must be drained out and send for cytological examination. Peritonial cavity and it is content carefully inspected, along under surface of diaphram ovarian capsule/ Omentam (Fig. 16.5). Bowel wall type of surgery, cytoreductive surgery, second look surgery means 3 cycle NACT—followed by reassessment for surgery again followed by adjuvant chemotherapy. Resurgical excession required after surgery. If residual tumor left and its size is more then 2 cm survival comes down this advisable is resurgical excession ideal surgery is TAH and B/L salpingo oophorectomy with omentectomy. Even if metastasis is found at laparotomy cytoreductive surgery is performed (like in neuroblastoma and renal cell Ca).

CHEMOTHERAPY

Response rate of modern chemotherapy regime is 60 to 80 percent in ovarian Ca response assessment done with subjective and objective (Ca-125). Nowadays postoperative chemotherapy. (Stage IA onwards) is standard of care. Should be follow-up with CT Scan, USG abdomen, TVS, Ca-125 estimation. We know the aggressive surgery (TAH and BSO pulse omencetomy is still) cornerstone in management of ovarian Ca, chemotherapy take care postoperative of micro and macrometastasis both.

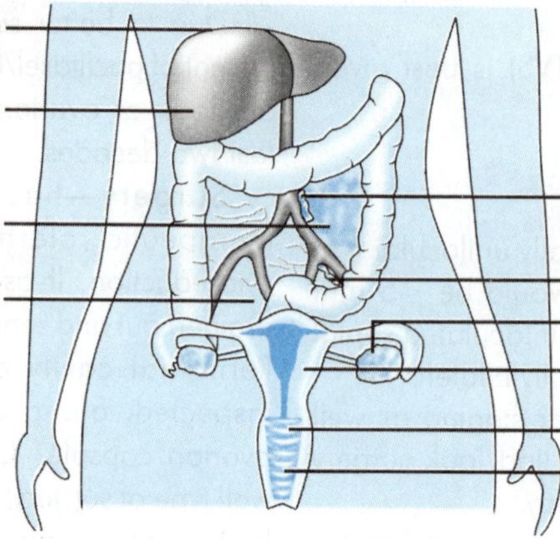

Fig. 16.5: Procedures required for surgical staging of ovarian cancer

Single Agent Vs Multiple Agent Merits and Demerits

Multiple agent advantages are decrease chances of drug resistence. Different drug have different type of mechanism of action, thus, increase response rate the disadvantage are toxicity is high, cost is high

1st. line (CAP) Cisplatin 75 mg/m^2 DI
Doxorubicin 40 mg/m^2 DI

Cyclophosfamide 750 mg/m^2 DI, with response rate 60 percent and increse median survival 24 months.

2nd line Paclitaxel 175 mg/m^2 DI
Cisplatine 100 mg/m^2 D2

With IInd liner response rate, 73 percent and medial survival is 38 months. Interperitonial chemotherapy based on ratinal that cytotoxic agent with low solubility and high molecular weight cleared from peritonial cavity very slowly thus high-dose chemoagent can be delivered in peritonium.

Complication of Intraperitoneal Chemotherapy

Occurs are :
1. Abdominal pain
2. Sepsis
3. Bowel adhesion.

DOSE INTENSE VS DOSE DENSE

Dose dense clinically practice in overian cancer and breast cancer, etc. conceptal dose dence are same standard dose of chemotherapy but less frequent interval (usually 2 weekly interval) give, rather high dose of chemically with some 3 weekly interval (Dose intance chemotherapy).

Risk Groups in Ovarian Cancers

1. Low-risk: Stage I, no residual disease and grade I
2. Intermediate, risk:
   a. Stage I, no residual, grade II-III
   b. Stage II, no residual, rage II-III
   c. Stage II, less than 2 cm residual, grade I-II
   d. Stage III, no residual or less than 2 cm residual, grade I.
3. High-risk:
   a. Stage II, less than 2 cm residual, grade III
   b. Stage III, no residual, or less than 2 cm residual grad II-III.

ROLE OF RADIOTHERAPY

Whole abdominal radiotherapy field used for ovarian cancer now commonly in use (Figs 16.6 and 16.7).

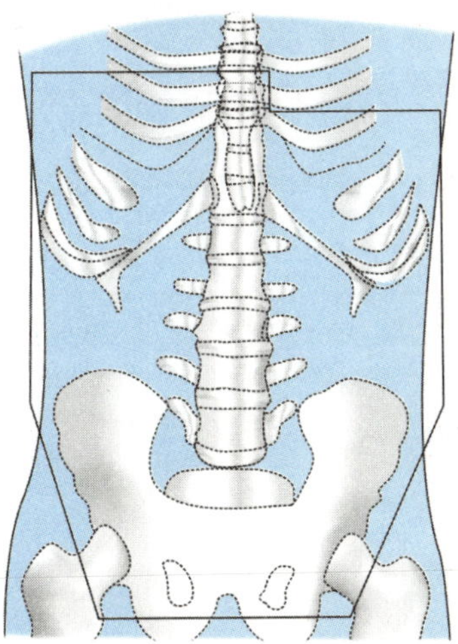

Fig. 16.6: Whole abdominal field used in ovarian cancer

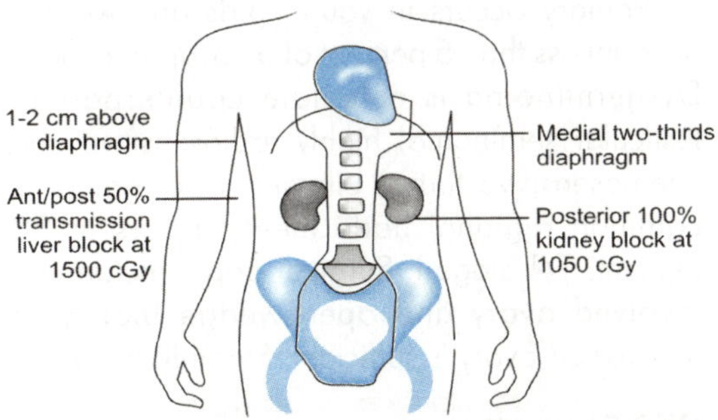

Fig. 16.7: Whole abdominal radiotherapy now obsolete

Role why declined because of advent of cisplatin/ paclitaxel based chemotherapy since we know surgery you cannot by pass and after surgery, if residual tumor more then 2 cm then radiotherapy. Is in effective to achieve local control and if residual less then 2 cm then modern chemotherapy provide excellent local control and tumor improved survival, in stage IA/IB once capsules not involved TAH and BSO and omentectomy produce. 5-year survival 90 percent.

IB onwards once capsule is involved post-surgery up 6 cycle chemotherapy is strongly advised.

Management of Germ Cell Tumor of Ovary

Dysgerminoma
Teratoma
Embryonal cell Ca
Choriocarcinoma
Yolk sac tumor (Endodermal sinus tumor)

Primary occurs in young girls and women accountless than 5 percent of all ovarian cancer. Dysgerminoma is a female counterpart of testicular seminoma, highly radiosensitive and chemosensitive tumor bilateral involvement is common regional node meets occurs in 20 percent. T/T stage I. Surgical oophorectomy of involved ovary and open wedge biopsy of uninvolved ovary is sufficient. Stage II, III, IV.

BEP Chemotherapy

Bleomycin 20 unit/m^2 D2
Cisplatin 20 mg/m^2 D1–D5
Etoposide 100 mg/m^2 D1 – D5

Followed with 25 Gy in 20 fractions of radiotherapy to mid plan of hemipelvis, If both ovary involved whole Pelvis RT.

Whole abdomen radiotherapy.

Indication in para-aortic lymphadenopathy. Peritoneal metastasis. 25 Gy/20# Whole abdomen followed by 10 Gy boost to primary site, treatment policy of other germ cell tumor like, Choriocarcinoma/yolk sac tumor/embryonal carcinoma is TAH and BSO and serial monitoring of β-hCG/LDH/α FP as well as 6 cycle of BEP chemotherapy since these tumor are not radio-sensitive thus, no role of radiotherapy.

Chapter 17

Endometrial Cancer

INTRODUCTION

Endometrial cancer refers to several types of malignancy which arise from the endometrium or lining of the uterus. Endometrial cancers are the most common gynecologic cancers in the United States, with over 35,000 women diagnosed each year in the US. The most common subtype, endometrioid adenocarcinoma, typically occurs within a few decades of menopause, is associated with excessive estrogen exposure endometrial hyperplasia and presents most often with vaginal bleeding. Endometrial carcinoma is the third most common cause of gynecologic cancer death (behind ovarian and cervical cancer). A total abdominal hysterectomy (surgical removal of the uterus) with bilateral salpingo-oophorectomy is the most common therapeutic approach (Fig. 17.1).

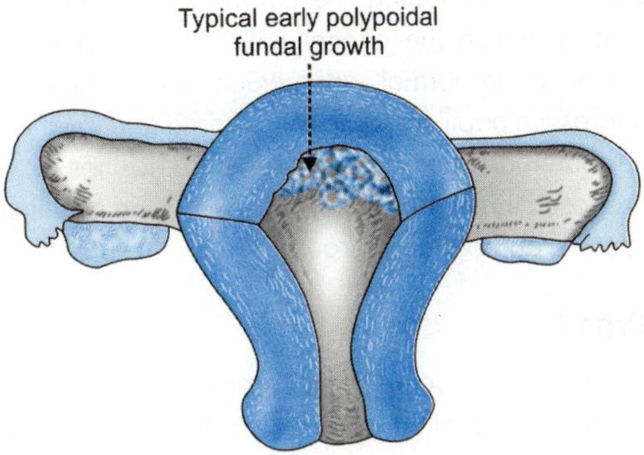

Fig. 17.1: Endometrial cancer

Endometrial cancer may sometimes be referred to as uterine cancer. However, different cancers may develop not only from the endometrium itself but also from other tissues of the uterus, including cervical cancer, sarcoma of the myometrium and trophoblastic disease. Endometrial cancer cammoly spread to various organs near by uterine like, fallopian tube, ovary, vaginal spread as well as to pelvic lymph nodes (Fig. 17.2).

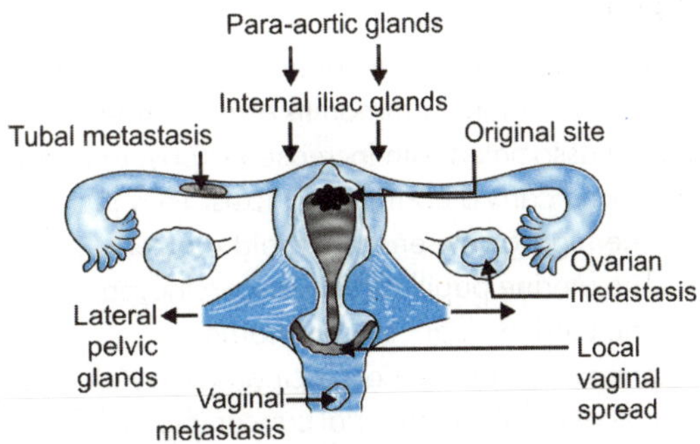

Fig. 17.2: Spread of endometrial cancer

CLASSIFICATION

Most endometrial cancers are carcinomas (usually adenocarcinomas), meaning that they originate from the single layer of epithelial cells which line the endometrium and form the endometrial glands. There are many microscopic subtypes of endometrial carcinoma, including the common endometrioid type, in which the cancer cells grow in patterns reminiscent of normal endometrium and the far more aggressive papillary serous carcinoma and clear cell endometrial carcinomas. Some authorities have proposed that endometrial carcinomas be classified into two pathogenetic groups:

Type I

These cancers occur most commonly in pre- and perimenopausal women, often with a history of unopposed estrogen exposure and/or endometrial hyperplasia. They are often minimally invasive into the underlying uterine wall, are of the low-grade endometrioid type and carry a good prognosis.

Type II

These cancers occur in older, postmenopausal women, are more common in African-Americans, are not associated with increased exposure to estrogen and carry a poorer prognosis. They include:

A. The high-grade endometrioid cancer.
B. The uterine papillary serous carcinoma.
C. The uterine clear cell carcinoma.

In contrast to endometrial carcinomas, histological classification of endometrial cancer (Fig. 17.3) the uncommon endometrial stromal sarcomas are cancers which originate in the nonglandular connective tissue of the endometrium. Uterine carcinosarcoma, formerly called malignant mixed müllerian tumor, is a rare uterine cancer which contains cancerous cells of both glandular and sarcomatous appearance—in this case, the cell of origin is unknown.

- Endometrial stromal sarcoma
- Uterine carcinosarcoma
- An endometrial adenocarcinoma invading the uterine muscle.

SIGNS AND SYMPTOMS

Vaginal bleeding and/or spotting in postmenopausal women. Abnormal uterine bleeding, abnormal menstrual periods. Bleeding between normal periods in premenopausal women in women older than 40: extremely long, heavy or frequent episodes of bleeding (may indicate premalignant changes). Anemia, caused by chronic loss of blood. (This may occur if the woman has ignored symptoms of prolonged or frequent abnormal menstrual bleeding). Lower abdominal pain or pelvic cramping. Thin white or clear vaginal discharge in postmenopausal women.

RISK FACTORS

High levels of estrogen, endometrial hyperplasia, obesity, hypertension, polycystic ovary syndrome, nulliparity (never having carried a pregnancy), infertility (inability to become pregnant), early menarche (onset of menstruation), late menopause

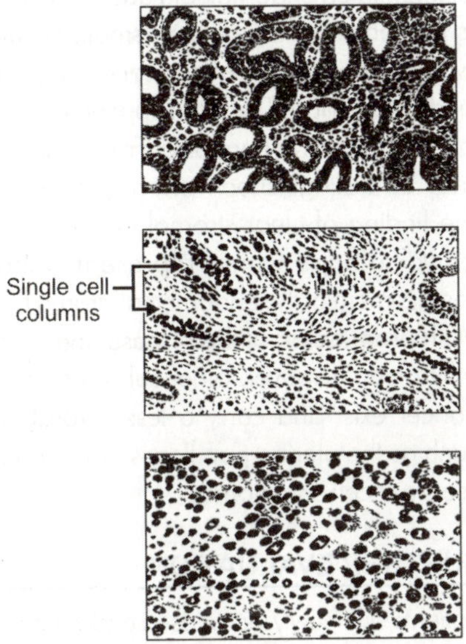

Fig. 17.3: Histology: The majority of tumors (60%) are pure adenocarcinomata. They can be divided into three groups according to the degree of glandular differentiation

(cessation of menstruation), endometrial polyps or other benign growths of the uterine lining, diabetes, Tamoxifen high intake of animal fat, pelvic radiation therapy, breast cancer ovarian cancer, heavy daily alcohol consumption (possibly a risk factor).

DIAGNOSIS AND CLINICAL EVALUATION

Routine screening of asymptomatic women is not indicated, since the disease is highly curable in its early stages. Results from a pelvic examination are frequently normal, especially in the early stages of disease. Changes in the size, shape or consistency of the uterus and/or its surrounding, supporting structures may exist when the disease is more advanced.

A pap smear may be either normal or show abnormal cellular changes.

Endometrial curettage is the traditional diagnostic method. Both endometrial and endocervical material should be sampled.

If endometrial curettage does not yield sufficient diagnostic material, a dilation and curettage (D&C) is necessary for diagnosing the cancer (Fig. 17.4).

Hysteroscopy allows the direct visualization of the uterine cavity and can be used to detect the presence of lesions or tumors. It also permits the

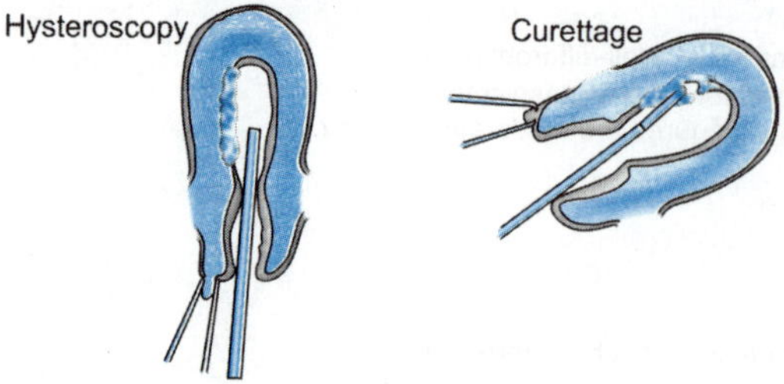

Fig. 17.4: Hysteroscopy and curettage to confirm diagnosis

doctor to obtain cell samples with minimal damage to the endometrial lining (unlike blind D&C).

Endometrial biopsy or aspiration may assist the diagnosis.

Transvaginal ultrasound to evaluate the endometrial thickness in women with postmenopausal bleeding is increasingly being used to evaluate for endometrial cancer.

Recently, a new method of testing has been introduced called the true test, offered through. It uses the small flexible tao brush to brush the entire lining of the uterus. This method is less painful than a pipelle biopsy and has a larger likelihood of procuring enough tissue for testing. Since it is simpler and less invasive, the true test can be performed as often, and at the same time as, a routine pap smear, thus, allowing for early detection and treatment. Ongoing research suggests that serum p53 antibody may hold value in identifying high-risk endometrial cancer.

ENDOMETRIAL ADENOCARCINOMA

The histopathology of endometrial cancers is highly diverse. The most common finding is a well-differentiated endometrioid adenocarcinoma, which is composed of numerous, small, crowded glands with varying degrees of nuclear atypia, mitotic activity and stratification. This often appears on a background of endometrial hyperplasia. Frank adenocarcinoma may be distinguished from atypical hyperplasia by the finding of clear stromal invasion, or "back-to-back" glands which represent nondestructive replacement of the endometrial stroma by the cancer. With progression of the disease, the myometrium is infiltrated. However, other subtypes of endometrial cancer exist and carry a less favorable diagnosis such as the uterine papillary serous carcinoma and the clear cell carcinoma.

FURTHER EVALUATION

Patients with newly-diagnosed endometrial cancer do not routinely undergo imaging studies, such as CT scans, to evaluate for extent of disease, since this is of low yield. Preoperative evaluation should include a complete medical history and physical examination, pelvic examination and rectal examination with stool Guaiac test, chest X-ray, complete blood count and blood chemistry tests, including liver function tests. Colonoscopy is recommended if the stool is Guaiac positive or the woman has symptoms, due to the etiologic factors common to both endometrial cancer and colon cancer. The tumor marker CA-125 is sometimes checked, since this can predict advanced stage disease.

STAGING

Endometrial carcinoma is surgically staged using the FIGO cancer staging system. Although the FIGO staging has recently been updated, the older staging described below is still commonly used.

1. *Stage IA:* Tumor limited to the endometrium
2. *Stage IB:* Invasion of less than half the myometrium
3. *Stage IC:* Invasion of more than half the myometrium
4. *Stage IIA:* Endocervical glandular involvement only
5. *Stage IIB:* Cervical stromal invasion
6. *Stage IIIA:* Tumor invades serosa or adnexa, or malignant peritoneal cytology
7. *Stage IIIB:* Vaginal metastasis
8. *Stage IIIC:* Metastasis to pelvic or para-aortic lymph nodes
9. *Stage IVA:* Invasion of the bladder or bowel
10. *Stage IVB:* Distant metastasis, including intra-abdominal or inguinal lymph nodes (Fig. 17.5).

TREATMENT

The primary treatment is surgical. Surgical treatment should consist of, at least, cytologic sampling of the peritoneal fluid, abdominal exploration, palpation and biopsy of suspicious lymph nodes, abdominal hysterectomy, and removal of both ovaries (bilateral salpingo-oophorectomy). Lymphadenectomy, or removal of pelvic and para-aortic lymph nodes, is sometimes performed for tumors that have high-risk features, such as pathologic grade 3 serous or clear-cell tumors, invasion of more than 1/2 the myometrium, or extension to the cervix or adnexa. Sometimes, removal of the omentum is also performed.

Abdominal hysterectomy is recommended over vaginal hysterectomy because it affords the opportunity to examine and obtain washings of the abdominal cavity to detect any further evidence of cancer.

Women with stage 1 disease who are at increased risk for recurrence and those with stage 2 disease are often offered surgery in combination with radiation therapy. Chemotherapy may be considered in some cases, especially for those with stage 3 and 4 disease. Hormonal therapy with progestins and antiestrogens has been used for the treatment of endometrial stromal sarcomas. The antibody herceptin, which is used to treat breast cancers that overexpress the HER2/neu protein, has been tried with some success in a phase II trial in women with uterine papillary serous carcinomas that overexpress HER2/neu.

COMPLICATIONS OF TREATMENT

Uterine perforation may occur during a D and C or an endometrial biopsy. Asherman's syndrome (intrauterine adhesions) may occur from D and C, resulting in infertility and an increased risk of future obstetric complications.

PROGNOSIS

Because endometrial cancer is usually diagnosed in the early stages (70 to 75 percent of cases are in stage 1 at diagnosis; 10 to 15 percent of cases are in stage 2; 10 to 15 percent of cases are in stage 3 or 4), there is a better probable outcome associated with it than with other types of gynecological cancers such as cervical or ovarian

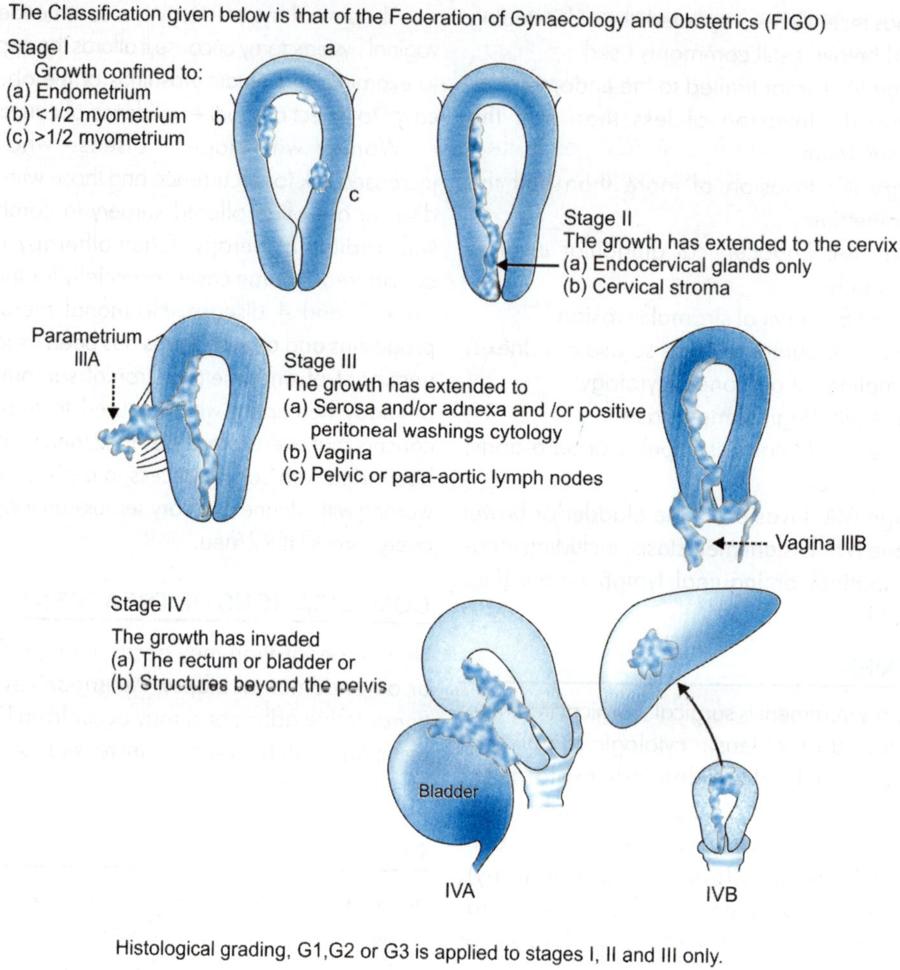

Fig. 17.5: Staging of endometrial cancer

cancer. While endometrial cancers are 40 percent more common in caucasian women, an African-American woman who is diagnosed with uterine cancer is twice as likely to die (possibly due to the higher frequency of aggressive subtypes in that population, but more probable due to delay in the diagnosis).

SURVIVAL RATES

The 5-year survival rate for endometrial cancer following appropriate treatments are:

- 75 to 95 percent for stage 1
- 50 percent for stage 2
- 30 percent for stage 3
- Less than 5 percent for stage 4.

Chapter

18 Hodgkin's Lymphoma

1. Five percent of childhood malignancy
2. Male:Female 2:1 in children, adults almost equal M:F
3. Mixed cellularity (MC) Hodgkin's disease is more common at younger ages
4. Clustering in some families
5. More common in immune deficiency patients (Ataxia-telangiectasia, HIV).

Epstein-Barr Virus, (EBV) has been implicated in the causation of HD by epidemiologic and serologic studies. Large proportion of HD patients have high titer of EBV-Ab titer, EBV genome in Reed-Sternberg cells by *in situ* hybridization EBV-positive genome are more frequently observed in children <10 years. Incidence of EBV-associated HD varies by ethnic background (93% Asians, 86% Hispanic, 46% Whites, 17% African-American).

IMMUNOPHENOTYPE

Antigen	*Lymphocytic predominance*	*Nodular sclerosis*	*Mixed cellularity*
LCA (CD45)	+	–	–
Ki-1 (CD30)	–(+)	+	+
LeuM1(CD15)	–	+	+
L26(CD20)	+	–(+)	–(+)

CLINICAL PRESENTATION

Signs and symptoms	*Percentage of patients*
Lymphadenopathy	90
Mediastinal mass	60
"B" symptoms	30 % Fever, weight loss, night sweats

LYMPHADENOPATHY

Hepatosplenomegaly, 25 percent most commonly involved lymph nodes are the cervical and supraclavicular in 75 percent (Fig.18.1), bone marrow is involved in 5 percent of patients.

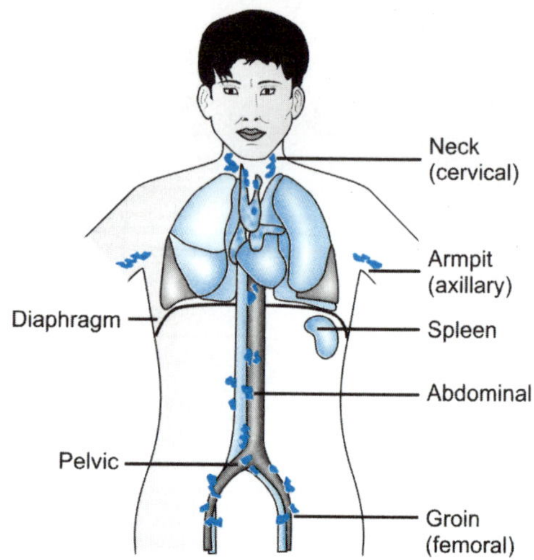

Fig. 18.1: Lymph node spread of Hodgkin's lymphoma

DIAGNOSTIC EVALUATION

Physical examination with measurement of lymph nodes, CBCD, ESR, renal and hepatic function, AP, LDH and serum ferritin

1. Lymph node biopsy.
2. CXR with measurement of mediastinal ratio.
3. CT scan of neck, chest, abdomen and pelvis.
4. Bone marrow biopsy.
5. Gallium scan in doubtful abdominal involvement and mediastinal involvement.
6. Echocardiogram.

ANN ARBOR STAGING CLASSIFICATION

Stage definition:

1. Involvement of a single lymph node region (I) or of a single extralymphatic organ or site (I_E).
2. Involvement of two or more lymph node regions on the same side of the diaphragm (II) or localized involvement of an extralymphatic organ or site and one or more lymph node regions on the same side of the diaphragm (II_E).
3. Involvement of lymph node regions on both sides of the diaphragm (III) which may be accompanied by involvement of the spleen (III_S) or by localized involvement of an extra-lymphatic organ or site (III_E) or both (III_{SE}).
4. Diffuse or disseminated involvement of one or more extralymphatic.

B symptoms: Fever >38°C for three consecutive days, drenching night sweats or unexplained loss 10 percent or more of weight the preceding 6 months (Table 18.1).

TREATMENT

Hodgkin's lymphoma is a highly curable disease with cure rates of >90 percent, appropriate treatment depends on risk features at time of diagnosis (risk adapted therapy), and therapy may be radiotherapy, chemotherapy or combined modality.

Table 18.1: Clinical groups and prognostic factors

Group	***Prognostic factors***
Very favorable	Stage I and age <40 and 'A' + ESR <50 + female and MT ratio* <0.35
Favorable	All other patients
Unfavorable	Age ≥ 50, or 'A' + ESR ≥50, or 'B' + ESR ≥30, or stage $11_{4/5\$}$, or MT Ratio ≥0.35

*MT ratio = size of mediastinal mass compared with transverse diameter of chest on chest X-ray

$ the subscript number denotes the number of nodal regions involved an adverse prognostic factor

ESR = erythrocyte sedimentation rate

1. Standard radiation dose of (36–40 Gy) produces unacceptable cosmetic and skeletal abnormalities in prepubertal children and high-risk of subsequent breast Ca in adolescent females, combined modality therapy using low dose radiation (15–25 Gy) is the most commonly used therapy
2. Evaluation of chemotherapy alone treatment is difficult because most reports describe outcome after nonrandom assignment
3. Unfavorable prognostic factors:
   a. Stage IIIB, IV
   b. B symptoms
   c. Bulky disease
   d. High ESR >5
4. Long-term effects of treatment should be taken into consideration: Radiotherapy field used in Hodgkin's lymphoma are, IFRT, (involve field radiotherapy) mediastinal field involving neck node and hilar, axillary and pectoral lymph node (Fig. 18.2).
   a. Treatment related second neoplasm's (e.g. AML, NHL and Ca breast), infertility, growth consideration, long-term organ dysfunction (e.g. thyroid, heart, lung), adolescent patients who have achieved maximum growth can be treated as adult patients.
5. Early stage HD: stage I and IIA.
6. It is not clear which combinations of treatment strategies are most effective at maintaining high cure rates and minimizing long-term squeal.
7. The Cochrane library: 2002, "Intervention for early Hodgkin's disease in children."

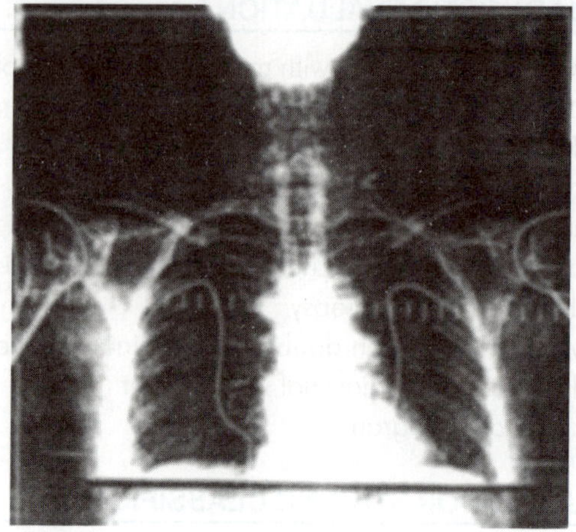

Fig. 18.2: Mediastinal field for radiotherapy

8. Four randomized controlled trials with 334 patients, There is little evidence from randomized clinical trials to evaluate the consensus approach of short course chemotherapy and local radiotherapy, significant failure rate when involved field irradiation is applied alone.
9. High ultimate survival in children with early stage HD, combined modality treatment: 2 to 4 courses of ABVD or hybrid regimen+ IF radiation with 20 to 25 Gy. Combination chemotherapy with a proven regimen without radiation is currently under clinical evaluation (CCG-5942) 235 patients received IF radiation and 266 patients with no RT. The 3 year EFS was 92.9 percent vs 86.1 percent. Patients who have PR after initial therapy will receive 4 courses of COPP.

Stage IIIA

Pediatric series support both the use of combined modality therapy and chemotherapy alone as initial management. Radiation therapy may be indicated in patients with bulky disease at presentation or for residual disease after chemotherapy RT alone is inappropriate. Combination chemotherapy alone 6 courses of ABVD patient who are slow responders (PR after 3 c) will be shifted to COPP or APPE.

Stage IV and Patients with B Symptoms

Combination chemotherapy is the treatment of choice, radiation therapy is sometimes added to areas of bulky disease, due to poor outcome of patients with stage IV they may benefit from enrollment in clinical trials, ABVD or MOPP/ABVD total of 8 courses. Slow responders will be individualized for APPE and radiation therapy± ABMT.

Recurrent/Refractory

Treatment failure: Primary refractory disease. {A} early relapse <1yr of complete remission, {B} late relapse, patients with primary refractory disease and those relapsing after 6 cycles of chemotherapy would benefit of chemotherapy followed by peripheral stem cell transplant. Chemotherapy regimens: high dose Ara-c+cisplatin or ifosfamide, carboplatin and etoposide. Gemcitabine has shown promising activity as a single agent.

Chapter 19 Non-Hodgkin's Lymphoma

This group of tumors includes a very wide spectrum of malignancy, from almost benign to highly aggressive disease.

PATHOLOGY

Epidemiology

Non-Hodgkin's Lymphomas (NHL) are responsible for 1.4 percent of all cancers and 0.4 percent of cancer deaths. The peak incidence is in the fifth and sixth decades. Children in developed countries are rarely affected. The incidence among children in developing countries is higher, particularly of high-grade Burkitt's lymphoma. Males are slightly more commonly affected than females. The sex ratio is 1.7:1.

Etiology

The cause of most NHL is unknown. The risk of developing NHL is increased in certain inherited genetic syndromes such as combined immunodeficiency syndromes and ataxia telangiectasia. Chromosomal defects have been identified in some types of NHL (14:18 translocation in follicular lymphoma and 8:14 translocation in Burkitt's lymphoma). However, these are acquired as part of tumor development, not inherited abnormalities.

Some NHL are associated with, though not necessarily caused by, viral infection. For examples, endemic Burkitt's lymphoma, originally described in East African children, is associated with infection by the Epstein-Barr virus (EBV). These children have evidence of antibodies to the viral antigen. EBV is unlikely, however, to be the sole causative agent of Burkitt's lymphoma since the virus is distributed worldwide, whereas the tumor is limited to areas where malaria is endemic. Malaria has therefore been suggested as a possible cofactor. Some NHL are caused by infection with the human T leukemia virus type 1 (HTLV-1).

Conditions in which the body's immune system is impaired predispose to the development of NH, particularly immunoblastic. Examples are rheumatoid arthritis, celiac disease, hypogammaglobulinemia and AIDS. There is a 60-fold excess of these tumors in patients who have undergone immunosuppressive drug therapy following organ transplantation.

Microscopic Features

NHL are typified by the monoclonal proliferation, in order of frequency, of B lymphocytes or T lymphocytes.

The wide variation in histological appearance of NHL and the difficulty in classifying many of them with certainty has led to a confusing variety of systems of pathological classification. The availability of modern immunohistochemical techniques to identify different cell types has contributed to the complexity. However, the basis of classification is to recognize the malignant cell and name it according to its normal counterparts.

In the UD the British National Lymphoma Investigation (BNLI) group and the Kiel classifications have been most commonly used. The Working formulation of the US National Cancer Institute and more recently the Revised European-American Lymphoma (REAL) classification are also popular. Much expertise is required to classify the NHL. High-grade NHL may be confused with a poorly differentiated carcinoma by the unwary. The management and prognosis of these two conditions is different. Referral of all cases to a specialist histopathologist for review before taking a decision on management is recommended.

BNLI Classification

The BNLI classification is based on morphological appearances. Its attraction to the clinician is the division into grade 1 and grade 2 disease which provides a comprehensible and practical guide to decision-making. The BNLI classification has the advantage of wide usage in the UK. The BNLI offers an excellent centralized service for review of pathology to centers participating in its studies (Fig. 19.1).

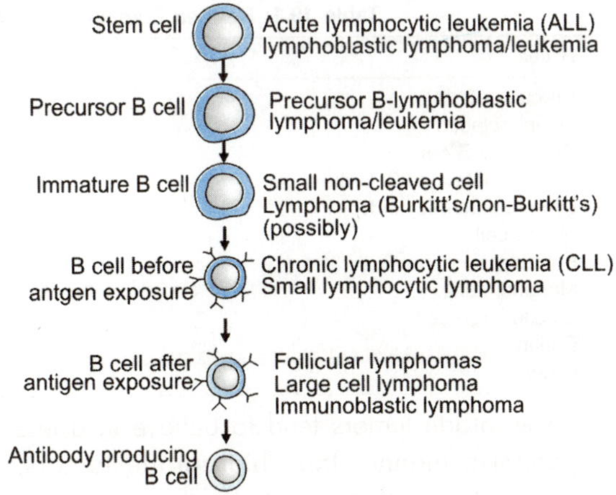

Fig. 19.1: B cell cancers by cell development

Kiel Classification

The Kiel classification is based on scientific principles and microscopic appearances. It also divides lymphomas into low or high-grade malignancy. Both the Kiel and another classification (Luck-Collins) take account of the T or B cell origin of the tumor.

Real Classification

The revised European-American lymphoma classification lists lymphoid neoplasms which are distinctive biological entities and which can be reproducibly diagnosed by hematopathologists (Table 19.1). This has been accepted and updated in the new World Health Organization classification.

Table 19.1: Revised European-American Lymphoma classification (simplified)

B cell	*T cell*
Precursor B cell	Precursor T cell
Lymphoblastic	Lymphoblastic
Peripheral B cell	Peripheral T cell
Small lymphocyte/CLL-like	CLL–like
Lymphoplasmacytoid	Mycosis fungoides
Mantle cell	Angioimmunoblastic
Follicular	Anaplastic large cell
Marginal zone	Unspecified
Diffuse large cell	Other
Burkitt	
Other	

Low–grade tumors tend to behave in a less aggressive manner than high-grade tumors. However, this applies more to B cell than to T cell lymphomas. In general, low-grade tumors tend to have smaller cells. High-grade tumors usually have larger cells, often multinucleate with prominent nucleoli. Some tumors contain a mixture of cells, which can make them difficult to classify.

Clinical Features

NHL differ in several respects from Hodgkin's disease. These differences are simplistically summarized in Table 19.2. In contrast to Hodgkin's disease, very few patients (10%) have localized disease at presentation. Systemic B symptoms are, common.

A further difference is the frequency of presentation (20%) with involvement of extranodal sites Table 19.3. The most common of these are in the head and neck, particularly in the lymphoid tissue of the tonsil, nasopharynx and base of tongue (Waldeyer's ring). Second in frequency is the gastrointestinal tract (stomach > small bowel > large bowel). Less common sites are the skin, thyroid, CNS, bone, and testis. Epitrochlear and mesenteric nodes and the bone marrow are only rarely involved by Hodgkin's disease but not infrequently by NHL, Para-aortic lymph node can also be involved in non-Hodgkin's lymphoma (Fig. 19.2).

Table 19.2: Comparison of clinical features of Hodgkin's disease and non-Hodgkin lymphoma

Feature	*Hodgkin's disease*	*Non-Hodgkin lymphoma*
Localized	+++	+
Nodal spread		
Contiguous	+++	+
Non-contiguous	+	+++
Bone marrow infiltration	±	++
CNS involvement	±	+

Investigations

The staging investigations for NHL are similar to those for Hodgkin's disease. An adequate biopsy is essential for proper histological examination and cell surface marker studies. There are, however the following differences:

Table 19.3: The relative frequency of non-Hodgkin's lymphoma types at the Department of Pathology Registry, NCI during the period 1998–2000 (n=1095)

Type	*%*	*Average Age*	*Male:Female*
B cell lymphomas			
Diffuse large B cell lymphoma	49	47.5	1.3:1
Burkitt's lymphoma	6.9	11.9	1.4:1
Small lymphocytic lymphoma	6	58.3	5.3:1
Follicular lymphoma	5.2	49.3	1.5:1
Plasmacytoma/Myeloma	4.8	52.1	1.1:1
Marginal zone lymphoma	4.5	44.1	1.3:1
Mantle cell lymphoma	4.3	52	2.1:1
Hairy cell leukemia	0.2	36	-
T cell lymphomas			
Lymphoblastic lymphoma	4.6	17	2.3:1
T cell lymphoma NOS	3.7	39.9	3.7:1
Anaplastic lymphoma	1.8	28.2	1.6:1
Mycosis fungoides	1	47.5	1.8:1
Unspecified	8	44.9	1:1
Total	**100**	**40.7**	**2.3:1**

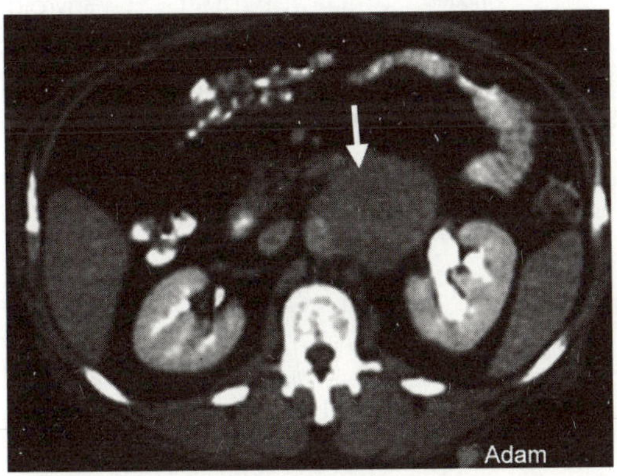

Fig. 19.2: Large para-aortic lymphadenopathy

1. Surface markers. A number of monoclonal antibodies to cell surface proteins made by these tumors are useful in determining whether they are of B or T cell origin. Most (about 85%) lymphomas are of B cell origin. Individual subtypes can be identified using immunocytochemical markers. Staining with antibodies against epithelial cell components (e.g. cytokeratins) usually identifies undifferentiated carcinomas, separating them from lymphomas.
2. CT scanning. Since NHL tend to be more generalized than Hodgkin's disease, CT scanning of the thorax and the abdomen is

The International Prognostic Index

Factor	*Adverse prognosis*
Age	≥60 years
Ann Arbor stage	III or IV
Serum LDH	Above normal
Number of extranodal sites of involvement	≥2
Performance status	≥ECOG 2 or equivalent

International Non-Hodgkin's Lymphoma prognostic factors Project, A predictive model for aggressive non-Hodgkin's lymphoma. *N Engl J Med* 1993; 329: 987–94.

preferred to lymphangiography. In those unfit for CT scanning of chest and abdomen because of advanced age or poor general medical condition, a chest radiograph and abdominal ultrasound provide simpler alternatives.

3. Bone marrow examination. A bone marrow aspirate and a small core of bone (trephine) should be examined for tumor infiltration. The trephine may be positive when the aspirate is negative. Marrow involvement is much commoner in low-grade (>60%) than high-grade (10–15%) NHL.
4. Staging laparotomy. This is not recommended since so few patients have localized disease. Many patients are elderly and unfit for surgery on medical grounds.

The following standard staging investigations are recommended.

1. Hematology
   a. Full blood count and ESR
   b. Bone marrow aspirate and trephine.
2. Biochemistry
   a. Liver function tests
   b. Serum immunoglobulins
   c. Serum urea, creatinine and electrolytes (including calcium)
   d. Serum uric acid.
3. Radiology
   a. Chest radiograph
   b. CT scan of thorax and abdomen to see extension of lymph node (Fig. 19.3).

Principles of Management

The management of NHL depends upon the age and general condition of the patient, the histology, the extent of the disease and whether the tumor is nodal or extranodal. NHL are generally, very sensitive to radiation and to chemotherapy.

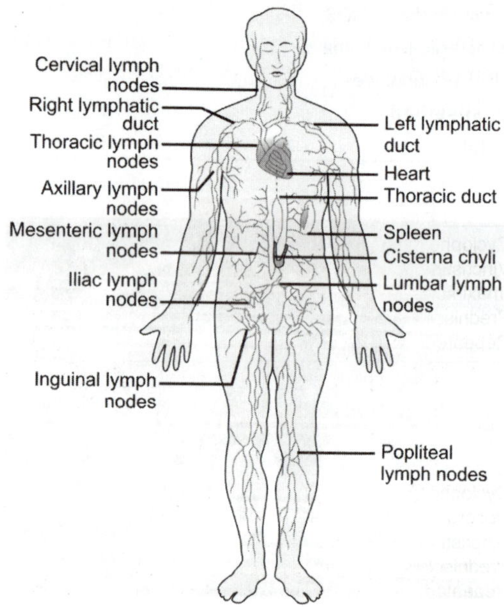

Fig. 19.3: Lymph node can be involved in non-Hodgkin's lymphoma

In general, widespread low-grade (BNLI grade 1, mostly REAL follicular B cell) tumors are treated with 'gentle' chemotherapy (chlorambucil with or without steroids) or slightly more aggressive combination chemotherapy (chlorambucil, vincristine (Oncovin) and prednisolone) CV (O) P; (Table 19.4). Radiotherapy at modest doses is used for localized disease.

High-grade (BNLI grade 2, mostly REAL diffuse large B cell) tumors usually require more aggressive combination chemotherapy, e.g. with cyclophosphamide, doxorubicin, vincristine (Oncovin) and prednisolone [CHOP] (Table 19.5). Radiotherapy at higher dosage than for low-grade tumors is required for truly localized (stage Ia) disease or for masses failing to resolve completely on chemotherapy.

1. Localized disease (stages I and II)

Table 19.4: CV (O)P regimen for low-grade non-Hodgkin lymphomas

Cyclophosphamide 750 mg/m^2 IV	Day 1
Vincristine (Oncovin) 1.4 mg/m^2 (maximum 2 mg) IV	Day 1
Prednisolone 40 mg/m^2 orally	Day 1–5
Repeated every 21 days (minimum 6 courses)	

Table 19.5: CHOP regimen for high-grade non-Hodgkin lymphomas

Cyclophosphamide 750 mg/m^2 IV	Day 1
Doxorubicin 50 mg/m^2 IV	Day 1
Vincristine 1.4 mg/m^2 (max. 2 mg) IV	Day 1
Prednisolone 50 mg/m^2 orally Day 1–5	
Repeated every 21 days (minimum 6 courses)	

Low-grade (grade 1)

For patients with localized stage I or II disease of low-grade histology local radiotherapy is generally recommended.

High-grade (grade 2)

Previously local radiotherapy alone was recommended for non-bulky (<2.5 cm) stage Ia disease of high-grade histology. Nowadays, it is standard practice to give an abbreviated course of chemotherapy followed by radiotherapy. In view of the frequent failure of radiotherapy to control bulky stage I and stage II disease, full-course cytotoxic chemotherapy is advised and may be followed by radiotherapy to the initial site of involvement. Combination chemotherapy is most commonly with the CHOP regimen (Table 19.5) subject to response and patient tolerance.

Results of Treatment

For low-grade stage I and II, local control is about 80 percent at 5 years; occasionally stage I disease is 65 percent at 5 years. Radiotherapy is less effective for high-grade bulky (>2.5 cm) stage I or stage II (Local control only 27% at 5 years). With chemotherapy before radiotherapy a 20 percent improvement is seen.

2. Widespread disease (stages III–IV) Low-grade

There is little evidence that treatment influences the natural history of stage III–IV disease of low-grade histology. Despite treatment, 75 percent of patients will relapse within 5 years. Since cure is unrealistic with current radiotherapy or chemotherapy, it is important to minimize the toxicity of treatment.

In general, in the absence of life-threatening disease (e.g. liver metastases, bone marrow failure, renal or cerebral involvement), asymptomatic patients should be kept under regular surveillance on an outpatient basis. Treatment is instituted with local radiotherapy or with chemotherapy if there is symptomatic progression or vital organs (e.g. kidneys) are threatened.

Chemotherapy

For symptomatic non-life-threatening disease, chlorambucil [0.2 mg/kg daily (maximum 10 mg)] with or without prednisolone (10–40 mg daily) can provide good control. To reduce the risk of leukem genesis and preserve adequate bone marrow tolerance to subsequent chemotherapy, if needed, treatment with chlorambucil should usually be stopped 3 months after a response has been achieved. Total duration of treatment should not exceed 6 months.

If disease progresses despite chlorambucil and /or steroids, more aggressive treatment is necessary. Combination chemotherapy such as cyclophosphamide, vincristine and prednisolone (CV (O) P) is advised (Table 19.4) to a total of six courses, if a useful clinical response is obtained. If not doxorubicin may be added.

New treatments are being evaluated especially in younger fitter patients, for example fludarabine (especially in combination chemotherapy), high-dose therapy (with interferon or anti-idiotypic antibodies such as rituximab-) (Fig. 19.4).

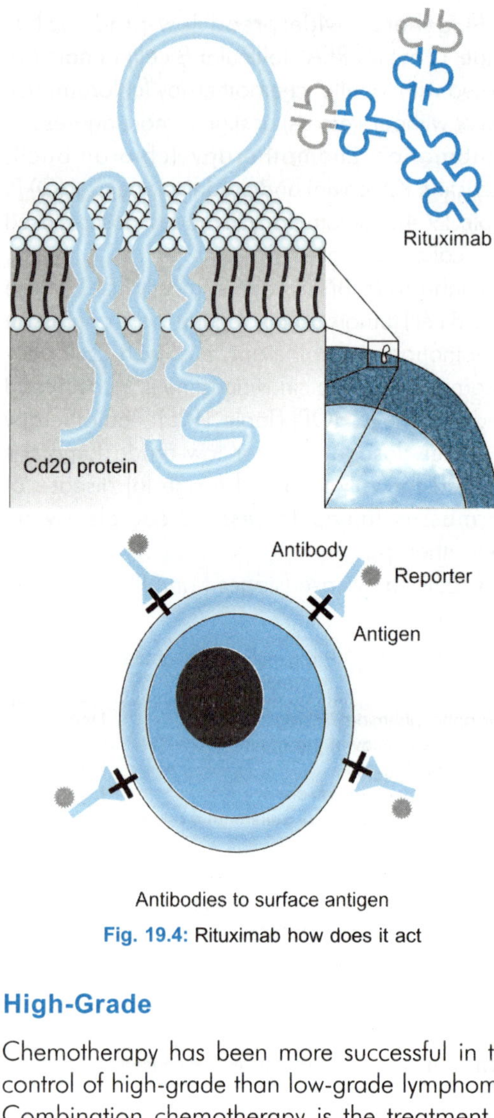

Fig. 19.4: Rituximab how does it act

High-Grade

Chemotherapy has been more successful in the control of high-grade than low-grade lymphoma. Combination chemotherapy is the treatment of choice. Of the available regimens, CHOP (Table 19.5) is still the gold standard (though more intensive forms of chemotherapy, such as high-dose chemotherapy, are currently being evaluated). Six courses are given, subject to response and patient tolerance. The most aggressive forms of high-grade disease (e.g. lymphoblastic) are often treated with leukemia type regimens and additionally with prophylactic CNS irradiation because of the high incidence of CNS involvement.

Result of chemotherapy for high-grade disease. Complete response rates of the order of 60 percent are achievable. Overall cure rate is about 40 percent.

Relapse

High dose chemotherapy with or without autologous stem cell 01 bone marrow transplantation should be considered for patients failing to respond or relapsing after CHOP chemotherapy. However, the probability of cure is low.

Radiotherapy

Localized disease (Low-grade)

Target Volume

Since NHL do not necessarily spread to contiguous nodes, local radiotherapy should be confined to the affected nodes, with a generous (e.g. 5 cm) margin. This is in contrast to regional (e.g. mental) radiotherapy in Hodgkin's disease where the cervical, mediastinal and axillary nodes are treated, even if only one of these sites is involved.

Technique

For the treatment of neck nodes, patients should be immobilized using a plastic shell lying supine with the neck extended as much as possible. A direct anterior field is simulated with the nodal mass marked by use of wire. The medial border is usually placed lateral to the spinal cord. Where the disease is extensive, an opposed posterior field may be required.

Where both the pelvic and para-aortic nodes are involved, an inverted Y technique is used (as in Hodgkin's disease).

For involved mediastinal nodes, it is not necessary to include the cervical, infraclavicular or axillary nodes as in the mental technique.

Dose and Energy

The energy chosen will vary according to the site of involvement. For superficial nodes in the neck or the groin, orthovoltage (250–300 kV) is often adequate. For bulky nodes megavoltage is advised.

Dose 30 Gy in 15 fractions over 3 weeks is adequate for low-grade lymphoma localized disease (high-grade).

Technique

This is similar to that for low-grade disease. Care should be taken to avoid delivering more than 40 Gy in 20 daily fractions to the spinal cord, either by excluding it from the field or shielding the cord with a central lead block placed over the spine.

Dose and Energy

A higher dose is required than for low-grade disease.

40 Gy applied (250–300 kV) or midplane dose (4–6 MV photons) in 20 daily fractions over 4 weeks.

Chapter 20

Gallbladder Cancer

The gallbladder is pear shaped 7.5 to 12.5 cm long with a normal capacity about 50 ml but capable of considerable amount of distension GB divided into fundus/body/neck.

1. Common bile duct = 7.5 cm large common hepatic duct and cystic duct union forms common bile duct which has divided into four parts
    a. Supraduodenal portion
    b. Retroduodenal portion
    c. Infraduodenal portion
    d. Intraduodenal portion

It opens obliquely through the wall of IInd part of duodenum where it is surrounded by sphincter of Oddi. This infraduodenal portion of CBD opens on a papilla of Vater (Fig. 20.1A). For gallbladder cancer diagnosis is confirmed usually by FNAC (Fig. 20.1B) or in early stage after surgery postoperative histopathological examination of specimen of gallbladder.

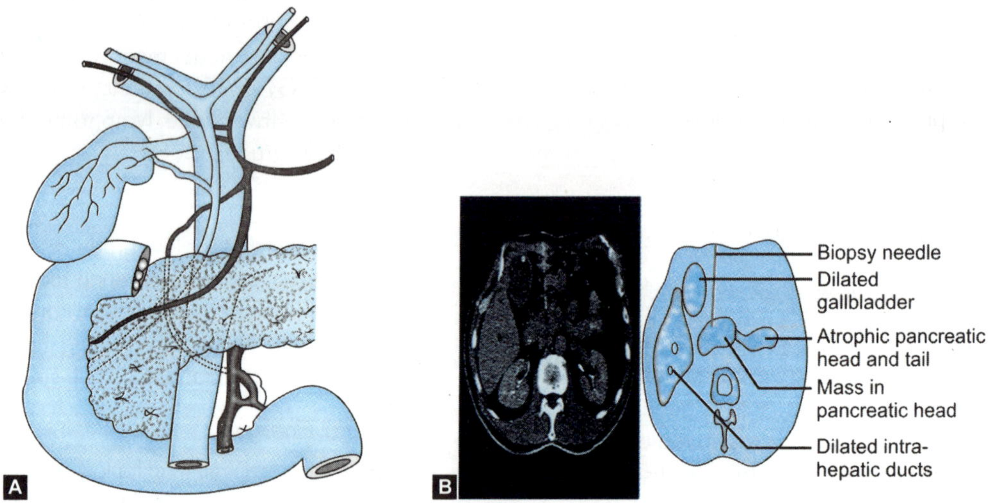

Figs 20.1A and B: (A) Anatomical relation of gallbladder; (B) FNAC CT guided to confirm diagnosis

ARTERY SUPPLY OF GALLBLADDER

1. Cystic artery supplies the gallbladder which is the branch of right hepatic artery.

   Lymphatic vessels of GB (subserosal and submucosal drain into cystic lymph node of Lund which lies in the fork created by the junction of cystic duct and common hepatic duct (Fig. 20.2). The subserosal lymphatics of GB also connected with subcapsular lymphatic channel of liver this is the reason why CAGB frequently spread to liver at the earliest. Liver exerts bile at the rate of 40 ml/ hr to GB.

2. Role of GB
   a. Act as reservoir
   b. Concentration of hepatic bile 5 to 10 times.

3. CAGB shows increased incidence with increase in age, peak incidence is in 7th decade of life. MF suction vary from 1:2 or 1:5. Geographically South India have lower incidence of CAGB. North or Central India have high incidence.

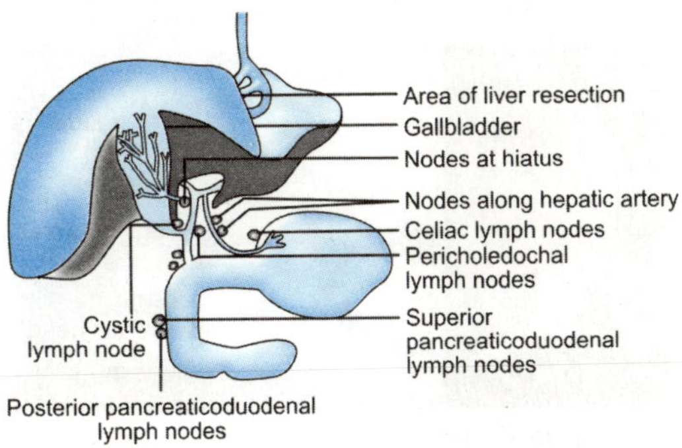

Fig. 20.2: Anatomy and regional lymph node

CAGB Etiology/Risk Factor

1. Most widely recognized risk factor for CAGB is cholelithiasis, the association between 70 to 98 percent of CAGB gallstone is present.
2. Cumulative risk of CAGB for a patient of gall-stone is not enough to justify prophylactic cholecystectomy for preventing CAGB.
3. CAGB with GB stone relation is that stone cause recurrent change to GB mucosa and bouts of acute/chronic inflammation of GB mucosa and generation of carcinogen in bile by action of bacteria.
4. Procelain gallbladder is a significant risk factor for CAGB (risk 12–61%) thus, there is course of procelain gallbladder prophylactic cholecystectom justified (procelain GB when wall of GB calcified).
5. Chronic typhoid carriers risk 6 times greater than general person to develop CAGB.
6. Ulcerative colitis increase risk for CAGB.
7. Adenomyomatosis of CAGB wall is risk for CAGB mainly in segmental type adenomyo-matosis (6.4%), diffuse type having risk in 3.4 percent cases.

PATHOLOGY OF CAGB

1. Adenocarcinoma of GB is commonest histology 85 percent to followed by squamous cell carcinoma—the adenoma squamous cell carcinoma in adenocarcinoma tubular variety is commonest variety.
2. Pattern of spread—Local infiltration and lymphatic spread are two commonest mode of spread.

3. Otherwise—Hematogenous spread, perineural spread, transperitoneal spread, intraductal spread.
4. Lymphatic drainage of gallbladder starts from an intramural plexus which is continuous through all layers of gallbladder wall, the plexus drain into large serosal lymphatic located along with inferior surface of gallbladder.

Histological Classification

1. Adenocarcinoma
2. Squamous cell carcinoma
3. Adenosquamous carcinoma
4. Clear cell carcinoma
5. Undifferentiated
6. Carcinoid tumors
7. Sarcomas
8. Melanoma
9. Lymphoma
   a. These lymphatic are drain into pericholedochal lymph node (along with the common bile duct) either directly or through cystic lymph node of Lund. Both these above lymph node drain into superior pancreaticoduodenal or retropancreatic node these node ultimately drain into celic gap of lymph node. The retroperitoneal LN drain ultimately into par-aortic LN. Per neural spread commonly seen in CAGB. Transperitoneal spread occur in late stage of disease manifest omental involvement and peritoneal seedlings/ascites Table 20.1.

Table 20.1 Pattern of spread

LN metastasis	50.7%	At autopsy CAGB patient show	
Lymphatic permeation	64.7%	Involvement of liver	90%
Venous invasion	46.6%	Regional LN	70%
Perineal spread	42%	Para-aortic LN	60%
		Bile duct involvement	60%
		SCF LN	33%

CLINICAL FEATURES

Majority of the patients present in stage III or IV. Usually CAGB case has been found to have very advance stage at presentation (Fig. 20.3) advance stage GB cancer.

Early CAGB imported and incidental discovery at operation or postoperative. HPE of GB. Local adenocarcinoma CAGB shows (Right upper quadrant abdominal pain, dyspepsia, anorexia, nausea, vomiting). Cholecystogram is a method is nowadays not common method to perform before gallbladder surgery (Figs 20.4A and B).

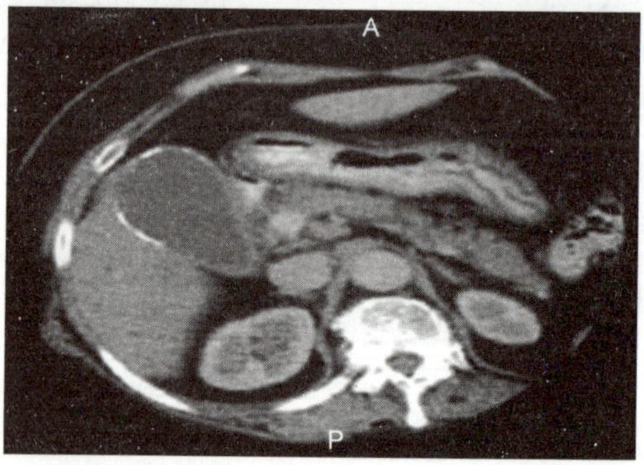

Fig. 20.3: CECT abdomen showing GB cancer

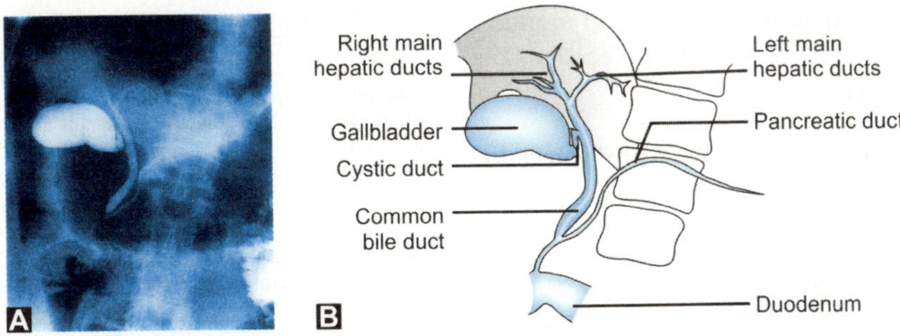

Figs 20.4A and B: (A) Cholecystogram; (B) Surgical anatomy of gallbladder

MANAGEMENT OF CAGB

Early stage tumor is curable by surgery with good long-term survival. Currently surgery is the primary modularity of curative treatment for early CAGB currently RT and chemo also used treatment improve the outcome in these patients.

SURGERY FOR CARCINOMA OF THE GALLBLADDER

1. To ensure the prolonged recurrence free survival surgical resection should include potential sites of microscopic tumor spread which are the adjacent liver bed draining LN cholecystogram.
2. Simple cholecystectomy done for the benign gallbladder disease.
3. In CAGB extended cholecystectomy has to be done. It comprises of enblock removal of GB, adjacent liver, portal lymphadenopathy.
4. Liver resection carried out with 2 to 5 cm margin and anatomical resection of segment IVb/V. More extensive liver resection is not required when direct infiltration of liver by tumor is absent.
   a. In CAGB we resects (during wedge resection of liver segment V and segment IV) but in CAGB with liver infiltration for direct infiltration of liver anatomical resection of segments IV, V and segment VI to be resected out.
   b. Infiltration of tumor in portal vein or hepatic artery is usually considered as criteria of nonresectability by most of the surgeons.

COMPLICATIONS AFTER SURGERY

Major complications are anastomotic leakage, liver failure, respiratory failure, intra-abdominal bleed with overall mortality seen in 5.3 percent cases. Major complication seen after surgery:

1. 48.3 percent complication in major hepatic resection
2. 21.9 percent in extended cholecystectomy
3. 12 percent in simple cholecystectomy

4. There is no significant difference in mortality rate in extended vs simple cholecystectomy (2.9 vs 2.3%).

Surgery for (Occult CAGB) Carcinoma *In Situ* (Tables 20.2 and 20.3)

Simple cholecystectomy is significant. T1a lesion of CAGB simple cholecystectomy 5-year survival up to 60 to 100 percent. For T1b lesion 5-year survival is 40 to 72 percent. If simple cholecystectomy carried out for disease infiltrating subserosal or serosal layer result are relatively poor. To avoid the problem of surprise diagnosis of CAGB after simple cholecystectomy when GB specimen send for HPE. It is recommended that all resected GB during operation for stone should be open and seen for examining carefully any tumor/polyp/GB wall thickening. Extended cholecystectomy is the answer when CAGB incidentally discovered during GB stone surgery.

Palliation Treatment

Contraindication to the surgery for CAGB: Multiple liver met's extensive liver infiltration ascitis, multiple peritoneal infiltration, tumor infiltrated to portal vein or hepatic artery. When surgery is not possible palliative treatment is only choice. Surgical palliation (ERCP) stenting to overcome obstructive jaundice or surgical intervention in duodenal/ colonic obstruction.

Table 20.2: Nevin's and TNM definitions CAGB

Nevins	*TNM*	*Definition*
I-Intramucosal	0	T1s-CIS
II-Extends to muscularis	I	T1a-invades mucosa; T1b-invades muscularis
III-Extends through the serosa	II	T2-invades perimuscular tissue, no extension beyond serosa
IV-Transmural involvement and cystic nodes involved	III	T3-perforates serosa or invades one organ (<2 cm into liver); regional nodes involved
V- Direct extension to liver	IV	T4->2 cm into liver or invades Two organs or second level nodes involved

Table 20.3: TNM staging system for gallbladder carcinoma

Primary tumor	
T1	Tumor invades the lamina propria or muscular layer Tumor invades the perimuscular connective tissue but not through
T2	Serosa
T3	Tumor perforates the serosa but <2 cm into liver
T4	Tumor extends >2 cm into liver or invades ≥2 adjacent organs
Regional lymph nodes	
N1	Tumor in cystic, parochial, or hilar lymph nodes Tumor peripancreatic, periduodenal, celiac, or superior mesenteric
N2	Lymph nodes
Distant metastases	
M1	Distant metastases
Stage	
1	T1, N0, M0
2	T2, N0, M0
3	T1, T2 or T3; N1, M0 T3, N0, M0
4A	T4
4B	N2 or M1

RADIOTHERAPY ROLE IN GALLBLADDER CANCER

After surgery recurrence of the disease in liver bed or regional lymph node metastasis thus logical to consider the RT as adjuvant treatment after surgical resection of GB. Postoperative radiotherapy after conservative surgery radiotherapy 45Gy/25 fraction provides median survival of 16 months. IORT also practice in CAGB single dose of 20 to 30 Gy given during surgery followed by EBRT 30 Gy. Palliative RT in nonoperable disease 2600 CGy usually given. Currently role of adjuvant postoperator. Radiotherapy is not very well defined Fig. 20.5.

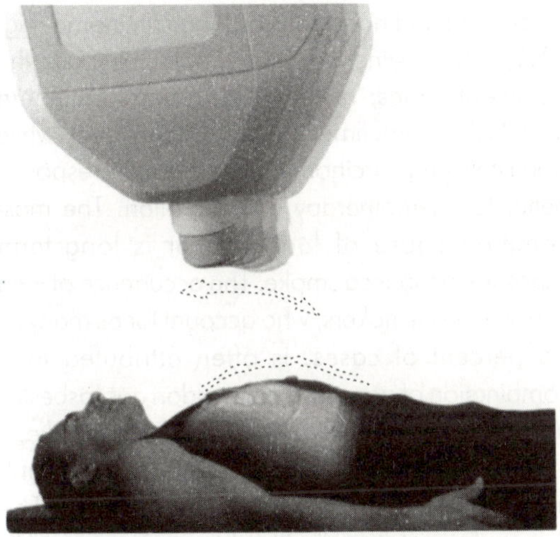

Fig. 20.5: Radiotherapy in GB cancer

Chemotherapy

1. 5 Fu/Mitomycin/Gemcitabine/Cisplatin having a promising result in nonoperable cases.
2. 5 Fu 500 mg/m^2 D1 to D5 4 weekly response rate 18 percent

Advantage	Disadvantage
Low-cost	Low response

3. FAM

5 Fu	600 mg/m^2 D_1 To D_3
Adriamycin	40 mg/m^2 D_2 3 weekly
Mitomycin	10 mg/m^2 D_1

Advantage	Disadvantage
High response rate 31 percent	highly toxicity

Modern chemo agent: Gemcitabine 1gm/m^2 D_1D_8 cisplatin 50 mg/m^2 D_2 3 weekly no advantage no toxicity and high response rate (50%) disadvantage high-cost incorrect infusion may lead to significant myelosuppression, overall with gemcitabine response rate noted 37 percent till now alonge with cisplatin, capecitabine also useful drug.

Chapter 21 Lung Cancer

INTRODUCTION

Lung cancer is a disease of uncontrolled cell growth in tissues of the lung. This growth may lead to metastasis, which is the invasion of adjacent tissue and infiltration beyond the lungs. The vast majority of primary lung cancers are carcinomas of the lung, derived from epithelial cells. Lung cancer, the most common cause of cancer-related death in men and women, is responsible for 1.3 million deaths worldwide annually, as of 2004. The most common symptoms are shortness of breath, coughing (including coughing with blood) and weight loss. The main types of lung cancer are small cell lung carcinoma and nonsmall cell lung carcinoma (Fig. 21.1). This distinction is important, because the treatment varies; nonsmall cell lung carcinoma (NSCLC) is sometimes treated with surgery, while small cell lung carcinoma (SCLC) usually responds better to chemotherapy and radiation. The most common cause of lung cancer is long-term exposure to tobacco smoke. The occurrence of lung cancer in nonsmokers, who account for as many as 15 percent of cases, is often attributed to a combination of genetic factors, radon gas, asbestos and air pollution, including secondhand smoke.

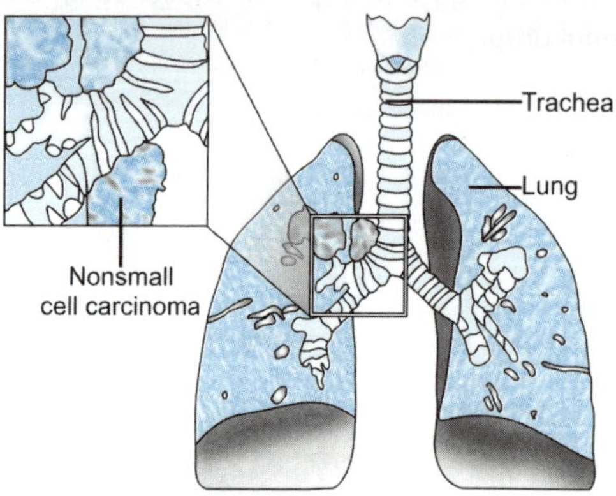

Fig. 21.1: Nonsmall cell carcinoma

Lung cancer may be seen on chest radiograph and computed tomography (CT scan). The diagnosis is confirmed with a biopsy. This is usually performed by bronchoscopy or CT-guided biopsy. Treatment and prognosis depend upon the histological type of cancer, the stage (degree of spread) and the patient's performance status. Possible treatments include surgery, chemotherapy and radiotherapy. Depending on the stage and treatment, the five-year survival rate is 14 percent.

Classification

The vast majority of lung cancers are carcinomas—malignancies that arise from epithelial cells. There are two main types of lung carcinoma, categorized by the size and appearance of the malignant cells seen by a histopathologist (Table 21.1) under a microscope: nonsmall cell (80.4%) and small cell (16.8%) lung carcinoma. This classification, based on histological criteria, has important implications for clinical management and prognosis of the disease.

Table 21.1: Frequency of histological types of lung cancer

Histological type	Frequency (%)
Nonsmall cell lung carcinoma	80.4
Small cell lung carcinoma	16.8
Carcinoid	0.8
Sarcoma	0.1
Unspecified lung cancer	1.9

NONSMALL CELL LUNG CARCINOMA (NSCLC)

The nonsmall cell lung carcinomas are grouped together because their prognosis and management are similar. There are three main subtypes: squamous cell lung carcinoma, adenocarcinoma, and large cell lung carcinoma. Accounting for 25 percent of lung cancers, squamous cell lung carcinoma usually starts near a central bronchus. A hollow cavity and associated necrosis are commonly found at the center of the tumor. Well-differentiated squamous cell lung cancers often grow more slowly than other cancer types. Adenocarcinoma accounts for 40 percent of lung cancers. It usually originates in peripheral lung tissue. Most cases of adenocarcinoma are associated with smoking; however, among people who have never smoked ("never-smokers"), adenocarcinoma is the most common form of lung cancer. A subtype of adenocarcinoma, the bronchioloalveolar carcinoma, is more common in female never-smokers and may have different responses to treatment.

SMALL CELL LUNG CARCINOMA (SCLC)

Small cell lung carcinoma (Fig. 21.2) (microscopic view of a core needle biopsy).

Small cell lung carcinoma is less common. Also called oat cell cancer, it tends to arise in the larger airways (primary and secondary bronchi) and grows rapidly, becoming quite large. The small cells contains dense neurosecretory granules (vesicles containing neuroendocrine hormones), which give this an endocrine/paraneoplastic syndrome association. While initially more sensitive to chemotherapy, it ultimately carries a worse prognosis and is often metastatic at presentation. Small cell lung cancers are divided into limited stage and extensive stage disease. This type of lung cancer is strongly associated with smoking.

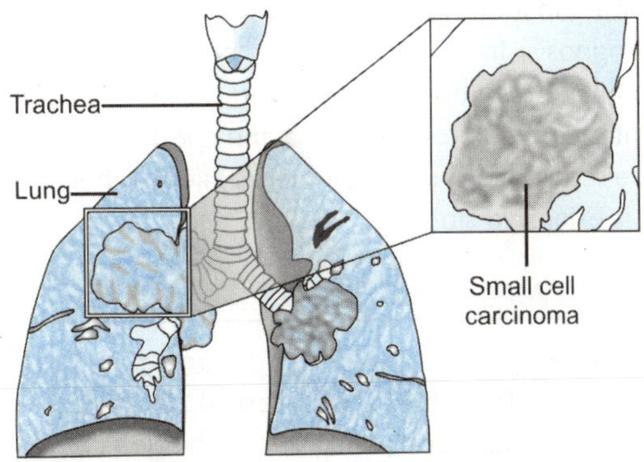

Fig. 21.2: Small cell lung carcinoma

Others

In infants and children, the most common primary lung cancers are pleuropulmonary blastoma and carcinoid tumor.

The lung is a common place for metastasis from tumors in other parts of the body. These secondary lungs cancers are identified by the site of origin; thus, a breast cancer metastasis to the lung is still known as breast cancer. They often have a characteristic round appearance on chest radiograph. In children, the majority of lung cancers are secondary (Fig. 21.3).

Primary lung cancers themselves most commonly metastasize to the adrenal glands, liver, brain and bone.

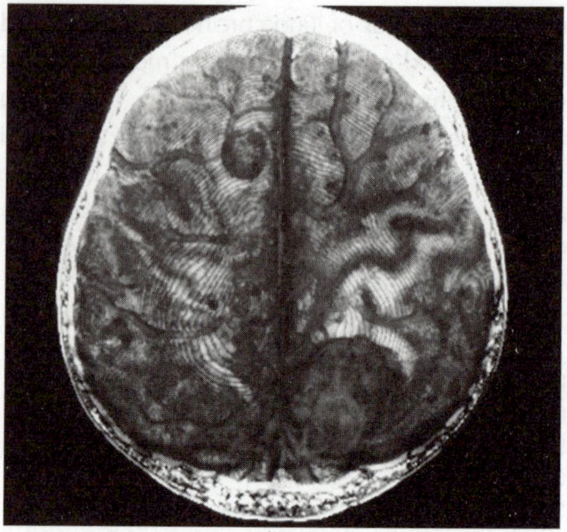

Fig. 21.3: Brain metastasis in lung cancer *(For color version, see Plate 1)*

Staging

Lung cancer staging is an assessment of the degree of spread of the cancer from its original source. It is an important factor affecting the prognosis and potential treatment of lung cancer. Nonsmall cell lung carcinoma is staged from IA ("one A"; best prognosis) to IV ("four"; worst prognosis). Small cell lung carcinoma is classified as limited stage, if it is confined to one-half of the chest and within the scope of a single radiotherapy field; otherwise, it is extensive stage.

SIGNS AND SYMPTOMS

Symptoms that suggest lung cancer include: Dyspnea (shortness of breath), hemoptysis (coughing up blood), chronic coughing or change in regular coughing pattern, wheezing, chest pain or pain in the abdomen, cachexia (weight loss), fatigue, and loss of appetite, dysphonia (hoarse voice) clubbing of the fingernails (uncommon) dysphagia (difficulty swallowing). If the cancer grows in the airway, it may obstruct airflow, causing breathing difficulties. This can lead to accumulation of secretions behind the blockage, predisposing the patient to pneumonia. Many lung cancers have a rich blood supply. The surface of the cancer may be fragile, leading to bleeding from the cancer into the airway. This blood may subsequently be coughed up. Depending on the type of tumor, so called paraneoplastic phenomena may initially attract attention to the disease. In lung cancer, these phenomena may include Lambert-Eaton myasthenic syndrome (muscle weakness due to autoantibodies), hypercalcemia, or syndrome of inappropriate antidiuretic hormone (SIADH). Tumors in the top (apex) of the lung, known as Pancoast tumors, may invade the local part of the sympathetic nervous system, leading to changed sweating patterns and eye muscle problems (a combination known as Horner's syndrome) as well as muscle weakness in the hands due to invasion of the brachial plexus.

Many of the symptoms of lung cancer (bone pain, fever and weight loss) are nonspecific; in the elderly, these may be attributed to comorbid illness. In many patients, the cancer has already spread beyond the original site by the time they have symptoms and seek medical attention. Common sites of metastasis include the brain, bone, adrenal glands, contralateral (opposite) lung, liver, pericardium and kidneys. About 10 percent of people with lung cancer do not have symptoms at diagnosis; these cancers are incidentally found on routine chest radiograph.

Causes

The main causes of any cancer includes carcinogens (such as those in tobacco smoke), ionizing radiation and viral infection. This exposure causes cumulative changes to the DNA in the tissue lining, the bronchi of the lungs (the bronchial epithelium). As more tissues become damaged, eventually a cancer develops.

Smoking

Following an increase in smoking in the population, the rate of lung cancer death increases. Smoking, particularly of cigarettes, is by far the main contributor to lung cancer. Across the developed world, almost 90 percent of lung cancer deaths are caused by smoking. In the United States, smoking is estimated to account for 87 percent of lung cancer cases 90 percent in men and 85 percent in women. Among male smokers, the lifetime risk of developing lung cancer is 17.2 percent; among female smokers, the risk is 11.6 percent. This risk is significantly lower in nonsmokers: 1.3 in men and 1.4 percent in women. Cigarette smoke contains over 60 known carcinogens, including radioisotopes from the radon decay sequence, nitrosamine and benzopyrene. Additionally, nicotine appears to depress the immune response to malignant growths in exposed tissue. The time a person smokes (as well as rate of smoking) increases the person's chance of developing lung cancer. If a person stops smoking, this chance steadily decreases as damage to the lungs is repaired and contaminant particles are gradually removed. In addition, there is evidence that lung cancer in never-smokers has a better prognosis than in smokers and that patients who smoke at the time of diagnosis have shorter survival times than those who have quit. Passive smoking—the inhalation of smoke from another's smoking—is a cause of lung cancer in nonsmokers. A passive smoker can be classified as someone living or working with a smoker as well. Studies have consistently shown a significant increase in relative risk among those exposed to passive smoke. Recent investigation of sidestream smoke suggests that it is more dangerous than direct smoke inhalation (Fig. 21.4).

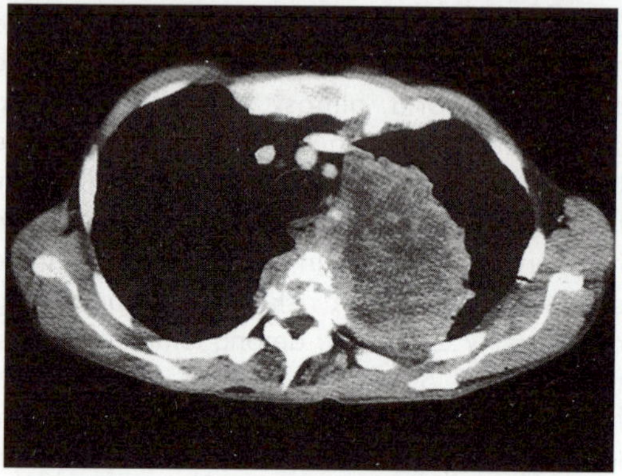

Fig. 21.4: CECT thorax showing left lung mass

CECT THORAX OF LUNG CANCER

Roughly ten to fifteen percent of lung cancer patients have never smoked. That means between 20,000 to 30,000 never-smokers are diagnosed with lung cancer in the United States each year. Because of the five-year survival rate, each year in the US more never-smokers die of lung cancer than do patients of leukemia, ovarian cancer, or AIDS.

Radon gas: Radon is a colorless and odorless gas generated by the breakdown of radioactive radium, which in turn is the decay product of uranium, found in the Earth's crust. The radiation decay products ionize genetic material, causing mutations that sometimes turn cancerous. Radon exposure is the second major cause of lung cancer, after smoking, Radon gas levels vary by locality and the composition of the underlying soil and rocks. For example, in areas such as Cornwall in the UK (which has granite as substrata), radon gas is a major problem, and buildings have to be force-ventilated with fans to lower radon gas concentrations. The United States Environmental Protection Agency (EPA) estimates that one in 15 homes in the US has radon levels above the recommended guideline of 4 picocuries per liter (pCi/L) (148 Bq/m^3). Lowa has the highest average radon concentration in the United States; studies performed there have demonstrated a 50 percent increased lung cancer risk, with prolonged radon exposure above the EPA's action level of 4 pCi/L.

Asbestos

Asbestos can cause a variety of lung diseases, including lung cancer. There is a synergistic effect between tobacco smoking and asbestos in the formation of lung cancer. In the UK, asbestos accounts for 2 to 3 percent of male lung cancer deaths. Asbestos can also cause cancer of the pleura, called *mesothelioma* (which is different from lung cancer).

Viruses

Viruses are known to cause lung cancer in animals and recent evidence suggests similar potential in humans. Implicated viruses include human papillomavirus, JC virus, simian virus 40 (SV 40), BK virus and cytomegalovirus. These viruses may affect the cell cycle and inhibit apoptosis, allowing uncontrolled cell division.

Particulate matter—Studies of the American Cancer Society cohort directly link the exposure to particulate matter with lung cancer. For example, if the concentration of particles in the air increases by only 1 percent, the risk of developing a lung cancer increases by 14 percent. Further, it has been established that particle size matters, as ultrafine particles penetrate further into the lungs.

PATHOGENESIS

Similar to many other cancers, lung cancer is initiated by activation of oncogenes or inactivation of tumor suppressor genes. Oncogenes are genes that are believed to make people more susceptible to cancer. Proto-oncogenes are believed to turn into oncogenes when exposed to particular carcinogens. Mutations in the *K-ras* proto-oncogene are responsible for 10 to 30 percent of lung adenocarcinomas. The epidermal growth factor receptor (EGFR) regulates cell proliferation, apoptosis, angiogenesis and tumor invasion. Mutations and amplification of EGFR are common in nonsmall cell lung cancer and provide the basis for treatment with EGFR-inhibitors. Her2/neu is affected less frequently. Chromosomal damage can lead to loss of heterozygosity. This can cause inactivation of tumor suppressor genes. Damage to chromosomes 3p, 5q, 13q and 17p are particularly common in small cell lung carcinoma. The p53 tumor suppressor gene, located on chromosome 17p, is affected in 60 to 75 percent of cases. Other genes that are often mutated or amplified are *c-MET*, *NKX2-1*, *LKB1*, *PIK3CA* and *BRAF*.

Several genetic polymorphisms are associated with lung cancer. These include polymorphisms in genes coding for interleukin-1, cytochrome P450, apoptosis promoters such as caspase-8 and DNA repair molecules such as XRCC1. People with these polymorphisms are more likely to develop lung cancer after exposure to carcinogens.

A recent study suggested that the MDM2 309G allele, is a low-penetrant risk factor for developing lung cancer in Asians.

Diagnosis

Performing a chest radiograph is the first step, if a patient reports symptoms that may suggest lung cancer. This may reveal an obvious mass, widening of the mediastinum (suggestive of spread to lymph nodes there), atelectasis (collapse), consolidation (pneumonia), or pleural effusion. If there are no radiographic findings but the suspicion is high (such as a heavy smoker with blood-stained sputum), bronchoscopy and/or a CT scan may provide the necessary information. Bronchoscopy or CT-guided biopsy is often used to identify the tumor type.

Abnormal findings in cells ("atypia") in sputum are associated with an increased risk of lung cancer. Sputum cytologic examination combined with other screening examinations may have a role in the early detection of lung cancer.

The differential diagnosis for patients who present with abnormalities on chest radiograph includes lung cancer as well as nonmalignant diseases. These include infectious causes such as tuberculosis or pneumonia, or inflammatory conditions such as sarcoidosis. These diseases can result in mediastinal lymphadenopathy or lung nodules and sometimes mimic lung cancers. Lung cancer can also be an incidental finding: a solitary pulmonary nodule (also called a coin lesion) on a chest radiograph or CT scan taken for an unrelated reason.

Prevention

Prevention is the most cost-effective means of fighting lung cancer. While in most countries industrial and domestic carcinogens have been identified and banned, tobacco smoking is still widespread. Eliminating tobacco smoking is a primary goal in the prevention of lung cancer and smoking cessation is an important preventive tool in this process, Most importantly, are prevention programs that target the young. In 1998 the master settlement agreement entitled 46 states in the USA to an annual payout from the tobacco companies. Between the settlement money and tobacco taxes, each state's public health department funds their prevention programs, although none of the states are living up to the Center for Disease Control's recommended amount by spending 15 percent of tobacco taxes and settlement revenues on these prevention efforts. Policy interventions to decrease passive smoking in public areas such as restaurants and workplaces have become more common in many Western countries, with California taking a lead in banning smoking in public establishments in 1998. Ireland played a similar role in Europe in 2004, followed by Italy and Norway in 2005, Scotland as well as several others in 2006, England in 2007, France in 2008 and Turkey in 2009. New Zealand has banned smoking in public places as of 2004. The state of Bhutan has had a complete smoking ban since 2005. In many countries, pressure groups are campaigning for similar bans. In 2007, Chandigarh became the first city in India to become smoke-free. India introduced a total ban on smoking at public places on Oct 2, 2008.

Arguments cited against such bans are criminalization of smoking, increased risk of smuggling and the risk that such a ban cannot be enforced. The long-term use of supplemental multivitamins—such as vitamin C, vitamin E and folate—does not reduce the risk of lung cancer. Indeed long-term intake of high doses of vitamin E supplements may even increase the risk of lung cancer.

The World Health Organization has called for governments to institute a total ban on tobacco advertising to prevent young people from taking up smoking. They assess that such bans have reduced tobacco consumption by 16 percent where already instituted.

Screening

Lung Cancer Screening

Screening refers to the use of medical tests to detect disease in asymptomatic people. Possible screening tests for lung cancer include chest radiograph or computed tomography (CT).

Treatment of Lung Cancer

Treatment for lung cancer depends on the cancer's specific cell type, how far it has spread and the patient's performance status. Common treatments include surgery, chemotherapy and radiation therapy.

Surgery

Gross appearance of the cut surface of a pneumonectomy specimen containing a lung cancer, here a squamous cell carcinoma (the whitish tumor near the bronchi).

If investigations confirm lung cancer, CT scan and often positron emission tomography (PET) are used to determine whether the disease is localized and amenable to surgery or whether it has spread to the point where it cannot be cured surgically.

Blood tests and spirometry (lung function testing) are also necessary to assess whether the patient is well enough to be operated on. If spirometry reveals poor respiratory reserve (often due to chronic obstructive pulmonary disease), surgery may be contraindicated. Surgery itself has an operative death rate of about 4.4 percent, depending on the patient's lung function and other risk factors. Surgery is usually only an option in nonsmall cell lung carcinoma limited to one lung, up to stage IIIA. This is assessed with medical imaging (CT, PET). A sufficient preoperative respiratory reserve must be present to allow adequate lung function after the tissue is removed. Procedures include wedge resection (removal of part of a lobe), segmentectomy (removal of an anatomic division of a particular lobe of the lung), lobectomy (one lobe), bilobectomy (two lobes), or pneumonectomy (whole lung). In patients with adequate respiratory reserve, lobectomy is the preferred option, as this minimizes the chance of local recurrence. If the patient does not have enough functional lung for this, wedge resection may be performed. Radioactive iodine brachytherapy at the margins of wedge excision may reduce recurrence to that of lobectomy. Video-assisted thoracoscopic surgery and VATS lobectomy have allowed for minimally invasive approaches to lung cancer surgery that may have the advantages of quicker recovery, shorter hospital stay and diminished hospital costs.

CHEMOTHERAPY

Small cell lung carcinoma is treated primarily with chemotherapy and radiation, as surgery has no demonstrable influence on survival. Primary chemotherapy is also given in metastatic non-small cell lung carcinoma.

The combination regimen depends on the tumor type. Nonsmall cell lung carcinoma is often treated with cisplatin or carboplatin, in combination with gemcitabine, paclitaxel, docetaxel, etoposide, or vinorelbine. In small cell lung carcinoma, cisplatin and etoposide are most commonly used. Combinations with carboplatin, gemcitabine, paclitaxel, vinorelbine, topotecan, and irinotecan are also used. in extensive-stage small cell lung cancer celecoxib may safely be combined with etoposide, this combination showed improve outcomes.

Adjuvant Chemotherapy for NSCLC

Adjuvant chemotherapy refers to the use of chemotherapy after surgery to improve the outcome. During surgery, samples are taken from the lymph nodes. If these samples contain cancer, the patient has stage II or III disease. In this situation, adjuvant chemotherapy may improve survival by up to 15 percent. Standard practice is to offer platinum-based chemotherapy (including either cisplatin or carboplatin). Adjuvant chemotherapy for patients with stage IB cancer is controversial, as clinical trials have not clearly demonstrated a survival benefit. Trials of preoperative chemotherapy (neoadjuvant chemotherapy) in resectable nonsmall cell lung carcinoma have been inconclusive.

Radiotherapy

Radiotherapy is often given together with chemotherapy and may be used with curative intent in patients with nonsmall cell lung carcinoma who are not eligible for surgery. This form of high intensity radiotherapy is called radical radiotherapy. A refinement of this technique is continuous hyperfractionated accelerated radiotherapy (CHART), in which a high dose of radiotherapy is given in a short time period. For small cell lung carcinoma cases that are potentially curable, chest radiation is often recommended in addition to chemotherapy. The use of adjuvant thoracic radiotherapy following curative intent surgery for nonsmall cell lung carcinoma is not well-established and is controversial. Benefits, if any, may only be limited to those in whom the tumor has spread to the mediastinal lymph nodes.

For both nonsmall cell lung carcinoma and small cell lung carcinoma patients, smaller doses of radiation to the chest may be used for symptom control (palliative radiotherapy). Unlike other treatments, it is possible to deliver palliative radiotherapy without confirming the histological diagnosis of lung cancer, sometimes for brain mets (Fig. 21.1) palliative radiotherapy 30 Gy in 10 fraction used.

Brachytherapy (localized radiotherapy) may be given directly inside the airway when cancer affects a short section of bronchus. It is used when inoperable lung cancer causes blockage of a large airway. Patients with limited stage small cell lung carcinoma are usually given prophylactic cranial irradiation (PCI). This is a type of radiotherapy to the brain, used to reduce the risk of metastasis. More recently, PCI has also been shown to be beneficial in those with extensive small cell lung cancer. In patients whose cancer has improved following a course of chemotherapy, PCI has been shown to reduce the cumulative risk of brain metastases within one-year from 40.4 to 14.6 percent.

Recent improvements in targeting and imaging have led to the development of extracranial stereotactic radiation in the treatment of early stage lung cancer. In this form of radiation therapy, very high doses are delivered in a small number of sessions using stereotactic targeting techniques. Its use is primarily in patients who are not surgical candidates due to medical comorbidities.

In recent years, various molecular targeted therapies have been developed for the treatment of advanced lung cancer. Gefitinib (Iressa) is one such drug, which targets the tyrosine kinase domain of the epidermal growth factor receptor (EGFR), expressed in many cases of nonsmall cell lung carcinoma. It was not shown to increase survival, although females, Asians, nonsmokers and those with bronchioloalveolar carcinoma appear to derive the most benefit from gefitinib.

Erlotinib (Tarceva), another tyrosine kinase inhibitor, has been shown to increase survival in lung cancer patients and has recently been approved by the FDA for second-line treatment of advanced non-small cell lung carcinoma. Similar to gefitinib, it also appeared to work best in females, Asians, nonsmokers and those with bronchioloalveolar carcinoma. The angiogenesis inhibitor bevacizumab, (in combination with paclitaxel and carboplatin), improves the survival of patients with advanced nonsmall cell lung carcinoma. However, this increases the risk of lung bleeding, particularly in patients with squamous cell carcinoma.

Advances in cytotoxic drugs, pharmacogenetics and targeted drug design show promise. A number of targeted agents are at the early stages of clinical research, such as cyclo-oxygenase-2 inhibitors the apoptosis promoter exisulind, proteasome inhibitors, bexarotene the epidermal growth factor receptor inhibitor cetuximab and vaccines. Future areas of research include ras proto-oncogene inhibition, phosphoinositide 3-kinase inhibition, histone deacetylase inhibition and tumor suppressor gene replacement.

Prognosis: Nonsmall cell lung carcinoma staging and Manchester score.

Prognostic factors in nonsmall cell lung cancer include presence or absence of pulmonary symptoms, tumor size, cell type (histology), degree of spread (stage) and metastases to multiple lymph nodes and vascular invasion. For patients with inoperable disease, prognosis is adversely affected by poor performance status and weight loss of more than 10 percent. Prognostic factors in small-cell lung cancer include performance status, gender, stage of disease and involvement of the central nervous system or liver at the time of diagnosis. For example, nonsmall cell lung carcinoma, prognosis is generally poor. Following complete surgical resection of stage IA disease, five-year survival is 67 percent. With stage IB disease, five-year survival is 57 percent. The five-year survival rate of patients with stage IV NSCLC is about 1 percent for small cell lung carcinoma, prognosis is also generally poor. The overall five-year survival for patients with SCLC is about 5 percent. Patients with extensive-stage SCLC have an average five-year survival rate of less than 1 percent. The median survival time for limited-stage disease is 20 months, with a five-year survival rate of 20 percent. According to data provided by the National Cancer Institute, the median age of incidence of lung cancer is 70 years and the median age of death by lung cancer is 71 years.

Chapter 22 Carcinoma Larynx

Larynx is a specialized organ that provides a protective sphincter at the inlet of the air passages and responsible for voice production. Larynx above open into laryngeal part of pharynx and below it is continuous with the trachea. Larynx situated infront of neck and lies opposite IIIrd to VIth cervical vertebra. Larynx has a cartilaginous framework supported by ligaments and muscles (Figs 22.1 and 22.2).

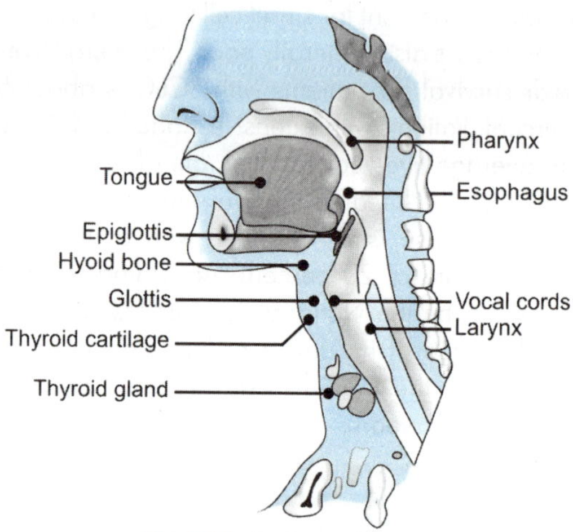

Fig. 22.1: Anatomy of larynx

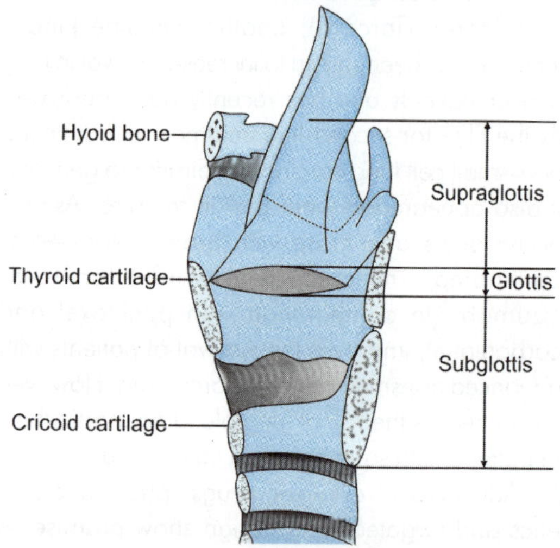

Fig. 22.2: Anatomical landmark in larynx

INDIRECT LARYNGOSCOPIC MIRROR VIEW (FIG. 22.3)

Posterolateral to the larynx on either side lies hypopharynx it extent from aryepiglottic fold at the level of hyoid bone to the inferior border of cricoid cartilage.

Larynx is divided into three parts:

1. Supraglottic larynx (epiglottis, arytenoid cartilage AE fold, false cord).

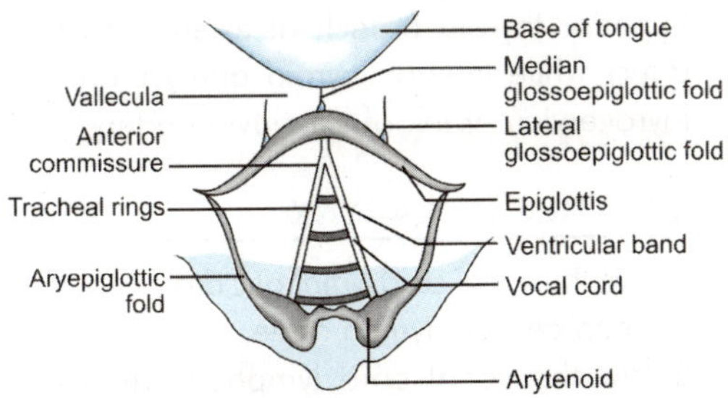

Fig. 22.3: Indirect laryngoscopic mirror view

2. Glottis larynx (true vocal cord) + ANT/Post-commissure.
3. Subglottic larynx lies 5 mm below the free margin of vocal cord in its mid point and 2 mm at the anterior commissure).

Note: Tumors of middle and anterior vocal cord with less than 1 cm extention usually may be easily resected without including cricoid.

TRANSGLOTTIC CARCINOMA

McGavran(1961), first used this term to define a tumor that crossed the ventricle and thus involved the glottis and supraglottis and in some cases subglottis. This topographic term was meant to describe the areas involved by carcinoma and did not imply site of origin. More recently Hao defined transglottic carcinoma as lesions that show supraglottic invasion from glottic region or that show evidence of paraglottic space involvement on radiologic pathologic examination.

The term transglottic carcinoma does not imply a site of origin. The current AJCC system of classification are based on site of origin and thus do not include a category for transglottic carcinoma.

Transglottic carcinoma are associated with highest rate of cervical metastasis with positive node in 52 percent of cases.

CONNECTIVE TISSUE BARRIERS OF THE LARYNX

(laryngeal compartments).

Rinke's Space

Mucosa overlying the vocal cords is loosely attached, there is a potential space extending submucosally for almost the whole length of the membranous cord is called Rinke's space.

Pre-epiglottic Space

In front of epiglottis a potential space lies which is rich in lymphatic channels commonly know as pre-epiglottic space. It is bounded superiorly by hyoepiglottic mucosa and vallecular mucosa, anteriorly by thyrohyoid membrane and thyroid cartilage and posteriorly by epiglottis and thyroepiglottic ligament. It communicates with paraglottic space laterally.

Paraglottic Space

The space is bounded medially by ventricles and laterally by thyroid cartilage, inferomedially by conus elasticus and superomedially by quadrangular membrane. Its significance is related to the ease with which tumors involving the ventricles or deeply panetrating glottic or supraglottic carcinoma may invade this space with potential risk of reaching subglottis or extending extralaryngeally.

PREMALIGNANT CONDITIONS OF LARYNX (TABLE 22.1)

Chronic laryngitis

Adult—Pappiloma larynx

Hyperkeratosis/leukoplakia.

LARYNX BLOOD SUPPLY/LYMPHATIC CHAIN/NERVE SUPPLY

1. Vocal cords have stratified squamous epithelium without submucus layer having poor blood supply and almost devoid of lymphatics.
2. Larynx supplied by superior/inferior thyroid arteries.

Table 22.1: Tumors of Larynx

Benign tumors		
i. Pappiloma	Multiple pappiloma most commonly in children, viral in origin tendency to regress at puberty site ANT-commissure	Solitary pappiloma most common adult common
ii. Hemangioma	C/F change invoice, respiratory difficulty. T/T repeated surgical	C/F hoarseness of voice T/T through D/L scopy excision
iii. Fibroma	Excision	of a growth, sent tissue of HPE since it is a premalignant
iv. Chondroma		condition

3. Superior thyroid branch of external carotid-artery while inferior thyroid artery branch of thyrocervical trunk of subclavian artery.

LYMPHATICS OF LARYNX

1. Above the vocal card lymphatic drains upwards to deep cervical lymph node.
2. Below the vocal cord lymphatic drains by pretracheal/paratracheal/lower deep cervical less often drains to superior mediastinal lymph node.
3. Vocal cord itself devoid of lymphatic channels.

NERVE SUPPLY

1. Sensory supply of the mucosa above vocal cord is by superior laryngeal nerve, same nerve is motor to cricothyroid muscle (palsy cause weakness in voice).
2. Mucosa below cord sensory as well as motor supply of all laryngeal muscles (except cricothyroid) by recurrent laryngeal nerve.

EPIDEMIOLOGY/ETIOLOGY

1. Larynx cancer is most common in male
2. Male female ratio is 12:1 for glottic cancer 4 : 1 for supraglottic carcinoma (Ca)
3. Glottic Ca seen in both the class rich class and poor class.

RISK FACTORS FOR LARYNX CANCER

1. Smoking—four-fold in development of larynx Ca (Figs 22.4A and B)

2. Alcohol
3. Tobacco chewing—lesser risk factor than smoking otherwise chewing tobacco is the risk of hypopharyngeal Ca.

OTHER RISK FACTOR FOR CA LARYNX

1. HPV infection of larynx
2. Previous irradiation

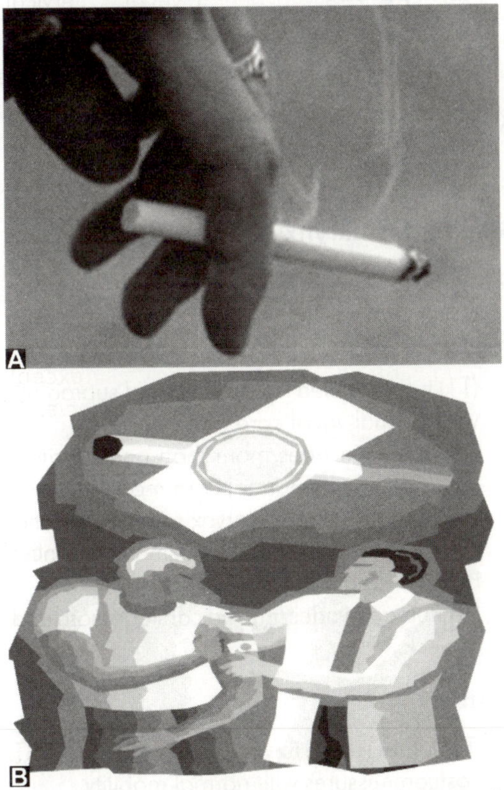

Figs 22.4 A and B: (A) Smocking is a major cause for lanyngeal cancer; (B) Doctor should ask the patient to stop it

3. Asbestos wood dust
4. Dietary deficiencies.

PATHOLOGY

- Most common squamous cell carcinoma (Ca) 95 percent
- SCC variants are spindle cell Ca verrucous Ca (well-differentiated-keratinizing epithelium)
- Adenosquamous Ca
- Sarcoma
- Laryngeal Ca accounts for 25 percent of all H/N cancers.

LOCAL AND DISTANT SPREAD OF LARYNX CA

Spread of larynx Ca mostly depend upon the anatomical location of growth.

GLOTTIC CA

Mostly tumor arises from free border of vocal cords growth mostly limited to ANT 2/3rds of vocal cord. Thus, ANT commissure involve in most of the cases when growth involves internal laryngeal muscles. Fixation of that side of cord occurs which is a poor prognostic factor.

Glottic Ca usually extend towards supraglottic region and thus percent of cervical LN involvement.

In 17 percent cases of glottic Ca opposite site of cord involvement occurs.

SUPRAGLOTTIC CA

Usually from postsurface of epiglottis or from false vocal cord/AE fold.

Commonly involve pre-epiglottic space anteriorly, may extent up to vallecula/but LAT extension involves PFF.

When growth limited up to supraglottic region main C/F will be throat pain hoarseness of voice.

But when growth extent and involve base of tongue (BOT)/pyriform sinus(PFF) dysphagia is a prominent feature.

Lesion arising from lingual surface of epiglottis considered as a extralaryngeal Ca and T/T like Ca BOT.

Subglottic Ca

It is a rare Ca of larynx less than 5 percent of total cases of larynx Ca comes under it. Subglottic region involve in downward extension of glottic Ca.

LYMPHATIC SPREAD

Glottic Ca

1. Vocal cord since devoid of lymphatic drainage age so, LN involvement in glottic Ca is less.
2. T1, T2 tumor without commissure involvement LN involvement is only less than 2 percent case.
3. But T1 T2 with anterior commissure involvement LN percent is little higher 5 to 10 percent.

Supraglottic Larynx

Since rich in lymphatics usually drains into level II/III lymph node (LN)

T1/T2 40 percent LN +ve

T3/T4 55 percent LN +ve

But if growth extending to BOT/Hypopharynx LN percent of involvement TN supraglottic is 70 percent or more overall occult metastasis in supraglottic larynx is around 35 percent.

Subglottic Larynx Ca

Subglottic Ca lymphatic drains into pretracheal/paratracheal/lower cervical LN, over 5 to 20 percent cases LN involvement.

Distant Spread

1. 10 percent cases of laryngeal Ca have distant mets. Distant mets is higher (50%) cases supraglottic Ca than glottic Ca (16%).
2. Distant spread involves (mediastinal, Lymph node, lung, liver, pleura, spleen, kidney).

Staging for Larynx Ca

UICC/AJCC-TNM 2002, followed presently.

Supraglottis

1. (T1) tumor limited to one subsite of supraglottis with normal vocal cord mobility.
2. (T2) tumor invades more than one subsite of supraglottis with normal cord mobility.
3. (T3) tumor limited to larynx with cord fixation or involve post cricoid area/medical wall of PFF/pre-epiglottic space.
4. (T4) tumor invades/thyroid cartilage/soft tissue of neck.

Glottis

1. (T1) tumor limited to vocal card or involve ANT/postcommissures with normal mobility
   T1a limited to one cord
   T1b involve both cord

2. (T2) tumor extend to supra or subglottic larynx with normal vocal cord mobility.
3. (T3) Tumor limited to Lx with vocal cord fixed.
4. (T4) Tumor invades/thyroid cartilage/ oropharynx/soft tissue of neck.

Subglottic

1. (T1) limited to subglottic Lx.
2. (T2) tumor extend to Lx with normal or impaired cord mobility.
3. (T3) tumor limited to Lx with vocal cord fixed.
4. (T4) tumor invades/thyroid/soft tissue neck.

Regional LN

- (N1) mets in single ipsilateral lymph node, 3 cm or less in any greatest dimension
- (N2)A mets in single ipsilateral LN $\geq$3 cm to 6 cm
- (N2)B multiple ipsilateral LN >3 cm to 6 cm
- (N2)C B/L neck node but no node more than 6 cm
- (N3) mets in LN more than 6 cm in maximum dimension
- This TNM system of classification is only an anatomical means of classification which does not takes account of tumor biological aggressiveness of several host factor
- So only TNM stage does not provide the best guide for T/T and prognosis for an individual patient
- Thus LCA (laryngeal cancer association) has done survey and given opinion about several factor which influence T/T outcome in laryngeal Ca
- Absence of extracapsular spread in LN
- Clear resection margin (is surgeon able to get adequate margin)
- Location of primary in glottic region rather in supra/subglottic region
- Cessation of smoking/alcohol intake.

Prognostic Factor for Larynx Ca

- Host factor
- Tumor factor
- Treatment factor.

Host Factor

- Age : Young age good prognosis
- Sex : Shows better response to T/T
- GC : Low KPS/poor nutritional status prognosis.

Tumor Factor

Size/site/location/cord fixation/LN status and its extracapsular spread. All influence T/T outcome, lymph node status is single most important prognostic factor.

T/T Factors

- After Sx patients those have +ve margin
- –ve Margin will have chances of recurrence
- Residual Tx after complication of RT is a poor prognostic sign.

CLINICAL PRESENTATION

- Hoarseness of voice main complain for glottic Ca, thus glottic Ca present early—good prognosis results

- Hoarseness and dysphagia, irritable cough, sometimes hemoptysis occurs in supraglottic Ca
- Dispnea/stridor are due to occlusion of airway by glottic or transglottic Ca in late stage
- Fullness/swelling in the anterior side of neck seen when growth infiltrates the cartilage/soft tissue of the neck
- Usually larynx moves laterally on vertebral column it produces a grating sensation called as laryngeal crepitus which normally elicited when growth extent in postcricoid region or in case of retropharyngeal lesion this is absent as the larynx pushed forwards and its movement over vertebral column do not occur.

Pretreatment Work-up for Larynx Ca

- Detail history
- Physical examination
- I/L examination
- D/L examination
- Clinical examination/palpation of Lx/neck, chest X-ray
- Radiography of the Lx → simple X-ray laryngogram, CT scan of neck.

Indirect Laryngoscopy

- You can see, BOT, valleculae, lingual aspect of epiglottis, by tilting mirror aryepiglottic fold/ arytenoid cartilage, false cord (vestibular band appear as dull red bands above the true vocal cords)
- Mobility of true vocal cord tested by asking patient to phonate-E
- We also see PFF, part of postpharyngeal wall.

Difficulties in Indirect Larynx Examination

- Patient not cooperative having GAG reflex local spray of lignocaine 10 percent may help
- Difficult in short neck person
- Difficult in children.

Structure that you Cannot See with I/L Examination

- Laryngeal aspect of epiglottis
- ANT commissure
- Subglottis region
- Cord mobility best seen with I/L examination.

Use of DL Scopy

- Performed in OT user Ga/LA
- With rigid/flexible fiberoptic endoscope. Visualization is superior with D/LS copy you can see laryngeal aspect of epiglottis ANT commissure, subglottis area that you cannot see with I/L examination in children you can make use of it
- DL scopy main and most commonly use for intubation of serious patient or in removal of foreign body in larynx or to take biopsy from lesion from larynx or removal of polyp/nodule at cord.

CONTRAINDICATION OF D/L SCOPY

- Cervical injuries when immobilization of neck required
- If patient having trismus/long incisor teeth/ than what should we do?
- **Flexible fiberoptic laryngoscopy :** This is to passed through nose into oropharynx with this can take larynx biopsy/photograph. **because of extensive growth (Fig. 22.5)**
- **Fiberoptic scope not possible to introduce of patient having severe deviated nasal septum (DNS) answer is CECT next to know extent of tumor/nodal status.**

RADIOGRAPHY IN LARYNGEAL CANCER

- Usually lateral view X-ray soft tissue of neck
- You can see destruction of cartilage/soft tissue swelling/position of tracheostomy tube in neck
- You can go for laryngogram with radioopaque dye it can pick up very small lesion like mucosal irregularity which you can not see by CT scan or may miss on D/L scopy.

CT SCAN

- CT scan of full neck reveals tumor as well as nodal status
- LAT-CT scout may be use for small localized filed for RT most important sign in CT for node positivity is central necrosis in node.

MANAGEMENT OF LARYNX CA

Main aim of T/T of larynx Ca to control primary site along neck node and to preserve voice if possible, curative modalities are **RT/SX**.

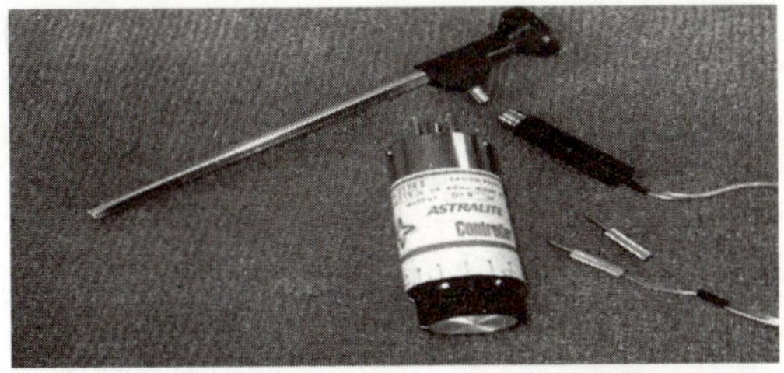

Fig. 22.5: Instruments use in laryngoscopy

GLOTTIC CA

In case of glottic dysplasia/leukoplakia complete stripping of mucosa is curative T/T and keep patient under follow with advise not smoke/ tobacco use.

CA *IN SITU*

Stripping of mucosa of cord again T/T of choice but here failure rate is 25 to 50 percent thus excisional biopsy (total tumor remove with adequate margin) answer of recurrence is radiotherapy. EBRT CO^{60} 5600 CGy in 28 fraction.

GLOTTIC CA T1/T2 LESION

T/T starts with when you are sure that either lesion is T1 or T2 not more than that RT is preferred modality in order to preserve voice surgery kept as salvage procedure.

Radiotherapy Failure Higher in Cases

- If tumor involves ANT commissure/or if cord is fixed (T3)
- Hence, in these type cases surgery is preferred inform of cordectomy or hemilaryngectomy but

after Surgery voice is week/hoarse but after RT voice quality is much superior laser surgery also use for T1, T2 lesion with success rate T1 – 80 to 90 percent, T2 – 65 to 70 percent.

GLOTTIC CA T3/T4 LESION

Advanced glottic Ca managed by Chemo/Radio/ Surgery all modalities.

RTOG PHASE-III TRIAL

- Chemo is an useful adjuvant to radical RT with 30 percent cure rate
- For organ (voice preservation surgery kept as reserve modality for radical radiotherapy failure cases (with further 30% cure rate) but after primary surgery, radiotherapy failure is high.

VETERANS AFFAIRS LARYNGEAL STUDY GROUP

- In this study stage-III/VI patient's of Larynx (SCC) given 3 cycle NACT (cisplatin/5 Fu) followed by radical RT other group was treated by total laryngectomy followed by chemo irradiation 2 year-survival in both group were almost equal (68%) but importantly Larynx was preserve in 64 percent patient given chemotherapy followed by radiotherapy
- In locally advanced lesion or subglottic extension (since high% of lower neck node involvement)
- Total laryngectomy followed by radical RT, post-operative RT is must in those group having. For laryngectomy commonly use incision are Gluck's and Sorrenson (Fig. 22.6)

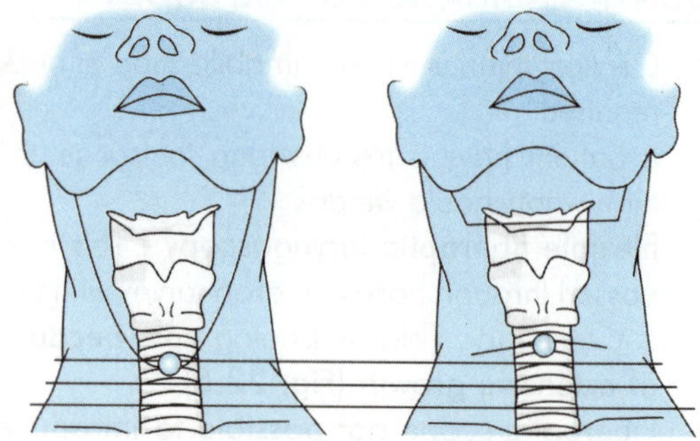

Fig. 22.6: Gluck's and Sorrenson incision for laryngectomy

- Patient's on tracheostomy because of recurrence from stoma site is high
- Extensive cartilage involvement
- Positive surgical margin, extracapsular spread, obvious morbidity after total laryngectomy is the loss of voice, for that, speech therapy/ device hand-held electrolarynx used.

RADIOTHERAPY

Sometimes in large laryngeal tumor there may be reactionary laryngeal edema develops even after I and II fraction of radiotherapy which can be dangerous if air inlet is already narrowed then it is better to perform elective tracheostomy prior to start of radical radiotherapy, field use for laryngeal radiotherapy (Figs 22.7A and B).

If tracheostomy tube is made-up of metal. It should be replaced by plastic tube in order to reduce scattered radiation which causes severe skin reactions.

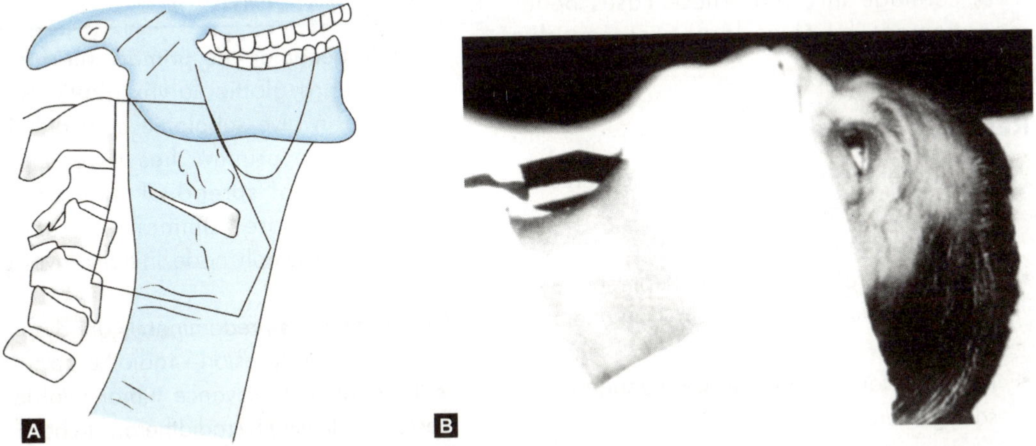

Figs 22.7A and B: (A) External radiotherapy boost portals in supraglottic larynx; (B) radiation portals

Scar site/tracheostomy stoma site to be covered with wet cotton bolus.

Factor which decrease radiotherapy control in T1/T2 lesion ANT commissure involvement subglottic extension.

AFTER RADIOTHERAPY

- Larynx edema most common 10 percent
- Larynx necrosis/coondritis 5 percent
- Subcutaneous fibrosis/skin of neck (called as woody neck)/facial/neck swelling.

RECURRENCE

- Tracheostomy stoma recurrence occur in less than 5 percent cases.

Radiotherapy Failure

Recurrence to very well delt by total laryngectomy but pharyngocutaneous fistula, carotid rapture are the dreaded complication, sometimes occur when surgery performed after RT.

MANAGEMENT OF SUPRAGLOTTIC LX

Change invoice pickedup very early in larynx Ca but in supraglottic larynx this case in different around 90 percent cases present in T3/T4 lesion with high percent of neck node involvement.

T1successfully treated by RT along with voice preservation.T2 late cases T3/T4 (subglottic extension, extensive PFF involvement cord fixity

+ve, cartilage involved. These cases better management by total laryngectomy plus radiotherapy.

Result

With radiotherapy alone in T1/T2 >75 percent

T3 40 to 70 percent

T4 30 percent

- Tumor control decrease with presence of lymph node fixed or more than 3 cm and cord is fixed.
- Radiation failure case can be managed with salvage surgery in 30 to 60 percent cases.

SUBGLOTTIC CA LARYNX

- It rarely becomes the primary site for Ca, mostly supra glottic Larynx/glottic Larynx extend to involve subglottic area only in 5 percent case primary lies here. Due to circumferential spread of tumor airway obstruction more common pretracheal/ prelaryngeal lymph node initially involve in these cases
- Clinical features predominantly are dyspnea/ stridar here early lesion—radiotherapy alone is the treatment. Advance tumor total laryngectomy followed by radiotherapy to be given.

Chapter 23

Nasopharynx Carcinoma (NPC)

Pharynx starts from base of skull to the upper end of esophagus at the level of six cervical vertebra. The pharynx is divided into three parts:

1. Nasopharynx
2. Oropharynx and
3. Laryngopharynx.
   a. This part of pharynx which lies above the soft palate and behind the nasal cavity is called nasopharynx. Nasopharynx is a roughly cuboidal structure. It measures 4.0 to 5.5 cm in its widest transverse diameter, 2.5 to 3.5 cm in this anteroposterior diameter and approximately 4.0 cm in height (Fig. 23.1).

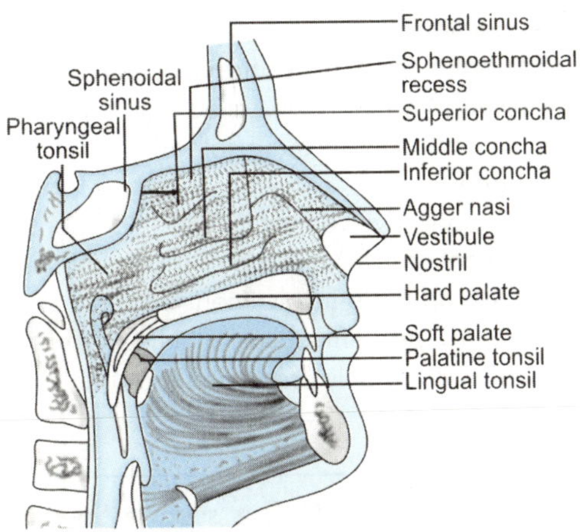

Fig. 23.1: Anatomy of nasopharynx

   b. **The foramen lacerum** lies wholly within boundaries of the nasopharynx and hence is an important route by which nasopharyngeal cancer can spread into the middle cranial fossa. It is in close anatomic relationship to the cavernous sinus and hence to the second, third, fourth, fifth and sixth cranial nerves. Basisphenoid and basiocciput form the roof of nasopharynx. The upper part of posterior wall is formed by anterior arch of the atlas. On the **lateral wall** are the pharyngeal openings of eustachian tube about 1.25 cm behind posterior end or inferior turbinate. Above and behind the tubal opening is a deep recess which is commonly a site for carcinoma and is called fossa of Rosenmuller. **Thus, the lateral wall of nasopharynx is the commonest site for the Ca nasopharynx (37%) and from the roof of nasopharynx (32%).**

NASOPHARYNGEAL TONSIL

It is collection of lymphoid tissue under the mucosa of nasopharynx situated at the junction of the roof and posterior wall of the nasopharynx. The collection disappears as the child starts growing. Hypertrophy of the lymphoid tissue is termed as **adenoids.** This lymphoid collection has no capsule. In the center of lymphoid mass is a depression called pharyngeal bursa. Thorwaldt's cysts, develop from the bursa. The collection of lymphoid tissue in the submucosa behind the opening of eustachian tube called as tubal tonsil.

Lymphatic drainage: The lymphatic tissues of pharynx and oral cavity are arranged in a ring like manner around the oropharyngeal inlet. The inner ring consists mainly of nasopharyngeal tonsil, peritubal lymphoid tissues, faucial tonsil and lingual tonsil. The efferents from this ring drain to lymph nodes situated around the neck forming the outer ring. This is called Waldeyer's ring (Figs 23.2 and 23.3).

The nasopharynx has a very rich lymphatic plexus, especially in the roof, posterior and the lateral walls.

The most important pathway is through the lateral pharyngeal wall to a small group of nodes

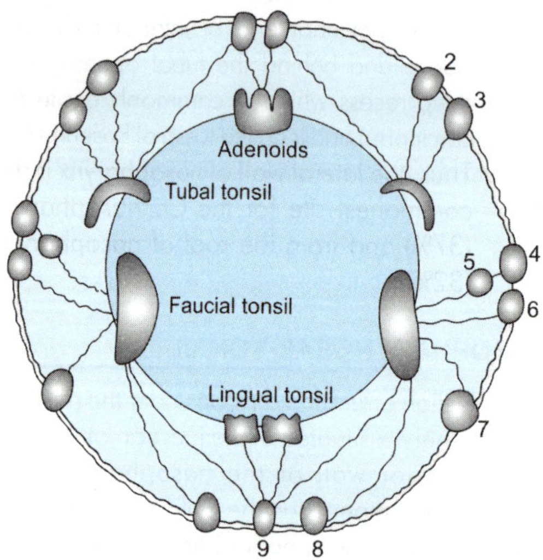

Fig. 23. 2: Waldeyer's ring of cervical lymph node

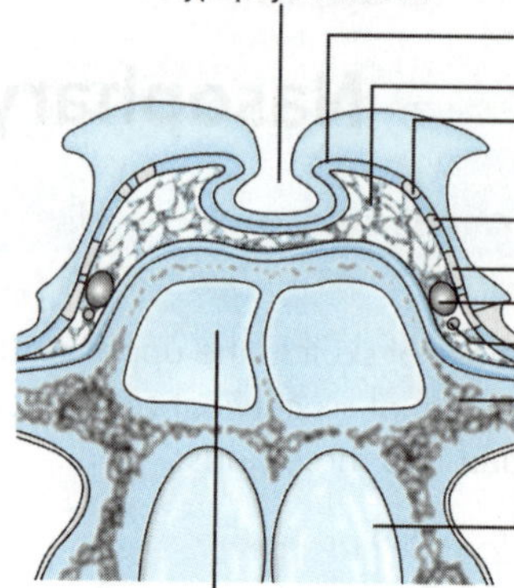

Fig. 23.3: Near by region of nasopharynx

lying near the base of skull in the space lateral to the pharynx called the parapharyngeal or retropharyngeal space. The upper most of these group is called the node of Rouviere. These nodal groups lies in close proximity to cranial nerves IX, X, XI and XII which run through the parapharyngeal space, enlargement of these lymph node causes above mention cranial nerves palsy.

Lymphatic from nasopharynx may directly involve level 2 lymph node called jugulodigastric nodes or indirectly through lateral pharyngeal lymph node.

Lymph node involvement in NPC in 85 percent to 90 percent cases. More than 50 percent cases bilateral lymph node involvement occurs.

20 to 40 percent cases of NPC lymphadenopathy will be only presenting features.

EPIDEMIOLOGY

- High incidence of NPC is seen in Southern China followed by Kenya and Hong Kong.

- Overall incidence of NPC is 0.1 percent worldwide.
- Rate in China rises from North to South 3 per lac to 25 lac per year.
- In India male female ratio is 3.4:1. High incidence of NPC in Southern China is due to smoke from wood ruff used by the boat people for cooking. Genetical determinant may also be the cause of NPC.
- Epstein-Bar virus relationship with NPC studied extensively and found that Epstein-Bar virus antibody known to be present in the maximum number of cases of NPC.
- The common age of presentation is 40 to 60 years of age. In compared to other head and neck region cancer NPC known to occur in younger age group.

Distant Mets

Most frequent site for distant mets is bone especially spine followed by lung and liver.

Clinical Features

- Nasal symptoms: Epistaxis/progressive nasal obstruction
- Aural symptoms: Because of blockage of Eustachian tube conductive deafness and frequent ASOM seen.
- Neurological features: Growth may cause destruction of base of skull and growth may extent upward intracranially through the foramen lacerum and involve 5th and 6th cranial nerve present in lateral wall of cavernous sinus.
- Overall cranial nerve palsy in NPC seen is 26 percent and trigeminal nerve is the commonest nerve to be involve in 15 percent **cases.** Involvement of maxillary division of 5th nerve leads to trigeminal neuralgia. Sixth nerve is earliest nerve to be involve and causes diplopia. Because it very closed to the foramen lacerum. But the 9, 10, 11 and 12 cranial nerve involvement occurs extracranially. Because after coming out of jugular foramen these 9, 10, 11 cranial nerve and 12th nerve after coming out from hypoglossal foramen. These above nerves runs in the close relation with lateral pharyngeal wall, where the tumor itself or enlarge lymph node at the base of skull. Compressed these nerves and palsies do occur. Laryngeal palsies pharyngeal wall/soft palate palsy.

Staging

- Committee (AJC) staging system (1998).
- **T1:** Tumor confined to the nasopharynx
- **T2:** Tumor extends to the soft tissue of oropharynx and/or nasal fossa.
- **T2a:** Without parapharyngeal extension
- **T3b:** Tumor invades bony structures and/or paranasal sinuses.
- **T4:** Tumor with intracranial extension and/or involvement of cranial nerves, infratemporal fossa, hypopharynx, orbit.
- **Nx:** Regional lymph node cannot be assessed.
- **No:** No regional lymph node metastasis.

- **N1:** Metastasis in a single ipsilateral lymph node(s), 6 cm or less in greatest dimension above supraclavicular fossa.
- **N2:** Bilateral metastasis in lymph node (s). 6 cm or less in greatest dimension, above supraclavicular fossa.
- **N3a:** Greater than 6 cm
- **N3b:** In the supraclavicular fossa
- **Mo:** No distant metastatis
- **M1:** Distant metastasis present.

Pathology

Ninty percent of NPC are epidermoid or undifferentiated carcinomas. Ten percent are NHL/extramedullary plasma cytomas/adenocarcinomas and adenoid cystic CA/malignant melanomas/rhabdomyosarcomas and chondromas. Nonkeratinizing undifferentiated Ca as a lymphoepithelioma is a highly malignant tumor of nasopharynx occur in younger age group and shows early distance metastasis. In lymphoepithelioma of nasopharynx distant mets 35 to 40 percent (common age 15–25), SCC of nasopharynx distant mets 23 percent.

Differential Diagnosis of Nasopharynx Tumors

- **NPC:** It is a friable proliferative lesion with high percentage of lymph node metastasis.
- **NHL**
- **Nasopharyngeal angiofibroma**—It is a benign but locally malignant tumor occurs in 10 to 25 years of age group mainly in male with recurrent episode of nasal bleeding/nasal obstruction. Treatment is excision of tumor is mass. Radiotherapy 30 to 35 Gy dose required.
- **Antroclonal polyp**—It is a gray pale nonfriable with smooth surface causes nasal obstruction history of chronic sinusitis

Pretreatment Work-up

- History and examination.
- Laboratory studies HMG/KFT/LFT.
- Chest X-ray-to r/o lung mets.
- X-ray base of skull (submentovertical view/waters' view) to demonstrate base of skull sphenoid sinus/nasopharynx.
- CECT neck and PNS—To see primary as well as lymph node in the neck and intracranial extension of NPC (Fig. 23.4).

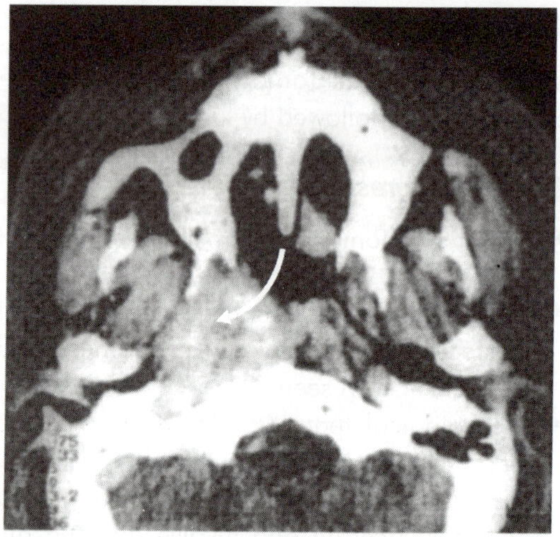

Fig. 23.4: CECT of PNS showing growth involving medial and lateral pterygoid plate

6. Bone scan if serum alkaline phosphatase is raised.

Treatment

Surgery is quit impractical due to it anatomical location since the tumor is adjacent to base of skull.

- Radiotherapy is the main stay of treatment volume includes primary as well as level I to IV lymph node on both side sometime and additional anterior field when the growth coming out anteriorly in the nasal fossa. The front half of orbit, optic chiasma brain stem should be shielded. to treat the lower neck node additional field required from the thyroid notch up to sternomanubrium joint with tracheal and lung block. Latest field exited cut 1/3rd clerical (Fig. 23.5). Because of the shoulder on either side the lateral field cannot give adequate dose is to lower neck node thus, anterior field require to treat paratracheal and paralaryngeal lymph node as well in super undutiful. The lateral field on either side should be tilted 5 to 80 to avoid radiation to contralateral eye and ipsilateral external/ middle ear. The treatment volume include:
  - Entire nasopharynx
  - Base of skull
  - Posthalf of nasal cavity
  - Postethmoidal sinus
  - Posthalf of orbit
  - Retropharyngeal LN
  - Pterygoid fossa
  - *When using the anterior field* the upper border of anterior field should not overlap with the lower border of lateral fields otherwise hot spot will be formed (Fig. 23.6).

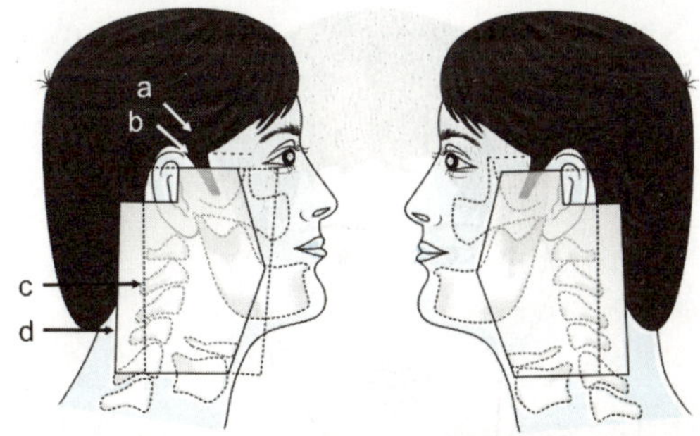

Fig. 23.5: Radiation field used for NPC. a. (For T3, T4, lesion) 4 cm above the zygomatic arch; b. (For T1, T2 lesion) 2 cm above the zygomatic arch; c. After 44 Gray (Anterior to cord); d. Whole neck leaving 1 cm soft tissue behind

Brachytherapy

- Primary use as a
- Boost treatment for primary after EBRT.
- Small local recurrence after EBRT.
- It is mainly used as a after loading catheter passed through the nasal cavity and dose 5 to 25 gray at the depth of 5 to 1 cm from Mucosa.

RESULT OF TREATMENT

- Nasopharyngeal carcinoma is a very radio-sensitive tumor, thus radiotherapy gives us excellent result. Average 5 years survival after RT full dose is **35 to 57 percent (average 40%)**, study says survival is better in younger age

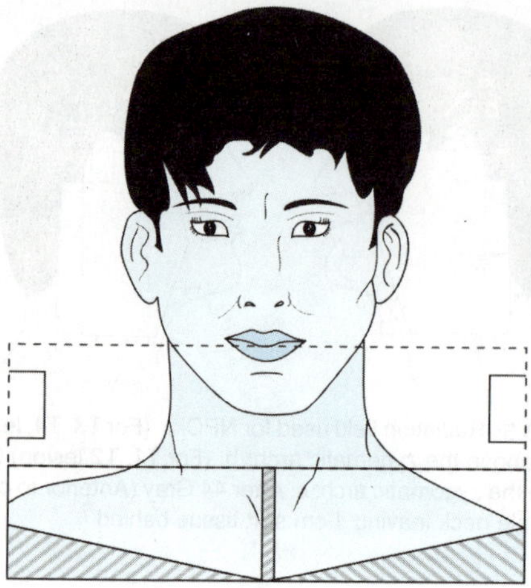

Fig. 23.6: Three field technique

group (5-year survival 45%) then older age group 5-year survival after RT 27 percent. Female show better response then male 61.2 vs 30.9 percent. Local recurrence in undifferentiated NPC vs SCC (10–12%) vs 30 to 33 percent. Because of the fact that undifferentiated NPC is more radiosensitive than SCC. Study says cranial nerve involvement does not have any significant effect on survival. Rather after full dose of RT 62 percent cases there is full recovery of cranial nerve palsy and 32 percent case partial recovery.

- Chemotherapy: Huang et al CT+RT patients have local recurrence 8.4 vs 15.7 percent local recurrence those who are treated with RT alone. Dimery study source in stage IV NPC local recurrence in 36 percent cases with RT alone treated patients vs 7 percent developed local recurrence those who are treated with concurrent cisplatin.

Chapter

24 Thyroid Cancer

There are about 37,000 new cases of thyroid cancer each year in the US, according to the National Cancer Institute. Females are more likely to have thyroid cancer at a ratio of three to one. Thyroid cancer can occur in any age group, although it is most common after age 30 and its aggressiveness increases significantly in older patients. The majority of patients present with a nodule on their thyroid that typically does not cause symptoms. Remember, over 99 percent of thyroid nodules are not cancer. But when thyroid cancer does begin to grow within the thyroid gland, it almost always does so within a discrete nodule within the thyroid. For vascular supply and antomy of thyroid gland (Figs 24.1A and B).

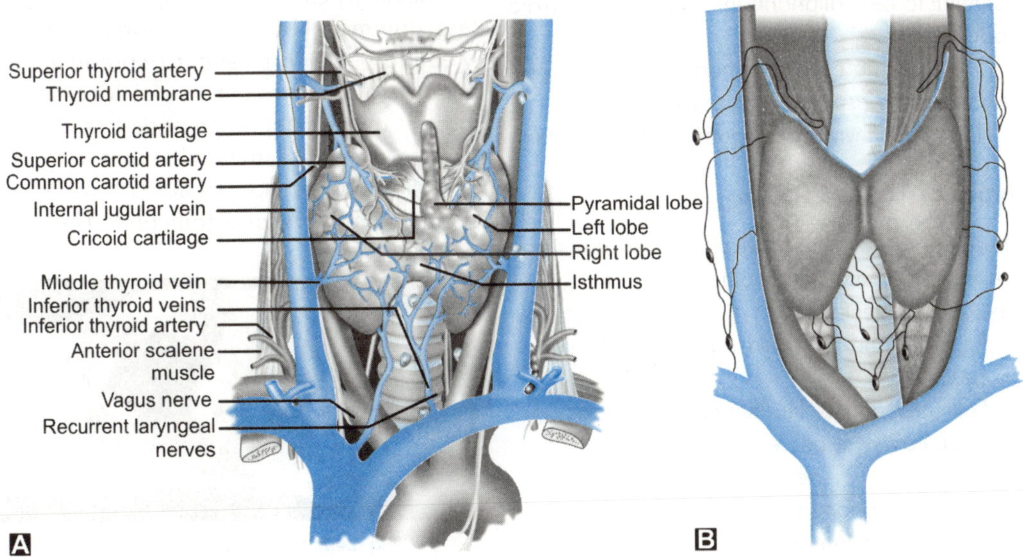

Figs 24.1 A and B: Anatomy of thyroid gland

Symptoms of Thyroid Cancer

Occasionally, symptoms such as hoarseness, neck pain and enlarged lymph nodes do occur in people with thyroid cancer. Although as much as 75 percent of the population will have thyroid nodules, the vast majority are benign. Young people usually do not have thyroid nodules, but as people age, they likely develop a nodule. By the time we are 80 to 90 percent of us will have at least one nodule.

Far less than 1 percent of all thyroid nodules are malignant. A nodule that is bold on scan is more likely to be malignant. Nevertheless, the majority of these are benign as well. You can read more information about thyroid nodules and their potential to be malignant: Introduction to thyroid nodules.

The work-up of thyroid nodules and the role of fine needle aspiration biopsy (FNA).

The role of thyroid ultrasound is also important.

Types of Thyroid Cancer

There are four types of thyroid cancer and some are more common than others. Thyroid cancer type and incidence.

Papillary and/or mixed papillary/follicular ~ 78 percent.

Follicular and/or Hürthle cell ~ 17 percent

Medullary ~ 4 percent

Anaplastic ~ 1 percent

Thyroid hormone replacement → All patients of differentiated tumor.

What's the Prognosis?

Most thyroid cancers are very curable. In fact, the most common types of thyroid cancer (papillary and follicular) are the most curable. In younger patients, both papillary and follicular cancers have a more than 97 percent cure rate if treated appropriately. Both papillary and follicular cancers are typically treated with complete removal of the lobe of the thyroid that harbors the cancer, in addition to the removal of most or all of the other side.

The bottom line is that most thyroid cancers are papillary thyroid cancer and this is one of the most curable cancers of all cancers that humans get. If treated correctly, the cure rate is extremely high.

Medullary cancer of the thyroid is significantly less common, but has a worse prognosis. Medullary cancers tend to spread to large numbers of lymph nodes very early commonly. It involves mediastinal lymph node (Fig. 24.2) and therefore require a much more aggressive operation than the more localized thyroid cancers, such as papillary and follicular. This cancer

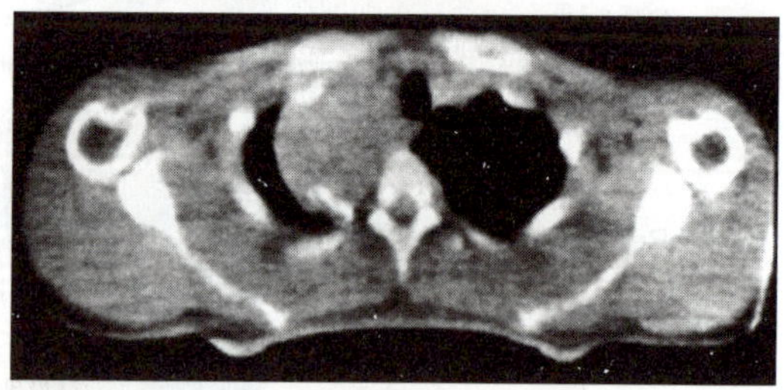

Fig. 24.2: Mediastinal lymphadenopathy

requires complete thyroid removal plus a dissection to remove the lymph nodes of the front and sides of the neck. The least common type of thyroid cancer is anaplastic which has a very poor prognosis. Anaplastic thyroid cancer tends to be found after it has spread and is incurable in most cases.

It is very uncommon to survive anaplastic thyroid cancer, as often the operation cannot remove all the tumor. These patients often require a tracheostomy during the treatment and treatment is much more aggressive than for other types of thyroid cancer—because this cancer is much more aggressive (Figs 24.3A and B).

WHAT ABOUT CHEMOTHERAPY?

Thyroid cancer is unique among cancers. In fact, thyroid cells are unique among all cells of the human body. They are the only cells that have the ability to absorb iodine. Iodine is required for thyroid cells to produce thyroid hormone, so they absorb it out of the bloodstream and concentrate it inside the cell.

Most thyroid cancer cells retain this ability to absorb and concentrate iodine. This provides a perfect "chemotherapy" strategy. Radioactive Iodine is given to the patient with thyroid cancer after their cancer has been removed. If there are any normal thyroid cells or thyroid cancer cells remain in the patient's body (and any thyroid cancer cells retaining this ability to absorb iodine), then these cells will absorb and concentrate the radioactive "poisonous" iodine. Since all other cells of our bodies cannot absorb the toxic iodine, they are unharmed. The thyroid cancer cells, however, will concentrate the poison within themselves and the radioactivity destroys the cell from within. No sickness, no hair loss, no nausea, no diarrhea, no pain.

Most, but not all, patients with thyroid cancer need radioactive iodine treatments after their surgery. This is important to know. Almost all, however, should have the iodine treatment if a cure is to be expected.

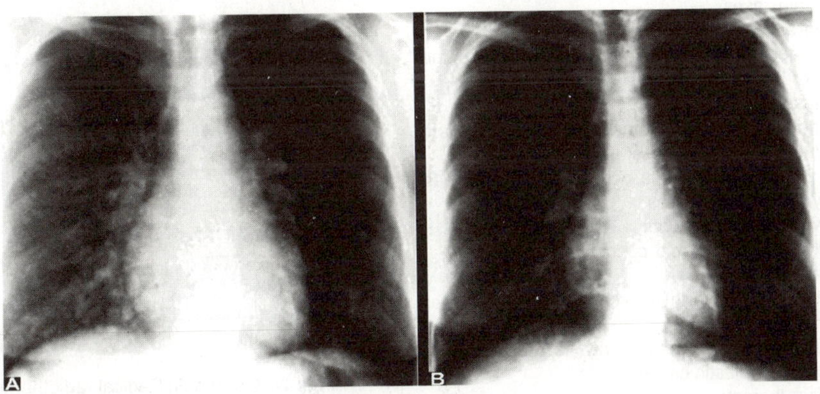

Figs 24.3A and B: Lung metastasis in thyroid cancer

Patients with medullary cancer of the thyroid usually do not need iodine therapy because medullary cancers almost never absorb the radioactive iodine. Some small papillary cancers treated with a total thyroidectomy may not need iodine therapy as well, but for a different reason.

These cancers (medullary and some small apillary cancers) are often cured with simple (complete) surgical therapy alone. This varies from patient to patient and from cancer to cancer. This decision will be made among the surgeons, the patient and the referring endocrinologist or internist. Remember, radioactive iodine therapy is extremely safe. If you need it, take it. Some time external beam radiotherapy also used in thyroid cancer, radiotherapy palliation use given in (Figs 24.4A and B).

INDICATION OF RADIOTHERAPY IN THYROID CANCER

1. Primary therapy of thyroid cancer if unresectable locally, particularly if ^{131}I does not concentrate in tumor
2. Bulky tumor (e.g. mediastinal disease) large enough that it is uncontrollable by ^{131}I alone
3. Residual bulky tumor in the central neck, tracheal and/or esophageal area or cervical nodal regions after thyroid surgery and removal of malignant cervical adenopathy that may not be controlled by ^{131}I alone
4. Skeletal metastases
   a. Concentration of ^{131}I small or absent
   b. Concern about a pathologic fracture, regardless of the degree of ^{131}I concentration
5. Brain metastases
6. Hepatic metastases if symptomatic or other treatment methods have been unsuccessful
7. Relief of pressure symptoms occurring in vital areas caused by soft tissue masses
8. Superior vena cava syndrome
9. Continually recurring thyroid cancer regardless of ^{131}I accumulation
10. Recurrent or metastatic thyroid cancer occurring after maximal ^{131}I therapy.
11. In sequence or conjunction with chemotherapy, particularly in anaplastic cancer
12. Preoperative therapy

Overview of Typical Thyroid Cancer Treatment

Thyroid cancer is usually diagnosed by sticking a needle into a thyroid nodule or removal of a worrisome thyroid nodule by a surgeon, overview of thyroid cancer treatment given in (Fig. 24.5).

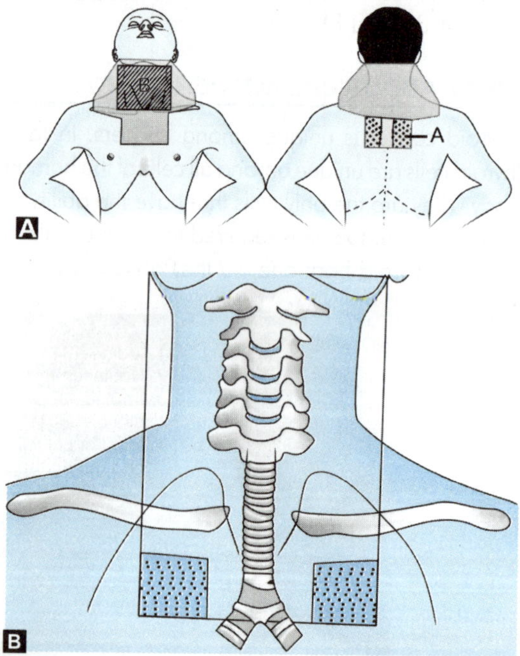

Figs 24.4 A and B: Radical radiotherapy field. Treatment field used for palliation in thyroid cancer

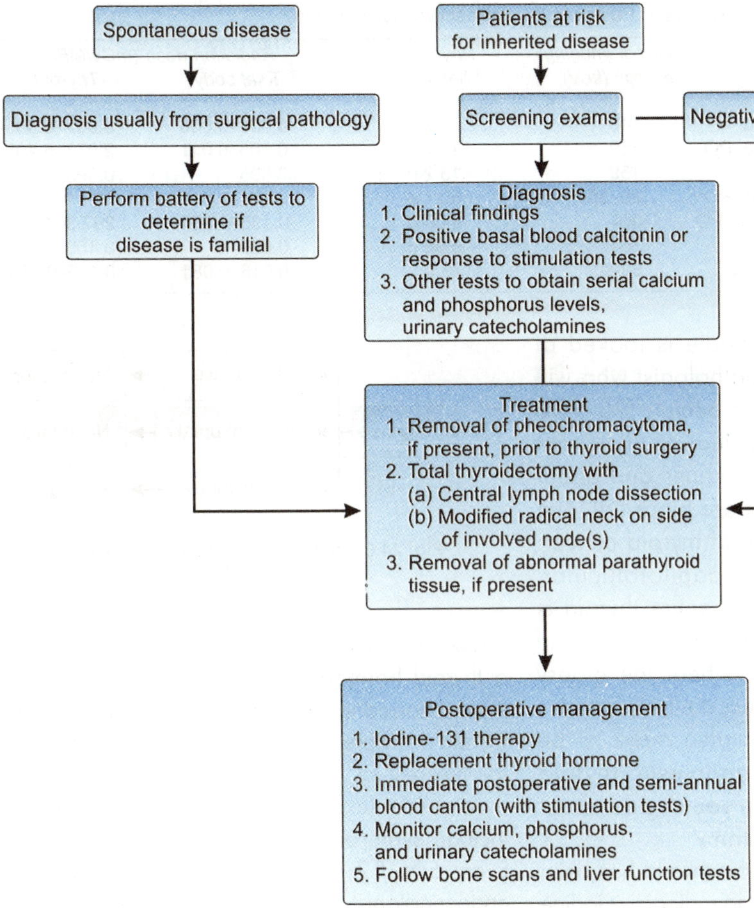

Fig. 24.5: Treatment tree for thyroid cancer

Table 24.1: Postoperative radioactive iodine therapy

Radionuclide	Dose	*Principal imaging energy (keV)*	*Physical half-life*	*Radiation dose (mGy/MBq)*	
				Total body	*Thyroid*
^{99m}Tc	185–370 MBq. IV	140	6.02 g	0.003–0.005	0.032–0.0054
^{123} I	3.7–14.8 MBq. PO	159	13.2 h	0.005–0.011	2.973–5.405
^{123} I-MIBG	370 MBq. IV	159	13.2 h	0.005	0.595
^{125} I	1.85–3.7 MBq. PO	28, 35	60.7 d	0.004–0.011	10.81–21.82
^{131} I	1.11–1.85 MBq. PO	364	8.06 d	0.135–1.081	297.3–432.4
^{131} I-MIBG	18.5 MBq. IV	364	8.06 d	0.027	9.459
^{201} Tl	37–111 MBq, IV	69-80	73 h	0.016–0.081	0.116–0.251

The removed thyroid nodule is looked at under a microscope by a pathologist who will then decide, if the nodule is benign (95–99% of all nodules that are biopsied) or malignant (less than 1 percent of all nodules and about 1–5 percent of nodules that are biopsied). The pathologist decides the type of thyroid cancer: papillary, follicular, mixed papilofollicular, medullary, or anaplastic. The entire thyroid is surgically removed; sometimes this is done during the same operation where the biopsy takes place. He/she will assess the lymph nodes in the neck to see if they also need to be removed. In the case of anaplastic thyroid cancer, your doctor will help you decide about the possibility of a tracheostomy.

About 4 to 6 weeks after the thyroid has been removed, the patient will undergo radioactive iodine treatment. This is very simple and consists of taking a single (Fig. 24.6 and Table 24.1) pill in a dose that has been calculated for the patient. The patient goes home and avoids contact with other people for a couple of days (so they are not exposed to the radioactive materials). A week or two after the radioactive iodine treatment the patient begins taking a thyroid hormone pill. No one can live without thyroid hormone, and if the patient does not have a thyroid anymore, he or she will take one pill per day for the rest of their life. This is a very common medication (examples of branded drug names include synthroid, levoxyl and armour thyroid). Every 6 to 12 months the patient returns to his endocrinologist for blood tests to determine if the dose of daily thyroid hormone is correct and to make sure that the thyroid tumor is not coming back. The frequency of these follow-up tests will vary greatly from patient to patient. Endocrinologists are typically quite good at this and will typically be the type of doctor that follows this patient long-term.

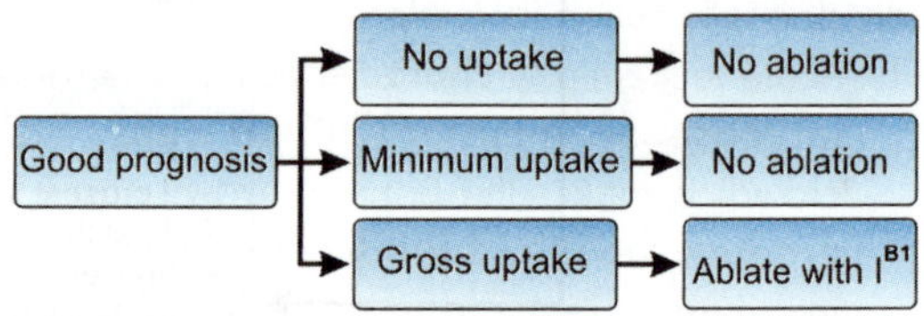

Fig. 24.6: After surgery I^{BI} ablation to be done

Chapter

25 Leukemia

CLASSIFICATION

leukemia is clinically and pathologically subdivided into a variety of large groups. The first division is between its *acute* and *chronic* forms:

1. *Acute leukemia* is characterized by the rapid increase of immature blood cells. This crowding makes the bone marrow unable to produce healthy blood cells. Immediate treatment is required in acute leukemia due to the rapid progression and accumulation of the malignant cells, which then spill over into the bloodstream and spread to other organs of the body. Acute forms of leukemia are the most common forms of leukemia in children.
2. *Chronic leukemia* is distinguished by the excessive build-up of relatively mature, but still abnormal, white blood cells. Typically taking months or years to progress, the cells are produced at a much higher rate than normal cells, resulting in many abnormal white blood cells in the blood. Whereas acute leukemia must be treated immediately, chronic forms are sometimes monitored for some time before treatment to ensure maximum effectiveness of therapy. Chronic leukemia mostly occurs in older people, but can theoretically occur in any age group.

Additionally, the diseases are subdivided according to which kind of blood cell is affected. This split divides leukemias into lymphoblastic or *lymphocytic leukemias* and myeloid or *myelogenous leukemias*:

1. In lymphoblastic or *lymphocytic leukemias*, the cancerous change takes place in a type of marrow cell that normally goes on to form lymphocytes, which are infection—fighting immune system cells. Most lymphocytic leukemias involve a specific subtype of lymphocyte, the B cell.
2. In myeloid or *myelogenous leukemias*, the cancerous change takes place in a type of marrow cell that normally goes on to form red blood cells, some other types of white cells, and platelets.

   Combining these two classifications provides a total of four main categories (Fig. 25.1 and Table 25.1):

   Within these main categories, there are typically several subcategories. Finally, hairy cell leukemia and T cell prolymphocytic leukemia are usually considered to be outside of this classification scheme.
3. *Acute lymphoblastic leukemia* (ALL) is the most common type of leukemia in young children.

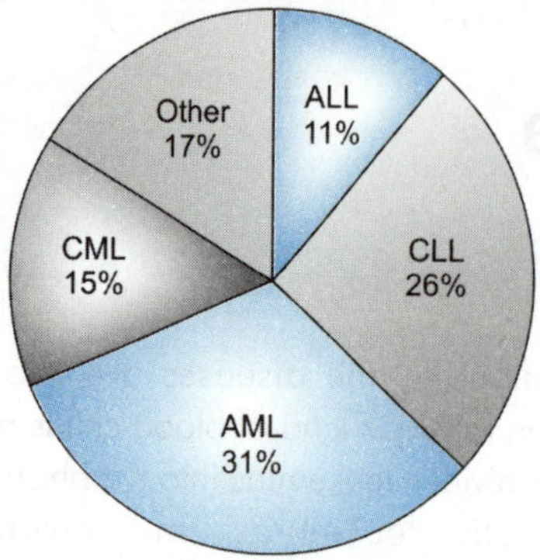

Fig. 25.1A: Percentage wise distribution of leukemia

This disease also affects adults, especially those age 65 and older. Standard treatments involve chemotherapy and radiation. The survival rates vary by age: 85 percent in children and 50 percent in adults. Subtypes include precursor B acute lymphoblastic leukemia, precursor T acute lymphoblastic leukemia, Burkitt's leukemia and acute biphenotypic leukemia.

4. *Chronic lymphocytic leukemia* (CLL) most often affects adults over the age of 55. It sometimes occurs in younger adults, but it almost never affects children. Two-thirds of affected people are men. The five-year survival rate is 75 percent. It is incurable, but there are many effective treatments. One subtype is B cell prolymphocytic leukemia, a more aggressive disease.
5. *Acute myelogenous leukemia* (AML) occurs more commonly in adults than in children, and more commonly in men than women. AML is treated with chemotherapy. The five-year survival rate is 40 percent. Subtypes of AML include acute promyelocytic leukemia, acute myeloblastic leukemia and acute megakaryoblastic leukemia.
6. *Chronic myelogenous leukemia* (CML) occurs mainly in adults. A very small number of children also develop this disease. Treatment is with imatinib (Gleevec) or other drugs. The five-year survival rate is 90 percent. One subtype is chronic monocytic leukemia.
7. *Hairy cell leukemia* (HCL) is sometimes considered a subset of CLL, but does not fit neatly into this pattern. About 80 percent of affected people are adult men. There are no reported cases in young children. HCL is incurable, but easily treatable. Survival is 96 to 100 percent at ten years.
8. T cell prolymphocytic leukemia (T PLL) is a very rare and aggressive leukemia affecting adults; somewhat more men than women are diagnosed with this disease. Despite its overall rarity, it is also the most common type of mature T cell leukemia; nearly all other leukemias

Table 25.1: Four major kinds of leukemia

Cell type	*Acute*	*Chronic*
Lymphocytic leukemia (or "lymphoblastic")	Acute lymphoblastic leukemia (ALL)	Chronic lymphocytic leukemia (CLL)
Myelogenous leukemia (also "myeloid" or "nonlymphocytic")	Acute myelogenous leukemia (AML)	Chronic myelogenous leukemia (CML)

involve B cells. It is difficult to treat and the median survival is measured in months.

9. Large granular lymphocytic leukemia may involve either T cell or NK cells; like hairy cell leukemia, which involves solely B cells, it is a rare and indolent (not aggressive) leukemia.

Signs and Symptoms

Common symptoms of chronic or acute leukemia. Damage to the bone marrow, by way of displacing the normal bone marrow cells with higher numbers of immature white blood cells, results in a lack of blood platelets, which are important in the blood clotting process. This means people with leukemia may easily become bruised, bleed excessively, or develop pinprick bleeds (petechiae). White blood cells, which are involved in fighting pathogens, may be suppressed or dysfunctional. This could cause the patient's immune system to be unable to fight off a simple infection or to start attacking other body cells. Because leukemia prevents the immune system from working normally, some patients experience frequent infection, ranging from infected tonsils, sores in the mouth, or diarrhea to life-threatening pneumonia or opportunistic infections. Finally, the red blood cell deficiency leads to anemia, which may cause dyspnea and pallor. Some patients experience other symptoms. These symptoms might include feeling sick, such as having fevers, chills, night sweats and other flu-like symptoms, or feeling fatigued. Some patients experience nausea or a feeling of fullness due to an enlarged liver and spleen; this can result in unintentional weight loss. If the leukemic cells invade the central nervous system, then neurological symptoms (notably headaches) can occur. All symptoms associated with leukemia can be attributed to other diseases. Consequently, leukemia is always diagnosed through medical tests.The word *leukemia*, which means 'white blood', is derived from the disease's namesake high white blood cell counts that most leukemia patients have before treatment. The high number of white blood cells are apparent when a blood sample is viewed under a microscope. Frequently, these extra white blood cells are immature or dysfunctional. The excessive number of cells can also interfere with the level of other cells, causing a harmful imbalance in the blood count, for diffrentiating normal blood cells versus leukemic cells plane (Figs 25.2 and 25.3).

Some leukemia patients do not have high white blood cell counts visible during a regular blood count. This less-common condition is called *aleukemia*. The bone marrow still contains cancerous white blood cells which disrupt the normal production of blood cells. However, the leukemic cells are staying in the marrow instead of entering the bloodstream, where they would be visible in a blood test. For an aleukemic patient, the white blood cell counts in the bloodstream can be normal or low. Aleukemia can occur in any of the four major types of leukemia and is particularly common in hairy cell leukemia.

Causes: No single known cause for all of the different types of leukemia exists. The known causes, which are not generally factors within the control of the average person, account for

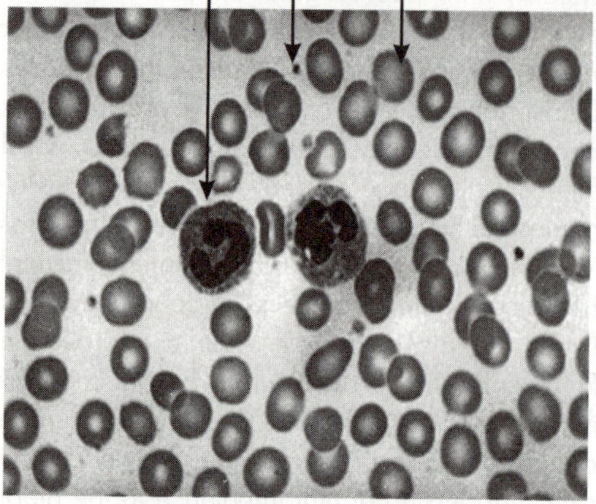

Fig. 25.2: Normal human blood
(For color version, see Plate 1)

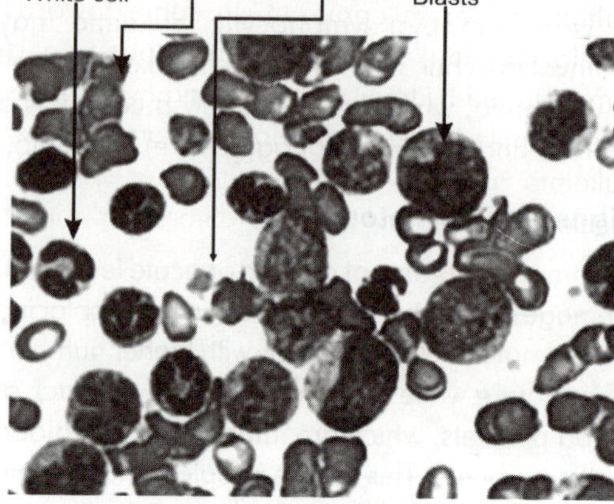

Fig. 25.3: Blood with leukemia
(For color version, see Plate 1)

relatively few cases. The different leukemias likely have different causes.

Leukemia-like other cancers, results from somatic mutations in the DNA. Certain mutations produce leukemia by activating oncogenes or deactivating tumor suppressor genes and thereby disrupting the regulation of cell death, differentiation or division. These mutations may occur spontaneously or as a result of exposure to radiation or carcinogenic substances and are likely to be influenced by genetic factors.

Among adults, the known causes are natural and artificial ionizing radiation, a few viruses such as human T-lymphotropic virus and some chemicals, notably benzene and alkylating chemotherapy agents for previous malignancies. Use of tobacco is associated with a small increase in the risk of developing acute myeloid leukemia in adults. Cohort and case-control studies have linked exposure to some petrochemicals and hair dyes to the development of some forms of leukemia. A few cases of maternal-fetal transmission have been reported. Diet has very limited or no effect, although eating more vegetables may confer a small protective benefit. Viruses have also been linked to some forms of leukemia. For example, certain cases of ALL are associated with viral infections by either the human immunodeficiency virus or human T-lymphotropic virus (HTLV-1 and -2, causing adult T cell leukemia/lymphoma). However, one report suggests exposure to certain germs may offer children limited protection against leukemia. Stage of leukemia development given in (Fig. 25.4).

Some people have a genetic predisposition. The affected people may have a single gene or multiple genes in common. In some towards developing leukemia. This predisposition is demonstrated by family histories and twin studies cases, families tend to develop the same kind of leukemia as other members; in other families, affected people may develop different forms of leukemia or related blood cancers. In addition to these genetic issues, people with chromosomal abnormalities or certain other genetic conditions have a greater risk of leukemia. For example, people with down syndrome have a significantly increased risk of developing forms of acute leukemia and fanconi anemia is a risk-factor for developing acute myeloid leukemia.

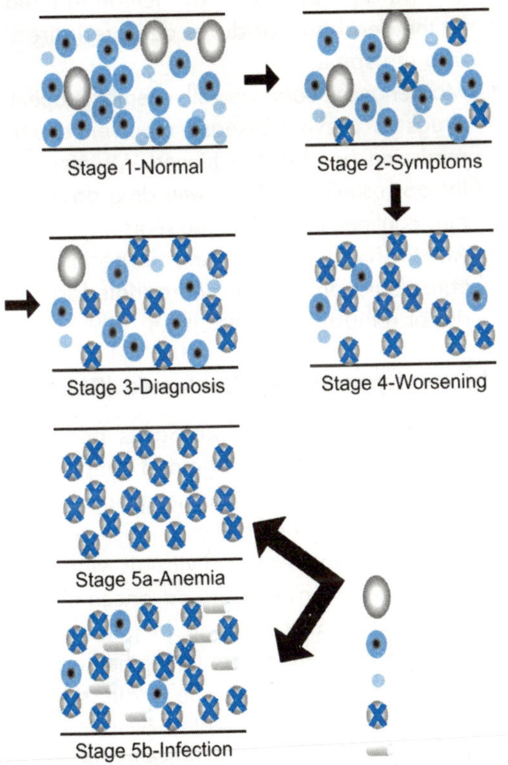

Fig. 25.4: From top 1: White blood cells; 2: RBC; 3: Platelet; 4: Blast cell; 5: Germ cell stage of leukemias development

Whether nonionizing radiation causes leukemia has been studied for several decades. The International Agency for Research on Cancer expert working group undertook a detailed review of all data on static and extremely low frequency electromagnetic energy, which occurs naturally and in association with the generation, transmission and use of electrical power. They concluded that there is limited evidence that high levels of ELF magnetic (but not electric) fields might cause childhood leukemia. Exposure to significant ELF magnetic fields might result in two-folds excess risk for leukemia for children exposed to these high levels of magnetic fields. However, the report also says that methodological weaknesses and biases in these studies have likely caused the risk to be overstated. No evidence for a relationship to leukemia or an other form of malignancy in adults has been demonstrated. Since exposure to such levels of ELFs is relatively uncommon, the World Health Organization (WHO) concludes that ELF exposure, if later proven to be causative, would account for just 100 to 2400 cases worldwide each year, representing 0.2 to 4.95 percent of the total incidence for that year until the cause or causes of leukemia are found, there is no way to prevent the disease. Even when the causes become known, they may not be readily controllable, such as naturally occurring background radiation and therefore not especially helpful for prevention purposes.

Treatment: Most forms of leukemia are treated with pharmaceutical medications, typically combined into a multidrug chemotherapy regimen. Some are also treated with radiation therapy. In some cases, a bone marrow transplant is useful.

Acute Lymphoblastic Leukemia (ALL)

Acute Lymphoblastic Leukemia Fraction Treatment

Management of ALL focuses on control of bone marrow and systemic (whole-body) disease. Additionally, treatment must prevent leukemic cells from spreading to other sites, particularly the central nervous system (CNS), e.g. monthly lumbar punctures. In general, ALL treatment is divided into several phases:

- *Induction chemotherapy* to bring about bone marrow remission. For adults, standard induction plans include prednisone, vincristine and an anthracycline drug; other drug plans may include L-asparaginase or cyclophosphamide. For children with low-risk ALL, standard therapy usually consists of three drugs (prednisone, L-asparaginase and vincristine) for the first month of treatment.
- *Consolidation therapy* or *intensification therapy* to eliminate any remaining leukemia cells. There are many different approaches to consolidation, but it is typically a high-dose, multidrug treatment that is undertaken for a few months. Patients with low—to average-risk all receive therapy with antimetabolite drugs such as methotrexate and 6-mercaptopurine (6-MP). High-risk patients receive higher drug doses of these drugs, plus additional drugs.
- *CNS prophylaxis* (preventive therapy) to stop the cancer from spreading to the brain and nervous system in high-risk patients. Standard prophylaxis may include radiation of the head and/or drugs delivered directly into the spine.
- *Maintenance treatments* with chemotherapeutic drugs to prevent disease recurrence once remission has been achieved. Maintenance therapy usually involves lower drug doses and may continue for up to three years.
- Alternatively, *allogeneic bone marrow transplantation* may be appropriate for high-risk or relapsed patients.

Chronic Lymphocytic Leukemia (CLL)

Decision-to-treat: Hematologists base CLL treatment upon both the stage and symptoms of the individual patient. A large group of CLL patients have low-grade disease, which does not benefit from treatment. Individuals with CLL-related complications or more advanced disease often benefit from treatment. In general, the indications for treatment are: falling hemoglobin or platelet count, progression to a later stage of disease, painful, disease-related overgrowth of lymph nodes or spleen, an increase in the rate of lymphocyte production.

Typical, treatment, approach: CLL is probably incurable by present treatments. The primary chemotherapeutic plan is combination chemotherapy with chlorambucil or cyclophosphamide, plus a corticosteroid such as prednisone or prednisolone. The use of a corticosteroid has the additional benefit of suppressing some related autoimmune diseases, such as immunohemolytic anemia or immune-mediated thrombocytopenia. In resistant cases, single-agent treatments with nucleoside drugs such as fludarabine, pentostatin, or cladribine may be successful. Younger patients may consider allogeneic or autologous bone marrow transplantation.

Acute Myelogenous Leukemia (AML)

Acute Myeloid Leukemia Treatment

Many different anticancer drugs are effective for the treatment of AML. Treatments vary somewhat according to the age of the patient and according to the specific subtype of AML. Overall, the strategy is to control bone marrow and systemic (whole-body) disease, while offering specific treatment for the central nervous system (CNS), if involved.

In general, most oncologists rely on combinations of drugs for the initial, *induction phase* of chemotherapy. Such combination chemotherapy usually offers the benefits of early remission and a lower risk of disease resistance. *Consolidation* and *maintenance* treatments are intended to prevent disease recurrence. Consolidation treatment often entails a repetition of induction chemotherapy or the intensification chemotherapy with additional drugs. By contrast, maintenance treatment involves drug doses that are lower than those administered during the induction phase.

Chronic Myelogenous Leukemia (CML)

Chronic Myelogenous Leukemia Treatment

There are many possible treatments for CML, but the standard of care for newly diagnosed patients is imatinib (Gleevec) therapy. Compared to most anticancer drugs, it has relatively few side effects and can be taken orally at home. With this drug, more than 90 percent of patients will be able to keep the disease in check for at least five years, so that CML becomes a chronic, manageable condition.

In a more advanced, uncontrolled state, when the patient cannot tolerate imatinib, or if the patient wishes to attempt a permanent cure, then an allogeneic bone marrow transplantation may be performed. This procedure involves high-dose chemotherapy and radiation followed by infusion of bone marrow from a compatible donor. Approximately 30 percent of patients die from this procedure.

Hairy Cell Leukemia (HCL)

Hairy Cell Leukemia Treatment

Decision to treat: Patients with hairy cell leukemia who are symptom-free typically do not receive immediate treatment. Treatment is generally considered necessary when the patient shows signs and symptoms such as low blood cell counts (e.g. infection-fighting neutrophil count below 1.0 K/μl), frequent infections, unexplained bruises, anemia, or fatigue that is significant enough to disrupt the patient's everyday life.

Typical Treatment Approach

Patients who need treatment usually receive either one week of cladribine, given daily by intravenous infusion or a simple injection under the skin, or six months of pentostatin, given every four weeks by intravenous infusion most cases, treatment will produce remission.

Other treatments include rituximab infusion or self-injection with Interferon-alpha. In limited cases, the patient may benefit from splenectomy (removal of the spleen). These treatments are not typically given as the first treatment because their success rates are lower than cladribine or pentostatin.

T cell Prolymphocytic Leukemia (T PLL)

Further information: T cell prolymphocytic leukemia Treatment.

Most patients with T cell prolymphocytic leukemia, a rare and aggressive leukemia with a median survival of less than one year, require immediate treatment T cell prolymphocytic leukemia is difficult to treat and it does not respond to most available chemotherapeutic drugs. Many different treatments have been attempted, with limited success in certain patients: purine analogs (pentostatin, fludarabine, cladribine), chlorambucil and various forms of combination chemotherapy (cyclophosphamide, doxorubicin, vincristine, prednisone [CHOP], cyclophosphamide, vincristine, prednisone [COP], vincristine, doxorubicin, prednisone, etoposide, cyclophosphamide, bleomycin [VAPEC-B]). Alemtuzumab (Campath), a monoclonal antibody that attacks white blood cells, has been used in treatment with greater success than previous options. Some patients who successfully respond to treatment also undergo stem cell transplantation to consolidate the response.

Juvenile Myelomonocytic Leukemia

Juvenile myelomonocytic leukemia treatment: Treatment for juvenile myelomonocytic leukemia can include splenectomy, chemotherapy and bone marrow transplantation.

Chapter

26 Neuroendocrine Tumor

Neuroendocrine tumors, or more properly gastro-enteropancreatic or gastroenteropancreatic neuroendocrine tumors (GEP-NETs), are cancers of the interface between the endocrine (hormonal) system and the nervous system.

THE NEUROENDOCRINE SYSTEM

The endocrine system is a communication system in which hormones act as biochemical messengers to regulate physiological events in living organisms. The nervous system performs the same functions using electrical impulses as messengers. The neuroendocrine system is the combination of those two systems, or more specifically, the various interfaces between the two systems. A GEP-NETs is a tumor of any such interface. More specifically, the endocrine system is primarily a network of glands that produce and secrete hormones, usually into the bloodstream. It also includes cells that are not part of glands: the diffuse neuroendocrine system, scattered throughout other organs.

A hormone is a chemical that delivers a particular message to a particular organ, typically remote from the hormone's origin. For example, the hormone insulin, secreted by the pancreas, acts primarily to allow glucose to enter the body's cells for use as fuel. The hormone gastric is secreted by the duodenum and the antrum of the stomach to tell the stomach to produce acids to digest food. Hormones can be divided into subtypes such as peptides, steroids and neuroamines. For some researchers, there is no clear distinction between peptide hormones and peptides; the hormones are simply longer than other peptides. In the context of GEP-NETs, the terms *hormone* and *peptide* are often used interchangeably.

Classification of GEP-NETs by Site of Origin and by Symptoms

A small intestine neuroendocrine tumor. The vast majority of GEP-NETs fall into two nearly distinct categories: carcinoids and pancreatic endocrine tumors (PETs). Despite great behavioral differences between the two, they are grouped together as GEP-NETs because of similarities in cell structure.

Systemic Features of Neuroendocrine Tumor

Siegfried Oberndorfer, in 1907, was the first person to distinguish clearly what we now call GEP-NETs from other forms of cancer. He gave the term "carcinoid" to these tumors, because they were so slow-growing that he considered them to be "cancer-like" rather than truly cancerous. In 1929, he reported that some such tumors were not so indolent—these he distinguished as what we now call PETs from what most authorities call carcinoids. Despite the differences between the two categories, some doctors, including oncologists, persist in calling all GEP-NETs "carcinoid", even into the twenty-first century. Pancreatic endocrine tumors (PETs) are also known as endocrine pancreatic tumors (EPTs) or islet cell tumors. PETs are assumed to originate generally in the islets of Langerhans within the pancreas–or, Arnold *et al.* suggest, from endocrine pancreatic precursor cells (Arnold et al 2004, 199 though they may originate outside of the pancreas. (The term *pancreatic cancer* almost always refers to *adenopancreatic cancer*, also known as *exocrine pancreatic cancer*. Adenopancreatic cancers are generally very aggressive and are not neuroendocrine cancers. About 95 percent of pancreatic tumors are adenopancreatic; about 1 or 2 percent are GEP-NETs.) PETs may secrete hormones (as a result, perhaps, of impaired storage ability) and those hormones can wreak symptomatic havoc on the body. Those PETs that do not secrete hormones are called *nonsecretory* or *nonfunctioning* or *nonfunctional* tumors. Secretary tumors are classified by the hormone most strongly secreted – for example, insulinoma, which produces excessive insulin and gastrinoma, which produces excessive gastrin (see more detail in the summary below).

Carcinoid tumors are further classified, depending on the point of origin, as foregut (lung, thymus, stomach and duodenum) or midgut (distal ileum and proximal colon) or hindgut (distal colon and rectum). Less than one percent of carcinoid tumors originate in the pancreas. But for many tumors, the point of origin is unknown. Carcinoid tumors tend to grow much more slowly than PETs. A carcinoid tumor may produce serotonin (5-HT), a biogenic amine that causes a specific set of symptoms including:

- Flushing
- Diarrhea or increase in number of bowel movements
- Weight loss
- Weight gain
- Heart palpitations
- Congestive heart failure (CHF)
- Asthma
- Acromegaly
- Cushing's syndrome

This set of symptoms is called *carcinoid syndrome* (Fig. 26.1). Although this serotonin secretion is entirely different from a secretory PETs' hormone secretion, carcinoid tumors with carcinoid syndrome are nevertheless sometimes called *functioning*, adding to the frequent confusion of carcinoids with PETs. Carcinoid syndrome is primarily associated with midgut carcinoids. A severe episode of carcinoid syndrome is called *carcinoid crisis*; it can be triggered by surgery or chemotherapy, among other factors. The mildest of the carcinoids are discovered only upon surgery for unrelated causes. These *coincidental carcinoids* are common; one study found that one person in ten has them. Neuroendocrine tumors other than coincidental carcinoids are rare. Incidence of PETs is estimated

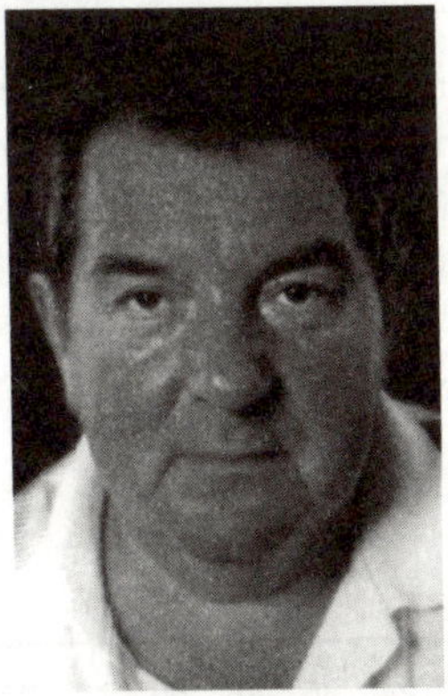

Fig. 26.1: Carcinoid feature flashing of face

at one new case per 100,000 people per year; incidence of clinically significant carcinoids is twice that. Thus, the total incidence of GEP-NETs in the United States would be about 9,000 new cases per year. But researchers differ widely in their estimates of incidence, especially at the level of the secretory subtypes (the various "omas"). In addition to the two main categories, there are even rarer forms of GEP-NETs. At least one form – neuroendocrine lung tumors – arises from the respiratory rather than the gastroenteropancreatic system. GEP-NETs found at various sites and their prognosis and survival given in (Fig. 26.2).

Nonhuman animals also suffer from GEP-NETs; for example, neuroendocrine cancer of the liver is a disease of dogs, and Devil facial tumor disease is a neuroendocrine tumor of Tasmanian Devils. Rufini *et al.* summarize: "Neuroendocrine tumors (NETs) are a heterogeneous group of neoplasms originating from endocrine cells, which are characterized by the presence of secretory granules as well as the ability to produce biogenic amines and polypeptide hormones. These tumors originate from endocrine glands such as the adrenal medulla, the pituitary and the parathyroids, as well as endocrine islets within the thyroid or the pancreas and dispersed endocrine cells in the respiratory and gastrointestinal tract. The clinical behavior of NETs is extremely variable; they may be functioning or not functioning, ranging from very slow-growing tumors (well-differentiated NETs), which are the majority, to highly aggressive and very malignant tumors (poorly differentiated NETs). Classically, NETs of the gastrointestinal tract are classified into 2 main groups: (1) carcinoids and (2) endocrine pancreatic tumors (EPTs)" (Rufini, Calcagni and Baum 2006). (Note that the definition of well-differentiated may be counter intuitive: a tumor is well-differentiated if its cells are similar to normal cells, which have a well-differentiated structure of nucleus, cytoplasm, membrane, etc.)

Ramage *et al.* provide a summary that differs somewhat from that of Rufini *et al.*: "NETs originate from pancreatic islet cells, gastroenteric tissue (from diffuse neuroendocrine cells distributed throughout the gut), neuroendocrine cells within the respiratory epithelium and parafollicullar cells distributed within the thyroid (the tumors being referred to as medullary carcinomas of the thyroid). Pituitary, parathyroid, and adrenomedullary neoplasms have certain common characteristics with these tumors but are considered separately" (Ramage et al 2005).

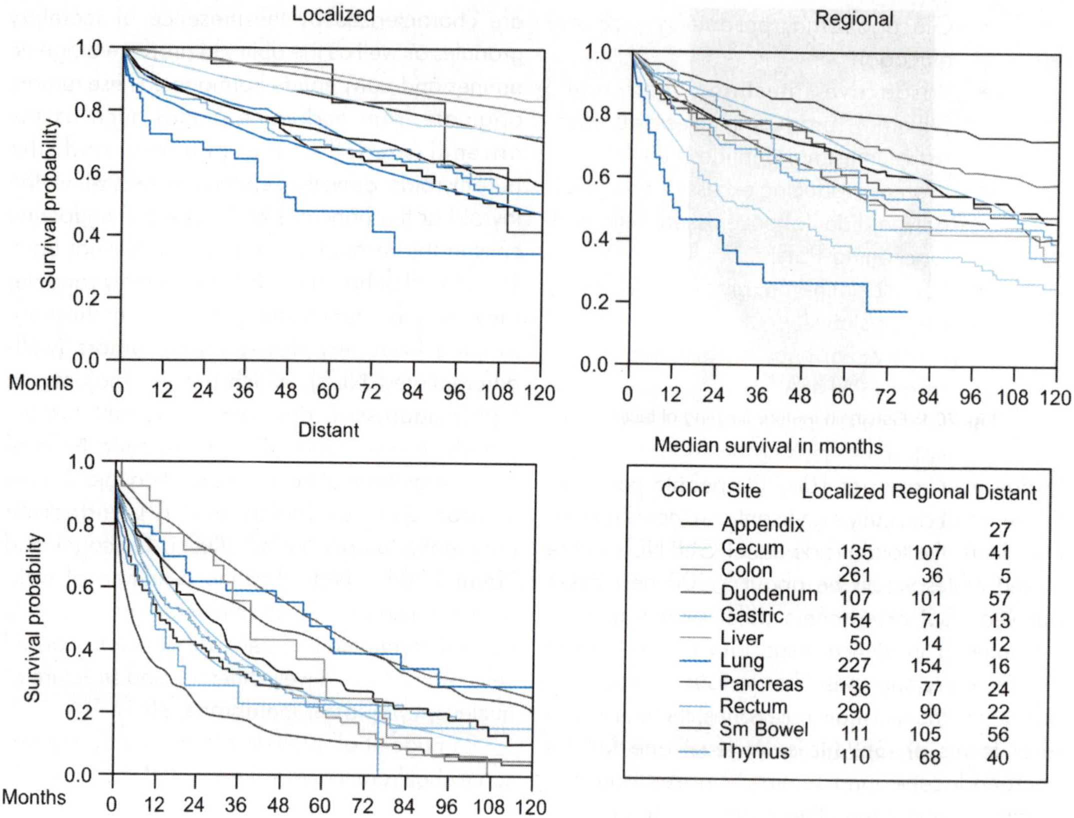

Median survival in months

Color	Site	Localized	Regional	Distant
—	Appendix			27
—	Cecum	135	107	41
—	Colon	261	36	5
—	Duodenum	107	101	57
—	Gastric	154	71	13
—	Liver	50	14	12
—	Lung	227	154	16
—	Pancreas	136	77	24
—	Rectum	290	90	22
—	Sm Bowel	111	105	56
—	Thymus	110	68	40

Fig. 26.2: Neuroendocrine tumor of various sites and its prognosis

Summary of Human GEP-NETs by Site of Origin and by Symptom

- Carcinoids (about two-thirds of GEP-NETs)
  - With carcinoid syndrome (about 10 percent of carcinoids)
  - Without carcinoid syndrome (about 90 percent of carcinoids)
- PETs (about one-third of GEP-NETs)
  - Nonfunctioning (15–30 percent of PETs)
  - Functioning (70–85 percent of PETs)
    - gastrinoma, producing excessive gastrin and causing Zollinger-ellison syndrome (ZES)
    - Insulinoma, producing excessive insulin

  - Glucagonoma, producing excessive glucagon
  - Vasoactive intestinal peptideoma (VIPoma), producing excessive vasoactive intestinal peptide (VIP)
  - PPoma, producing excessive pancreatic polypeptide (often classed with nonfunctioning PETs)
  - Somatostatinoma, producing excessive somatostatin
  - Watery diarrhea, hypokalemia-achlorhydria (WDHA)
  - CRHoma, producing excessive corticotropin-releasing hormonse (CRH)
  - Calcitoninoma, producing excessive calcitonin
  - GHRHoma, producing excessive growth-hormone-releasing hormone (GHRH)
  - Neurotensinoma, producing excessive neurotensin
  - ACTHoma, producing excessive adrenocorticotropic hormone (ACTH)
  - GRFoma, producing excessive Growth hormone-releasing factor (GRF)
  - Parathyroid hormone–related peptide tumor
- Rare GEP-NETs
  - Medullary carcinoma of the thyroid
  - Merkel cell cancer (trabecular cancer)
  - Small-cell lung cancer (SCLC)
  - Large-cell neuroendocrine carcinoma (of the lung)
  - Extrapulmonary small cell carcinomas (ESCC or EPSCC)in general
  - Neuroendocrine carcinoma of the cervix
  - Multiple endocrine neoplasia type 1 (MEN-1 or MEN1) (usually nonfunctioning) (also causing ZES)
  - Multiple endocrine neoplasia type 2 (MEN-2 or MEN-2)
  - Neurofibromatosis type 1
  - Tuberous sclerosis
  - von Hippel-Lindau (vHL) disease
  - Neuroblastoma
  - Pheochromocytoma
  - Paraganglioma
  - Neuroendocrine tumor of the anterior pituitary
  - Carney's complex, etc.

Classification of GEP-NETs by Cell Characteristics

The diverse and amorphous nature of GEP-NETs has led to a confused, overlapping and changing terminology. In general, aggressiveness (malignancy), secretion (of hormones) and anaplasia (dissimilarity between tumor cells and normal cells) tend to go together, but there are many exceptions, which have contributed to the confusion in terminology. For example, the term *atypical carcinoid* is sometimes used to indicate an aggressive tumor without secretions, whether anaplastic or well-differentiated.

In 2000, the World Health Organization (WHO) revised the classification of GEP-NETs, abandoning the term *carcinoid* in favor of *neuroendocrine tumor* (NET) and abandoning *islet cell tumor* or *pancreatic endocrine tumor* for *neuroendocrine carcinoma* (NEC). Judging from papers published into 2006, the medical community is accepting this new terminology with great sluggishness. (Perhaps one reason for the resistance is that the WHO chose to label the least aggressive subclass of neuroendocrine neoplasm with the term—*neuroendocrine tumor*—widely used previously either for the superclass or for the generally aggressive noncarcinoid subclass).

Klöppel *et al.* have written an overview that clarifies the WHO classification and bridges the gap to the old terminology (Klöppel, Perren and Heitz, 2004). In this article we conform to the old terminology.

Summary of Classification by Cell Characteristics (the WHO Classification)

- Superclass:
  - Öberg, WHO, Klöppel *et al.*: gastro-enteropancreatic neuroendocrine tumor (GEP-NET)
- Subclass 1 (less malignant)
  - Öberg: carcinoid
  - WHO: neuroendocrine tumor (NET)
  - Klöppel *et al.* well-differentiated neuroendocrine tumor (NET) (carcinoid)
  - This article: carcinoid
- Subclass 2 (more malignant)
  - Öberg: endocrine pancreatic tumor
  - WHO: neuroendocrine carcinoma (NEC)
  - Klöppel *et al.*: well-differentiated neuroendocrine carcinoma (NEC) (malignant carcinoid)
  - This article: pancreatic endocrine tumor (PET) or endocrine pancreatic tumor (EPT) or islet cell tumor or noncarcinoid GEP-NET
- Subclass 3 (most malignant)
  - WHO:poorly-differentiated neuroendocrine carcinoma
  - Klöppel *et al.*: poorly-differentiated neuroendocrine carcinoma (high-grade malignant carcinoid)
- Subclass 4 (mixed)
  - WHO: mixed endocrine/exocrine tumor
- Subclass 5 (miscellaneous)
  - WHO: rare neuroendocrine-like lesions

GEP-NETs are also sometimes called *APUDomas*, but that term is now considered to be misleading, since it is based on a discredited theory of the development of the tumors.

METASTASES AND MALIGNANCY

In the context of GEP-NETs, the terms *metastatic* and *malignant* are often used interchangeably GEP-NETs are often malignant, since the primary site often eludes detection for years, sometimes decades—during which time the tumor has the opportunity to metastasize. Researchers differ widely in their estimates of malignancy rates, especially at the level of the secretory subtypes (the various "-omas").

The most common metastatic sites are the liver, the lymph nodes and the bones. Liver metastases are so frequent and have such prominent blood supply that for many patients, they dominate the course of the cancer. For a patient with a nonsecretory PET, for example, the primary threat to life may be the sheer bulk of the tumor load in the liver (Fig. 26.3).

Diagnosis

CT-scans, MRIs, sonography (ultrasound) and endoscopy (including endoscopic ultrasound) are common diagnostic tools. Symptoms from hormone secretions or from carcinoid syndrome, or measures of the corresponding hormones in the blood, can aid in diagnosis. CT scans using contrast medium can detect 95 percent of tumors over 3 cm in size and no tumors under 1 cm (University of Michigan Medical School) According to Arnold et al "Many tumors are asymptomatic even in the presence of metastases" (Arnold et al. 2004, 197).

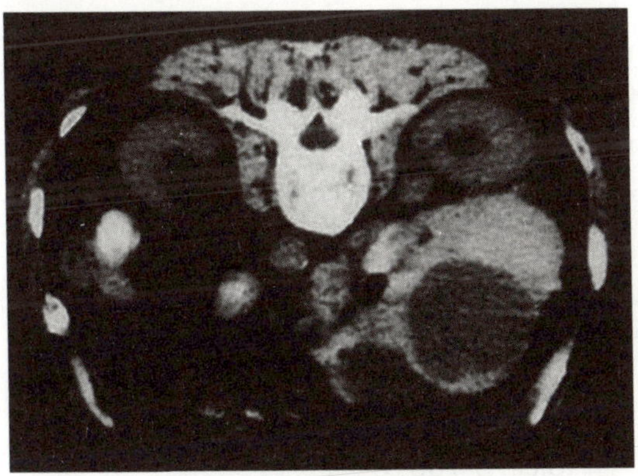

Fig. 26.3: Liver metastasis

Cells that receive hormonal messages do so through receptors on the surface of the cells. For reasons that are not understood, many neuroendocrine tumor cells possess especially strong receptors; for example, PETs often have strong receptors for somatostatin, a very common hormone in the body. We say that such tumor cells *overexpress* the somatostatin receptors (SSTRs) and are thus *avid for* the hormone; their *uptake* of the hormone is strong. This avidity for somatostatin is a key for diagnosis – and it makes the tumors vulnerable to certain *targeted therapies*, described below.

However, the half-life of somatostatin in circulation is under three minutes, making it useless for diagnosis and targeted therapies. For this reason, synthetic forms of somatostatin are used instead; the earliest was octreotide, first marketed, by Sandoz as Sandostatin, in 1988. The synthetic forms are typically called *somatostatin analogs* (*somatostatin analogues*), but according to the US Food and Drug Administration (FDA), the proper term is *somatostatin congeners*. (In this article we conform to the old terminology, as the medical community has been slow to adopt the term *congener*.) The analogs have a much longer half-life than somatostatin and other properties that make them more suitable for diagnosis and therapy.

The diagnostic procedure that utilizes a somatostatin analog is the octreoscan, also called somatostatin receptor scintigraphy (SRS or SSRS): a patient is injected with octreotide chemically bound to a radioactive substance, often indium-111; for

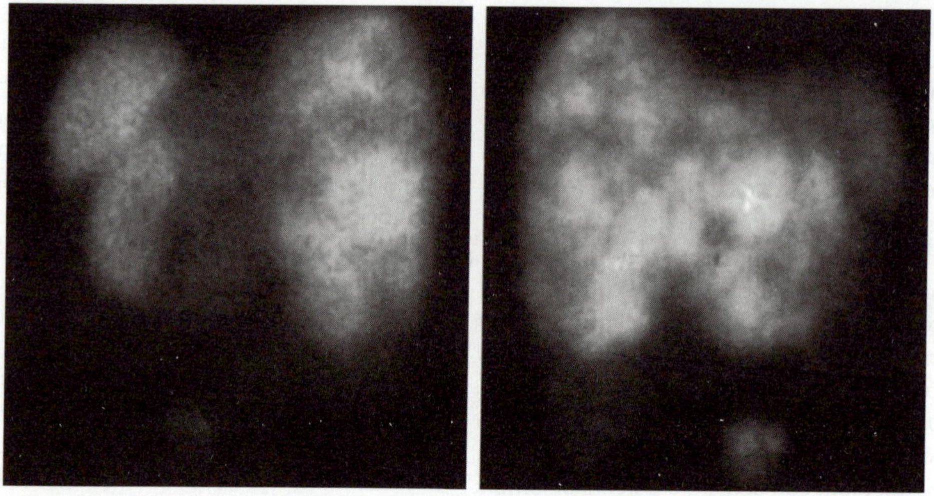

Fig. 26.4: Octreotide radiolabeled scan

those patients whose tumor cells are avid for octreotide, a radiation-sensitive scan *Neuro-endocrine tumor of various sites* can then indicate the locations of the larger lesions. An octreoscan is a relatively crude test that generates subjective results (Fig. 26.4). A gallium-68 receptor PET-CT, integrating a PET image with a CT image, is much more sensitive than an octreoscan, and it generates objective (quantified) results in the form of a standardized uptake value (SUV).

Fluorodeoxyglucose (FDG)-PET is not useful in diagnosis of GEP-NETs. As Warner says, "Most GEP NETs do not image with fluorodeoxyglucose PET" (Warner 2005, 7). According to Öberg, new PET "tracers such as C-5-hydroxy-L-tryptophan show very high sensitivity for detection of tumors, higher than for somatostatin receptor scintigraphy" (Öberg 2005b, The list of potential markers for GEP-NETs is long. Aside from the hormones of secretory tumors, the most important markers are:

- Chromogranin A (CgA)
- Achaete-scute homolog 1 (ASCL1)
- Urine 5-hydroxy indole acetic acid (5-HIAA) (grade C)
- Neuron-specific enolase (NSE, gamma-gamma dimer)
- Synaptophysin (P38) and other markers include
- Synaptobrevin (VAMP-1)
- Synapsin (1A, 1B, 2A, 2B)
- SV2
- Protein P65
- Protein S-100
- Protein gene product (PGP) 9.5

- Intermediate filaments (cytokeratins, vimentin, neurofilaments)
- Protein 7B2
- Chromogranin B (secretogranin I)
- Chromogranin C (secretogranin II)
- Pancreastatin
- Vasostatin
- Cytochrome b561
- Leu-7 (hnk-1)
- Calcitonin
- Human chorionic gonadotropin-alpha (hCG-α)
- Human chorionic gonadotropin-beta (hCG-β)
- Thyroid function tests (TFTS)
- Parathyroid hormone (PTH)
- Calcium
- Prolactin
- {Alpha}-fetoprotein
- Carcinoembryonic antigen (cea)
- β-human chorionic gonadotrophin (β-hCG) (grade D)
- Cgrp
- Grp
- Pyy
- hCG-α
- N peptide k
- Neurokinin a
- Serotonin
- Neurotensin
- Motilin
- Substance p
- Histamine
- Catecholamines
- Dopa
- Various rarer peptide hormones
- Synaptotagmin
- HISL-19

and newer (as of 2005) markers include

- N-terminally truncated variant of heat shock protein 70 (Hsp70)
- CDX-2, a homeobox gene product
- Neuroendocrine secretory protein-55

Aside from their use in diagnosis, some markers can track the progress of therapy while the patient avoids the detrimental side-effects of CT scan contrast.

Therapy

According to Warner, the best care, at least for noncarcinoid GEP-NETs, is provided by "an active [as opposed to wait-and-see] approach using sequential multimodality treatment" delivered by a "multidisciplinary team, which also may include a surgeon, endocrinologist, oncologist, interventional radiologist and other specialists". This recommendation is based on his view that, except for most insulinomas, "almost all" PETs "have long-term malignant potential"—and in sixty percent of cases, that potential is already manifest. "Indeed, the most common cause of death from PETs is hepatic [that is, liver] failure" (Warner 2005, 4).

Two tricky issues in evaluating therapies are durability (is the therapy long-lasting?) and stasis (are the tumors neither growing nor shrinking?). For example, one therapy might give good initial results – but within months the benefit evaporates.

And another therapy might be disparaged by some for causing very little tumor shrinkage, but be championed by others for causing significant tumoristasis.

Surgery and Chemotherapy

Surgery is the only therapy that can cure GEP-NETs. However, the typical delay in diagnosis, giving the tumor the opportunity to metastasize, makes most GEP-NETs ineligible for surgery (non-resectable).

There is "no established standard therapy for the liver metastasis of pancreatic endocrine tumors" (Sato et al. 2000). The most common nonsurgical therapy for all GEP-NETs is chemotherapy, although chemotherapy is reported to be largely ineffective for carcinoids, not particularly durable (long-lasting) for PETs and inappropriate for PETs of nonpancreatic origin. When chemotherapy fails, the most common therapy, in the United States, is more chemotherapy, with a different set of agents. Some studies have shown that the benefit from one agent is not highly predictive of the benefit from another agent, except that the long-term benefit of any agent is likely to be low. Strong uptake of somatostatin analogs is a negative indication for chemo.

Symptomatic Relief

There are two major somatostatin-analog-based targeted therapies. The first of the two therapies provides symptomatic relief for patients with secretory tumors. In effect, somatostatin given subcutaneously or intramuscularly "clogs up" the receptors, blocking the secretion of hormones from the tumor cells. Thus, a patient who might otherwise die from severe diarrhea caused by a secretory tumor can gain additional years of life.

Specific counter-hormones or other hormone-blocking medications are sometimes also used to provide symptomatic relief.

Hormone-delivered Radiotherapy – PRRT

The second of the two major somatostatin-analog-based targeted therapies is called *peptide receptor radionuclide therapy* (PRRT), though we might simply call it *hormone-delivered radiotherapy*. In this form of *radioisotope therapy* (RIT), radioactive substances (called *radionuclides* or *radioligands*) are chemically *conjugated* with hormones (peptides or neuroamines); the combination is given intravenously to a patient who has good uptake of the chosen hormone. The radioactive labeled hormones enter the tumor cells and the attached radiation damages the tumor and nearby cells. Not all cells are immediately killed this way. The process of tumor cells dying as result of this therapy can go on for several months, even up to two years. In patients with strongly overexpressing tumor cells, nearly all the radiation either gets into the tumors or is excreted in urine. As Rufini *et al.* say, GEP-NETs "are characterized by the presence of neuroamine uptake mechanisms and/or peptide receptors at the cell membrane and these features constitute the basis of the clinical use of specific radiolabeled ligands, both for imaging and therapy" (Rufini, Calcagni, and Baum, 2006.

The use of PRRT for GEP-NETs is similar to the use of iodine-131 as a standard therapy (in use since 1943) for nonmedullary thyroid tumors (which are not GEP-NETs). Thyroid cells (whether normal or neoplastic) tend to be avid for iodine and nearby cells are killed when iodine-131 is infused into the bloodstream and is soon attracted to thyroid cells. Similarly, overexpressing GEP-NET cells (neoplastic cells only) are avid for somatostatin analogs and nearby cells are killed when radionuclides attached to somatostatin analogs are infused into the bloodstream and are soon attracted to the tumor cells. In both therapies, hormonal targeting delivers a much higher dose of radiation than external beam radiation could safely deliver.

As of 2006, PRRT is available in at least dozen medical centers in Europe. In the USA it is FDA-approved and available at Excel Diagnostics/The RITA Foundation at 9701, Richmond Avenue, Houston, Texas, but using a radionuclide, indium-111, that is much weaker than the lutetium-177 and the even stronger yttrium-90 used on the European continent. In the UK, only the radionuclide metaiodobenzylguanidine (I-MIBG) is licensed (but GEP-NETs are rarely avid for MIBG). In Canada, there are two centers that offer GEP-NET patients treatment with radioisotope therapy; at the London Health Sciences Center in London, Ontario (Indium 111 and 131ImIBG) and at the Cross Cancer Institute in Edmonton, Alberta (131ImIBG). Patients can be treated (with lutetium-177) in The Netherlands, at the Erasmus Medical Center. PRRT with lutetium or yttrium is now here an "approved" therapy, but the German health insurance system, for example, covers the cost for German citizens.

PRRT using yttrium or lutetium was first applied to humans about 1999. Practitioners continue to refine their choices of radionuclides to maximize damage to tumors, of somatostatin analogs to maximize delivery, of chelators to bind the radionuclides with the hormones (and chelators can also increase uptake) and of protective mechanisms to minimize damage to healthy tissues (especially the kidneys).

Hepatic Artery-delivered Therapies

One therapy for liver metastases of GEP-NETs is hepatic artery embolization (HAE). Larry Kvols, of the Moffitt Cancer Center and Research Institute in Tampa, Florida, says that "hepatic artery embolization has been quite successful. During that procedure a catheter is placed in the groin and then threaded up to the hepatic artery that supplies the tumors in the liver. We inject a material called embospheres [tiny spheres of glass or resin, also called *microspheres*] into the artery and it occludes the blood flow to the tumors and in more than 80 percent of patients the tumors will show significant tumor shrinkage" (Kvols 2002). HAE is based on the observation that tumor cells get nearly all their nutrients from the hepatic artery, while the normal cells of the liver get about 75 percent of their nutrients (and about half of their oxygen) from the portal vein, and thus can survive with the hepatic artery effectively blocked.

Another therapy is hepatic artery chemoinfusion, the injection of chemotherapy agents into the hepatic artery. Compared with systemic chemotherapy, a higher proportion of the chemotherapy agents are (in theory) delivered to the lesions in the liver hepatic artery chemoembolization (HACE), sometimes called transarterial chemoembolization (TACE), combines hepatic artery embolization with hepatic artery chemoinfusion: embospheres bound with chemotherapy agents, injected into the hepatic artery, lodge in downstream capillaries. The spheres not only block blood flow to the lesions, but by halting the chemotherapy agents in the neighborhood of the lesions, they provide a much better targeting leverage than chemoinfusion provides.

Radioactive microsphere therapy (RMT) combines hepatic artery embolization with radiation therapy – microspheres bound with radionuclides, injected into the hepatic artery, lodge (as with HAE and HACE) in downstream capillaries. This therapy is also called *selective internal radiation therapy*, or *SIRT*. In contrast with PRRT, the lesions need not overexpress peptide receptors. (But PRRT can attack all lesions in the body, not just liver metastases.) Due to the mechanical targeting, the yttrium-labeled microspheres "are selectively taken up by the tumors, thus preserving normal liver" (Salem et al. 2002)

Other Therapies

Radiofrequency ablation (RFA) is used when a patient has relatively few metastases. In RFA, a needle is inserted into the center of the lesion and current is applied to generate heat; the tumor cells are killed by cooking. Cryoablation is similar to RFA; an endothermic substance is injected into the tumors to kill by freezing. Cryoablation has been considerably less successful for GEP-NETs than RFA. Interferon is sometimes used to treat GEP-NETs; its use was pioneered by Dr Kjell Öberg at Uppsala. For GEP-NETs, interferon is often used at low doses and in combination with other agents (especially somatostatin analogs such as octreotide). But some researchers claim that Interferon provides little value aside from symptom control.

As described above, somatostatin analogs have been used for about two decades to alleviate symptoms by blocking the production of hormones from secretory tumors. They are also integral to PRRT. In addition, some doctors claim that, even without radiolabeling, even patients with nonsecretory tumors can benefit from somatostatin analogs, which purportedly can shrink or stabilize GEP-NETs. But some researchers claim that this "cold" octreotide provides little value aside from symptom control. Finally, therapies based on growth factor inhibitors are in the experimental stage. These inhibitors of epidermal growth factor receptors (EGFRs), of vascular endothelial growth factor receptors (VEGFRs) and of angiopoietin-related growth factor (AGF) include imatinib, sunitinib, temozolomide, thalidomide, sorafenib, and panitumumab.

Section-D

RADIATION ONCOLOGY

Chapter 27

Radioactivity

RADIOACTIVITY

Radioactive materials are really to be handle with care not with fear (Fig. 27.1). Some of the proton-neutron combinations are not stable, they have excess energy which is constantly redistributed among nucleon (proton+neutron) by mutual collisions thus one of the particle may gain enough energy to escape from nucleus and makes nucleus to achieve state of lower energy emission of particle may leave nucleus in excited state and nucleus will continue slipping down to lower energy state by emitting particles until stable state achieved, this phenomenon in which radiation is produced by nucleus of the atom is said to be radioactivity and nucleus said to be radioactive. With passage of time of parent nuclei progressively decrease called radioactive decay change from one radioactive nucleus to another daughter nucleus called disintegration radioactive. Disintegration is completely uncontrollable and unalterable by any known physical or chemical methods. Radioavtive decay produces range of electromagnetic waves with different frequency (Fig. 27.2). During radioactive disintegration many instances daughter nucleus

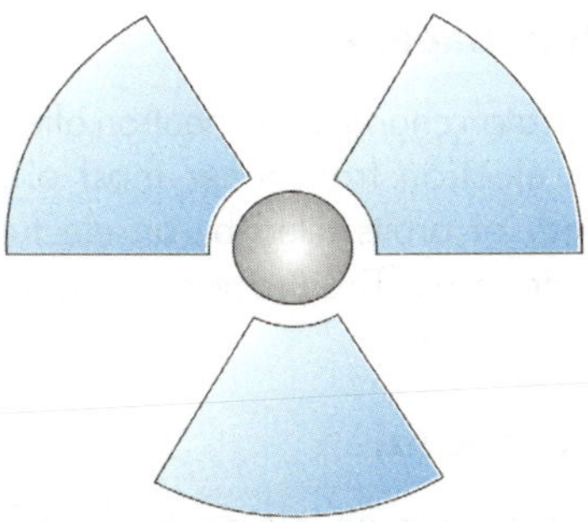

Fig. 27.1: Caution-sign of radioactive materials

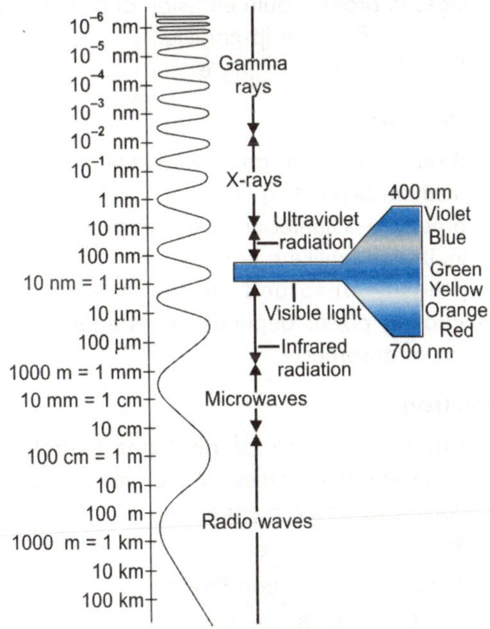

Fig. 27.2: Type of electromagnetic waves *(For color version, see Plate 2)*

is stable but there are cases in which daughter nucleus is also radioactive, and in some cases radioactive nucleus series formed called radioactive families.

Radioactive nuclides commonly decay with

a. β-particle
b. Positron
c. γ-rays
d. Annihilation radiation capture
e. K-electron capture
f. α-particle
g. Isomeric transitions

β-Particle

Nuclei having too many neutrons than neutron changes in proton couth emission of β-particles

$_0n^1$ —® $_1P^1$ + $_{-1}{}^{\circ}e$ (β-particle)

Exp $_{15}P^{32}$ —® $_{16}S^{32}$ + $_{-1}{}^{\circ}e$

Propertiesm

1. β-particle have a range few centimeters in a medium depending upon.
2. β-particle is lighter in mass thus produce less ionization (unlike a particle).

   β-easily absorbed in the medium its penetrating power depends on its energy and density of absorber.

Positron

Nuclei with lack of neutrons (which is equivalent to an excess of protons) may gain stability by positron emission.

$_1P^1$ —® $_1n^{1+}$ + $_{+1}{}^{\circ}e$

Proton Neutron Positron

Exp $_6C^{11}$ —® $_5B^{11}$ + $_{+1}{}^{\circ}e$

It's less common than β-particle emission

Gamma Rays (γ)

1. It is never emitted directly γ-rays emission is always preceded by some particle emission (such as α, β, etc.)
2. If nucleus still have excess energy after (a, b) particle emission is said to be in excited state and excess energy released in form of γ-ray. The γ-rays are like X-rays.
   a. Highly penetrating.
   b. They possess no charge no mass.
   c. They produce indirect ionization.

   $_{27}Co^{60}$ —® $_{28}N1^{60}$ + $_{-1}{}^{\circ}e$ +g (photon)
3. Here excited nickel nucleus is the source of γ-rays but their emission is so rapid that they are conveniently regarded as a part of cobalt decay scheme.

Annihilation Radiation Capture

1. In rare cases positrons quickly combine with electrons and both particles disappear and their masses converted into two photon of electromagnetic radiation.
2. This is called annihilation radiation.

K-Electron Capture

Here proton changes into neutron after capture of an electron from inner most orbits, the vacancy of orbits filled by an electron from just outer orbit. This process accompanied by X-ray radiation.

Alpha Particle (α)

Higher atomic no elements (Z>82) more commonly decay with emission of alpha particle (2 proton, 2 neutron) identical to nucleus of helium atom

$_{88}Ra^{226}$ —® $_{86}Rn^{222}$ + $2He^{4}$

Radon is also radioactive and emits.

Properties

1. α-particle mass is four time that of hydrogen M nucleus.
2. Because of large mass they are densely ionizing but larger mass makes it less penetrating.

Isomeric Transitions

In some cases, the excited nucleus after β-emission may be nearly stable state for minutes, hours or days the isomer behaves as a separate radioactive material decay by isomeric transition with emission of γ-rays only.

Mo —® -B + TcM

Tc 99   140 KeV γ-ray

Properties

Radioactive nuclei

Emission < Charged particle / Photons

1. Charge particles and photon are capable in producing ionization that means they penetrate or pass any material, if they are capable to remove electron from the atoms.
2. Since ionization requires energy thus particles are brought to rest and photons disappear.
3. Greater the charge on particle more ionizations it produces in unit length.
4. Ionization density is also inversely proportional to the velocity of the particle.
5. At the beginning of its track the particle is travelling at its fastest thus, less ionization density as the speed comes down it produces rather greater amount of ionization per unit length called **"Bragg Curve"** bragg phenomenon.

Bragg Curve

It also indicates that particle have definite range maximum Ionization occurs where (distance). Bragg peak of charge particle (like proton) utilized in pituitary tumor by utilizing its **Bragg Peak.** Advantage of this type of treatment is minimal or no exit dose beyond Bragg Peak. Gradual and finally steep build up of ionization density along with the track of the particle.

Radioactive Decay

1. Decay means gradual reduction of the number of parent nuclei with passage of time.
2. Different substances decay at different rates, rates of decay does not change with temperature, pressure or old and freshly prepared material.
3. Decay follow exponential law:

$$N = N_0 e^{-\lambda t}$$

N – Number of present atoms

N_0 – Number of initial atoms

D(λ) – Decay constant

t – Time lapse.

Half-life: Time required for half of the activity of the atom originally present to decay (Table 27.1).

Table 27.1: Half-life and radiation

Half-life	*Radiation*	
$_{27}Co$	® 5.3 Years	beta and gamma rays
$_{53}I^{131}$	® 8 Days	——do——
Cesium®	® 30 Years	——do——
Radium	® 1620 Years	—Alfa partial

is the chance or the likelihood that an atom will change in a second is usually called the transformation constant will be different, in different radioactive nuclei greater the value of l greater the chance of decay.

Radioactive Material

Radioactivity was first observed in natural uranium by Becquerel in 1896. 1934 Curie discovered that normal element could be rendered radioactive by suitable bombardment with nuclear particles this was called artificial radioactive. There are four sources of radioactive materials:

1. Natural radioactive materials.
2. Radioactivity induced by neutron bombardment.
3. Radioactivity induced by proton bombardment.
4. By fission products.

Natural Radioactive Material

Most of the natural radioactive materials have atomic numbers more than 80. For example: uranium, thorium, actinium. Natural radioactive material with atomic number less than 81 is an isotope of potassium^{40}, K^{40}. A β- and γ-rays emitter is found in about 0.01 percent of natural potassium.

Uranium 238 (U 238) radioactive decay

Type of radiation	Nuclide	Half-life
	Uranium-238	4.5×10^9 years
α	Thorium-234	24.5 days
β	Protactinium-234	1.14 minutes
β	Uranium-234	2.33×10^5 years
α	Thorium-230	8.3×10^4 years
α	Radium-226	1590 years
α	Radon-222	3.825 days
α	Polonium-218	3.05 minutes
α	Lead-214	26.8 minutes
β	Bismuth-214	19.7 minutes
β	Polonium-214	1.5×10^{-4} seconds
α	Lead-210	22 years
β	Bismuth-210	5 days
β	Polonium-210	140 days
α	Lead-206	stable

Radioactivity Induced by Neutron Bombardment

1. Being uncharged neutron are able to enter nuclei relatively easily, this is the most prolific method of producing artificial radioactivity. Result of o^{n1} Bombardment is 'h-g'. Reaction means neutron enters the nucleus and energy liberated in form of γ-rays.
   Exp $_{27}Co^{59} + {}_0n^1$ —® $_{27}Co^{60}$ + γ-rays

2. Since the product having same atomic number as the parent substance it is impossible to separate them chemically.
3. Nuclear reactor (Fig. 27.3) are use for producing radio nuclides (reactor).

Radioactivity Induced by Proton Bombardment

Being positive charge proton entry into nucleus is difficult than that of a neutron, so proton has to have extra energy to achieve desired penetration for this purpose. Proton is accelerated to high energy in the machine called a cyclotron.

1. Most common result of proton bombardment is capture of proton and ejection of neutron.

   ${}_{16}S^{32} + 1P^{1}$ ® $\rightarrow {}_{17}Cl^{34} + {}_{0}n^{1}$

   a. Here Cl isotope is radioactive since it has fewer neutrons than stable isotope so it gives out positron.

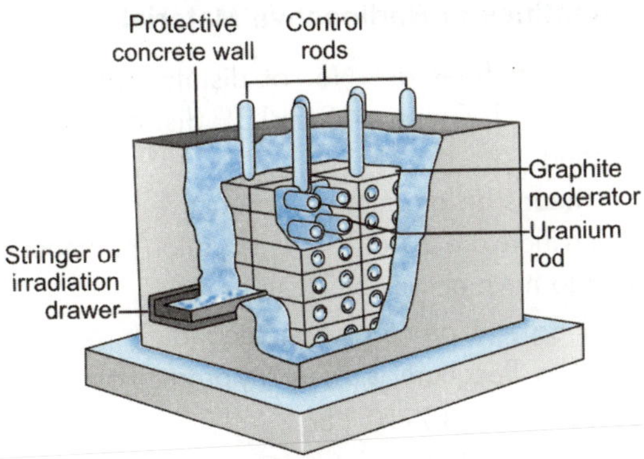

Fig. 27.3: Nuclear reactor

   b. Since product of above reaction (Cl^{34}) is different from irradiated material S^{34} thus, pure sample can be collected since S^{34} and Cl^{34} can be separated chemically.

RADIOACTIVITY BY NUCLEAR FISSION

1. It has been found that weight of nucleus is smaller than the sum of the individual masses of the protons and neutron difference having been given out as energy when nucleus was formed ® → "Difference called mass defect."

   ${}_{92}Cl^{235} + {}_{0}n^{1}$ ® $\rightarrow {}_{55}Cs^{137} + {}_{37}Rb^{97} + {}_{0}n^{1} + {}_{0}n^{1}$ + Energy
   ↓ ↓
   (Radioactive)

2. Point to be noted that one neutron was required for the fission and two neutrons emerged out of this reaction thus, giving possibility of chain reaction. Each fission only produce minute amount of energy but soon due to chain reaction (Fig. 27.4) considerable amount would be released in rapidly expending manner this

   Process ® → leads to atomic explosion

Natural uranium made-up of

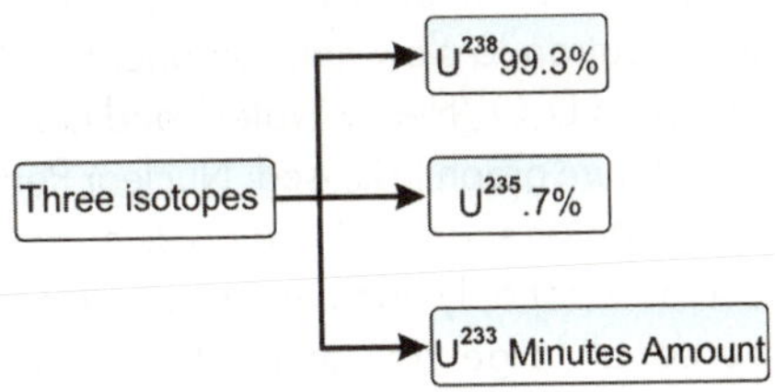

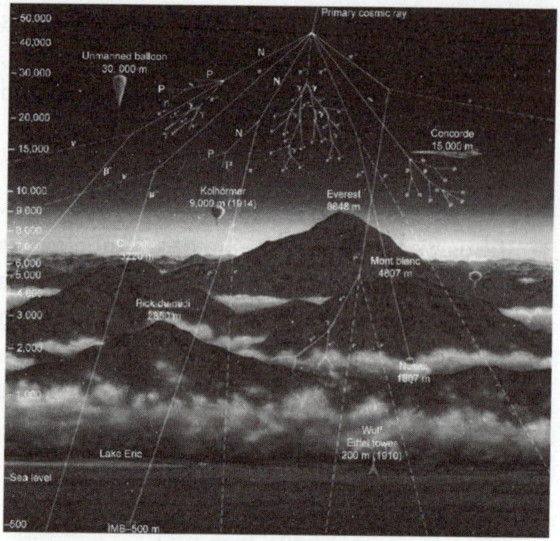

Fig. 27.4: Chain reaction

3. When neutron enters U^{235} nucleus fission always result but when neutron enters U^{238} nucleus in many cases U^{239} will be formed owing relative abundance of U^{238}. This capture of neutron may bring chain reaction to the end, if energy to be generated method has to be adopted to eliminate U^{238} or its neutron capturing property.
4. We solve this problem by using property of U^{238} so some method to be found to make these neutron to slow neutron agent here are deuterium D_2O "Heavy Water" and carbon in form of pure graphite is used. Nuclear Reactor/ Pile ® Major source of radioactive isotopes. Reactor is not only gives energy but it is also a source of large no. of neutron thus, the substances desired to irradiate with neutron can be placed reactor long drawers or stringers. In nuclear reactor source of neutron is spontaneous fission of uranium, neutron also present in cosmic radiation which is continuously bombard our world.

Radioactive Equilibrium

We know no, of radioactive nuclei decaying depends on the number present and therefore initially very few decay because few are present as the stock increases the "No." decaying increases and eventually a state is reached when the no decaying equals. The number of few radioactive nuclei being produced. A state of equilibrium is then attained.

Growth and Decay of Radioactive Isotope

Here we see after 2t½ decay would be one quarter and growth would be three quarters.

Quantities of Radioactive Material

Activity defines as "No. of disinter ration per second" 1 Curie = $3.7 x 10^{10}$ disintegration/ second

Means an amount of radioactive material in which there are $3.7 x 10^{10}$ disintegration per second said to have activity of 1 Curie.

1. 1 Bq = 1 disintegration/second

   Thus, Becquerel is a very tiny amount of activity.
2. I Curie = $3.7 x 10^{10}$ Bq

   Absorbed dose of 1 Gy=1J/Kg=10^7erg 10^3g=100 rad radiation.

Use of Radioactivity

1. For treatment purpose in radiotherapy.
2. Detection of emission of radiation can be used to reveal the presence of the isotope in any material it can be use for therapeutic as well as diagnostic purpose.

   For example: Bone scanning by radioactive substances.

1. ***Radioactive bone scanning*** (Diagnostic use)
2. ***Radioiodine use in follicular Ca of thyroid and in thyrotoxicosis as well*** (Therapeutic use).

   Specific active means activity/gm

   Specific active of Co^{60} = 200 ci/gm.

Radioactive Bone Scanning

Radioactive elements use in bone scanning mainly ^{99}TCM-Phosphates Complex, Sr^{85} (Strontium) especially in bone metastasis there are increased blood flow and increased osteoid tissue formation with high mineral turnover. This can be demonstrated by locally increased concentration of gamma emitting isotope by use of gamma camera by taking multiple overlapping views. Thus, positive bone scan seen before X-ray changes in bone. Simple X-ray shows no abnormality until more than 50 percent of bone mineral has been destroyed so metastasis may be present even in absence of X-ray changes. Increased radioactivity displayed as hot spot on scan. Bone scan use in other nonmalignant condition such as abscesses, aseptic necrosis of bone, pagets disease of bone, arthropathies, in very anaplastic tumor,^{99TCM} phosphate complex injected IV scanning per form 1 to 4 hours. After IV injection (5 to 10 MCI dose). Bladder must be empty before pelvis to be scanned as 40 percent of given dose excreted through urine within first four hours after injection thus pelvic lesion likely to be obscured by overlying bladder activity. Bony metastasis in Ca prostate may be present despite normal acid phosphates and alkaline phosphates level, thus bone scanning in Ca prostate is very important.

Use of Radioactivity

1. Treatment purpose in radiotherapy.
2. Detection of emission of radiation can be use to reveal the presence of isotope in material, it can be use as therapeutic as well as diagnostic purpose.

Bragg Curve of Ionization by a Charged Particles

After traveling some distance charged particle velocity decrease energy thus ionization increased.

Chapter

28 Measurement of X-ray

Many years after the discovery of X-rays and γ-rays. They have been used empirically in medicine, later on realized that this approach was dangerous mainly in radiotherapy and up to some extent in diagnostic radiology. Method of X-ray production (Fig. 28.1).

Thus, Means of measuring X-rays/γ-rays had to be found in terms of unit of X-rays quantity defined and accepted. The magnitude of the biological effect desirable in case therapy and undesirable in case of diagnosis. It depends upon how much radiation energy is absorbed by irradiated material. X-ray dosimetry is the measurement of energy absorbed in any material particularly in different tissues of the body.

THE BIOLOGICAL EFFECTS—DEPENDS UPON

- Quantity of absorbed energy
- Volume of tissue irradiated
- Pattern of absorbed energy distribution
- Length of time over which radiation is given
- Type of tissue
- Quality of the radiation
  - Direct measurement in the irradiated person is impracticable thus, a material to be taken, which nearly as possible simulate the material of interest.

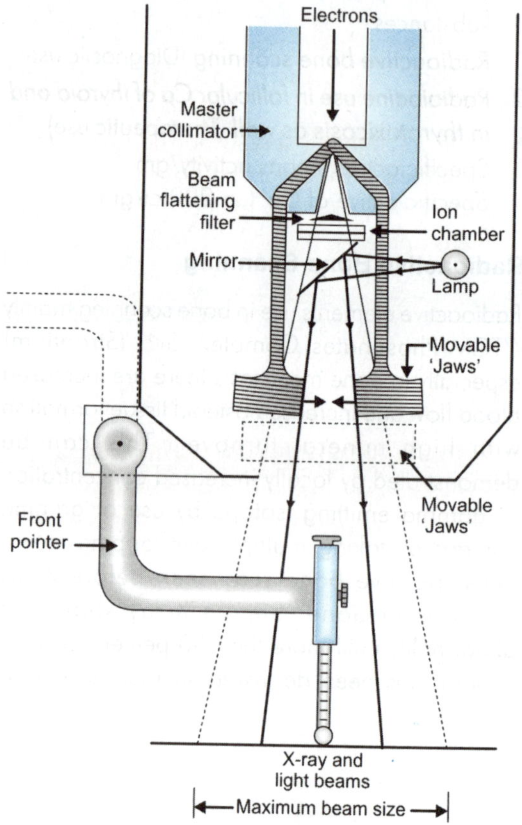

Fig. 28.1: X-ray production

Any measuring system must have certain criteria, system should be

- *Reproducible:* Obtainable in constant from any were any time.
- *Repeatable:* Repeated measurement of same amount of radiation should given same reading.
- *Sensitive:* Small amount should be enough to obtain acceptable reading.
- *Objective:* As far as possible personal subjective.
- *Linear:* Judgment should not be involved in obtaining an answer. Response should be simply proportional to the quantity being measurement.

REQUIREMENTS OF X-RAY DOSIMETER

- It should be capable of measuring from ***very small*** to ***very large*** amount of radiation.
- It is important that the variation of absorption with radiation energy in the test material should be nearly as possible the same as for the material of interest. This can be achieved, if two substances have same atomic number and electron density at any energy they will absorbed amount of energy per gram.
- The ionization of air internationally accepted basis of standard X-ray dosimetry.
- *Ionization of air:* We know ionization is a major product of the energy absorption process and therefore to measure ionization is essentially to measure energy absorption.

AIR IS CHOSEN

- Atomic number of air (average of several component) is 7.64 and and muscle is 7.42, so that energy absorbed/gram of muscle tissue will be same as per gram of air.
- Readily available and its composition is universally almost constant thus, is reproducible and repeatable.
- It is sensitive.
- Answer can be read of a meter dial thus, no personal judgment (Objective).
- Electron density of air and soft tissue is 3×10^{23}/gm. Ionization of air does not run parallel at all type of radiation qualities with the ionization and absorption per gram in materials of different atomic number. ***For example,*** radiation energy absorption in bone (Z»13) on basis of air ionization is more complex matter.
- **Roentgen:** This definition came in 1937. Roentgen is that amount of X-ray/γ-ray radiation such that the associated corpuscular emission per .001293 gram of air, (Weight of icc of air at 0°C and 760 mm) produces in air ions carrying 1 esu of charge of either sign. Here corpuscular emission refers to the photoelectron, Compton electron, pair production electrons set in motion by primary interaction between radiation photons and the air. If total charge librated by electrons originating in icc of air amounts to is then the air has been exposed to **1 roentgen** (Applicable only for X-ray/γ-ray energy up to 3 Mev). Thus, roentgen

is the amount of radiation but it does not measure the energy taken from that amount of radiation which is what we really want hence forth in 1962. Roentgen shall be unit of exposure and rad is the unit of absorbed dose.

Limitation of Roentgen

- It does not indicate directly absorbed dose in bone (due to higher atomic number of bone Z»B in compression to that of air and soft tissue (7.64 and 7.42).
- It cannot be use for beta rays/or neutron only can be used for only X-rays/γ-rays

  Exposure (X) is defined by

$$X = \frac{\Delta Q}{\Delta M}$$

Where is ΔQ is sum of all electrical charges of all the ions of one sign produced in air ΔM is the mass of volume of air in which all the electrons libeated by photon are completely stopped in air IR = 2.58×10^{-4} coulomb/kg of air **rad**: Since exposure dose not fulfill the purpose of measuring absorbed energy. But we want to measure absorbed dose. Thus, unit of absorbed dose is **rad** 1 rad = 100 ergs/gM, 1 ion pair = 33.7 eV, so the roentgen measures amount of radiation incident upon material and the rad is the amount of energy absorbed as a result of this exposer. To measure the rad we measure the exposure in roentgens and then calculate the rads. Through known factors which depends of the material irradiated and the radiation energy. This easy for soft tissue but complex for material like bone. Gray is the unit of absorbed dose, 1 Gray = 100 rad, 1 Gy = 1J/Kg = 10^7 Ery/10^3 gm= 100 rad, now we know the methods of dosemetry are generally indirect, so measure exposure by ionization in air and from this calculate absorbed dose in any other material.

OTHER MEASURING METHODS

We know standard measurement is ionization of air. But many effects of radiation can be use as detectors of radiation and up to some extent as measuring methods.

Biological Methods

Earliest attempt of X-ray measurement were based on erythema production.

The threshold erythema dose (TED) was amount of radiation which would produce reddening of skin in 80 percent those expose. But this effect has lots of variation person-to-person. Thus, repeatability was no high.

Chemical Methods

Here oxidation of ferrous sulfate to ferric sulfate use as a dose meter (called Frike dosimeter). It can use very large amount of radiation but not small amount of radiation. Thus, was not sensitive. Purity of chemical was important for the precise effect.

Physicochemical Methods

Photographic effect of X-ray on film, because use blackening produced in proportional to the radiation energy absorbed, but blackening also depends upon development condition and type of radiation quality other fact is that film contains element of high atomic number than that of low atomic number soft tissue.

Physical Methods

Fluorescence

- Intensity of visible light emitted by a fluorescent material depends primarily on the amount of energy absorbed by it therefore also on the intensity of X-ray falling upon it. Thus, fluorescence would therefore to offer method of measuring radiation dosage since measurement of visible light is quite straight forward.
- But material use in radiology (Zinc sulfide or calcium tungstate) contains elements of high atomic number so that the variation with radiation energy of this absorption will be very different from that of soft tissue.
- So we can use such as anthracene or one of the number of transparent plastics. Florence when irradiated with X-ray and also have atomic number close to air and soft tissue using a photo multiplier tube to amplify effect of tiny amount of light.
- This method is sensitive, repeatability is good but dose not have high reproducibility.

Thermoluminescence

A very wide range of dose can be measure by using the thermoluminescent. Phenomenon lithium fluoride use for this has, an AN close to that of soft tissue therefore the variation with radiation energy absorption. Both material will be very similar tiny capsules can readily be inserted into body cavities sites not normally accessible to more conventional measuring method. Relative values of doses at a number of sits can be readily obtained like fluorescence thermoluminescence depends on tiny amount of impurities in the crystalline material thus it is not possible to produce a universally constant material.

Calorimetry

Energy deposited in any material is to measure the heat generated due to slowing down of the primary electrons and product of many of the radiation induced chemical reactions. But amount of heat generated are extremely small thus requirement is most careful and sensitive techniques.

Standard Free Air Chamber

In free air chamber the ionization produced in air by the irradiation of a known amount of air must be measured. This free air chamber is principally confined to National Standard Laboratory (Fig. 28.2). X-ray from the focal spot of an X-ray tube is collimated by circular diagram of area A. The collimated beam inters the ionization chamber. Here interaction of X-ray with air produces ion pair. These ion pair travels in all directions. Electrons produced by the photon beam in specified volume must spend all their energy by

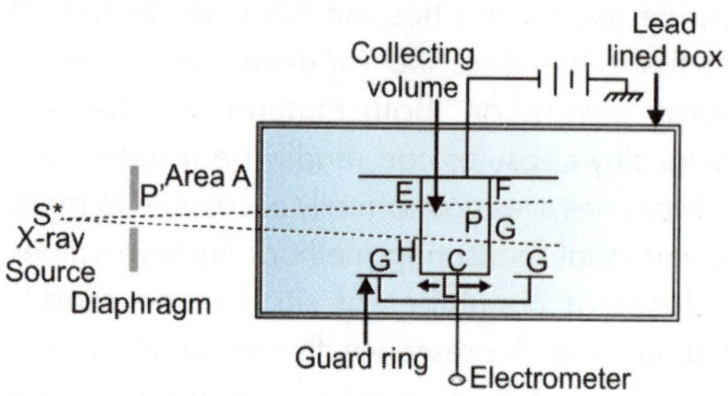

Fig. 28.2: The ionization chamber

ionization of air between the plates. This can occur only when range of electron liberated by the incident photon is less than the distance between each plate and specified volume.

Lead line box ions produced in EFGH volume collected by electrodes C of length connected to positive potential. Guarding arrangement is placed to keep field parallel at the edge of electrodes. **Plate spacing** requirement is that the distance of each plate form the beam should be greater than the fastest electron generated, thus every electron expands all its energy in air and produces all the ionization of which it is capable rather than colliding with the plate whilst still having some energy.

Voltage Applied between the Plates

With voltage application +ve and –ve ions combine thus, voltage applied and electric field generated by—voltage, — in the amount of liberated charge collected since — in voltage more it prevent its recombination but a state will come when if you increase voltage there would be no increase in collection because every ion being formed collected.

So it is require that free ion chamber applied voltage should be such as produced saturation condition.

The Charge Produced in Collected and Measured by Electrometer

$$(P)X = \frac{\Delta Q}{PAL}$$

Exposure at **P**

ΔQ total charge collected

P is density of the air

A is the area of diaphragm aperture

L is the length of electrode collector plate, CD is the uniform field so any ions from in section A, B, C, D no other will be attracted to plate CD and measured by E. When matter these electron

X-ray voltage	Photoelectron	Compton electron	Plate used	Separation
100 kV	12 cm	10%	.5 cm	90 (12 ~ SM)
200 kV	37 cm	.4%	4.6 cm	99.6
100 kV	290 cm	0	220 cm	100 (4 meter)

produce hundreds of ionization before being brought to rest. For example, 100 keV photo electron travel 12 cm in air and produce 3000 in ionization (100 keV) Compton electron set in motion and travel 1 cm in air and produce nearly 500 ionization. Ions collected from zone A, B, C, D may be produced by primary electron originating outside A, B, C, D called G electron. Electron entering A, B, C, D but produce effect outside the collecting zone some of their effect will be lost. Such tracks called lost (L) electron. In practice gain and lost described will be equal thus, ions collected by plate CD measure by electrometer, as being the ionization produced by the electron arising from the irradiation of volume represented by A, B, C, D. For equal lost and gain electron in the zone of interest provided that before arriving at collecting volume the beam has traversed a thickness of air which is least equal to the range of most energetic electron the beam can produce.

TLD SYSTEM OF EXPOSURE MEASUREMENT

Temperature and Pressure taking into Account

- Practically ionization chambers that are an open chamber thus, temperature and pressure must be taken into account and their difference from normal temperature and pressure NTP (760 mm and 0° C). Thus, if reading **M** found then true reading (X) is given by departmental chamber. The free air chamber exit in small number in the world is used as standard and a standardizing instrument but it is not suitable for use in X-ray department (large size). It cannot measure dose within patient. It cannot measure dose of radiation received by radiographer during his or her work for the purpose the use TLD system to monitor exposure of radiography, physicist, radiation oncologist during working in the close proximity of radiotherapy equipments (Fig. 28.3).

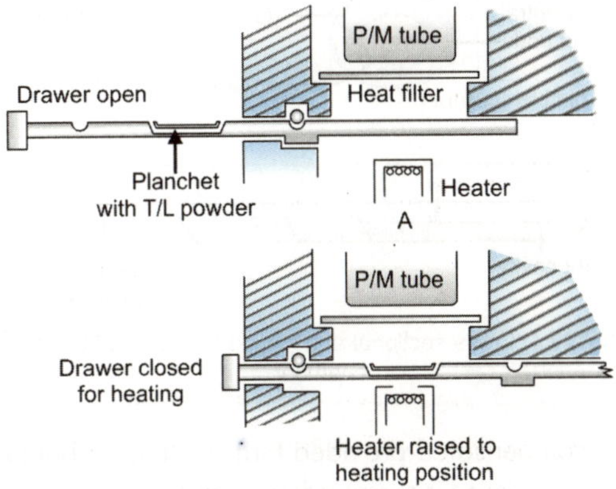

Fig. 28.3: TLD system of exposure measurement

- This thimble chamber must standardize at intervals against the standard free air ion chamber (Fig. 28.4). The volume of thimble chamber (.33 to 3 cc) here in thimble chamber ionization taken in small circumscribed volume. Large majority of electron tracks start inside will produce much of their ionization beyond its confines while tracks majority in number will originate outside the volume of interest. Lost and gain electron can be

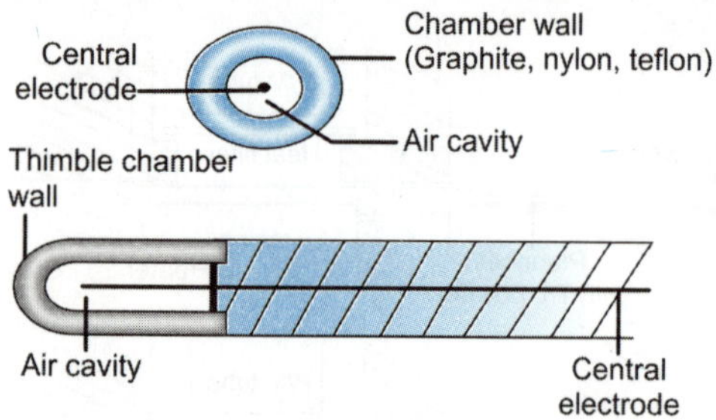

Fig. 28.4: Cross-sectional and longitudinal view of thimble chamber

compensated provided that air volume being considered is surrounded by air to a maximum thickness® to the maximum range of electron. If all ionization in little volume collected and measure we can get exposure. Since great bulk of ionization produce in the volume arises from electron which is liberated in its surrounding air. Now, the situation with in the volume would not be altered in surrounding air out to the range R were solidified to give wall to the air volume. Due to low atomic number of graphite (z=6), thus the wall materials tends to contribute less ionization than would in air wall. This can be compensated by using central electrode aluminium (z=13).

CHAMBER SIZE

Large volume = larger charge amount can measure anyway. But for small volume requirement of sensitive electrometer required like air 1 R (exposure) gives in 1 esu® 1 cc air charge 1 R in 1000 cc of air gives 1000 esu.

MEASURING SYSTEM

Exposure Meter (Dosimeter)

Exposure Rate Meter (Dose Rate Meter)

Voltage supplied by: Battery must be high enough to saturate the ionization chamber and about 200 volt per cm of gap between central electrode and wall are usually provided. In exposure meter reading increase continuously as long as the irradiation continues because that instrument adding up the charges librated. However, this not in case exposure rate meter. Here, reading comes fastly up to appropriate value assuming the radiation rate is constants and stays at the value number matter, how long the exposure continues (Figs 28.5A and B).

Practically: Exposure meter and exposure rate meter present in same instrument. Both the instrument connected to ionization chamber with long leads, so that ionization chamber can be expose to radiation chamber reading can be take from outside the zone of radiation.

WALL THICKNESS

Condition is that has to be fulfilled before an ionization chamber measures roentgens is that its wall thickness must be at least equal to maximum range of electrons produced by the radiation that is being measured. Now that thickness will be different for radiation energies. It is usual to have wall which is about 1 mm thick since the handling is easy and it can be use for radiation up to about

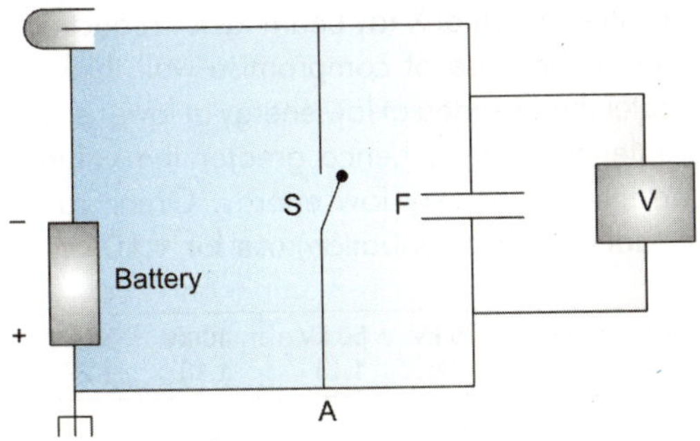

Fig. 28.5A: Exposure meter

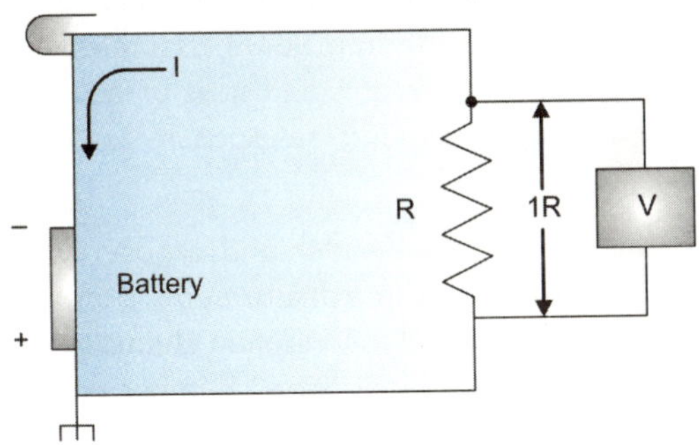

Fig. 28.5B: Exposure rate meter

300 kV. Perspex or other plastic caps are use to supplement the wall thickness for higher energy radiations.

Effect of Wall Thickness on Measured Ionization

Wall thinner than E contributes too few electrons. Whilst if the thickness is greater than E, then measured effect is reduced because of attenuation of beam in the wall. Wall attenuation effect will be marked at low energies.

Calibration

The response of a radiation meter to give exposure or exposure rate depending on a factor:

- Air volume
- Wall thickness
- Material of wall and central electrode
- Sensitivity of electrical measuring system.
  – In calibration, the instrument readings compared with free air standard chamber and reading multiplied with calibration factor to give roentgens these calibrations should be use different for different radiation quality at which the instrument is likely to be used. It should be repeated at 2 yearly intervals to check the constancy of equipment. Side-by-side meter should be check at local level at monthly /2 monthly interval. Such check is carried out by placing the ionization chamber to some radioactive source of a known radiation exposure rate. Above stated factors given by standardizing laboratory for departmental meter. For higher energy, Compton effect produced and we know Compton effect in dependent of material used in chamber wall and central electrode, thus instrument will be more incentive. It will give reading slightly increased value.

At low energy: Photo electric effect produced max. effect since we photo electric effect varies with a z^3 (AN) thus wall material and central electrode becomes very important in correction factor indicating that the instrument become more sensitive for low energy radiation. Other factor is wall attenuation of X-ray beam factor reduction is reversed because of compromise wall thickness greater than needed at low energy at lower energy greater this effect, hence greater the value of correction. For very low energy, Grenz rays – special chamber (ionization) use for <10 kV.

Generating voltage	300 kV	200 kV	175 kV	150 kV	100 kV	75 kV	50 kV	40 kV	30 kV
Multiplying factor	1.02	1.02	1.01	1	1.02	1.06	1.13	1.18	1.27

Chapter 29 Principles of Radiation Therapy

Father of radiotherapy named after discovery of X-ray by Sir WC Roentgen (Fig. 29.1). Physical considerations ionizing radiation is the energy that during absorption causes the ejection of an orbital electron. A large amount of energy is associated with ionization. Ionizing radiation can be electromagnetic or particulate. Electromagnetic radiation may be considered as a wave and as a packet of energy (a photon). The packet of energy is large enough to cause ionizations, and these are distributed unevenly trough tissues, examples of

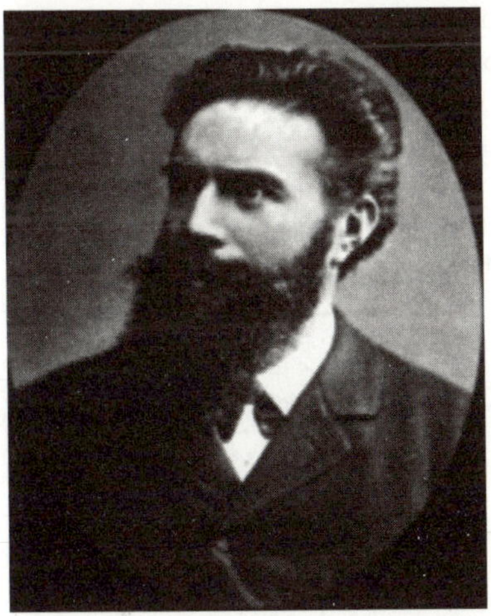

Fig. 29.1: Sir WC Roentgen Father of radiotherapy

particulate radiations are the subatomic particles: electrons, protons, alpha particles neutrons and atomic nuclei. All of these have been experimentally considered or are being used in radiation therapy.

Electromagnetic Radiation

Electromagnetic radiation consists of roentgen and gamma radiation. They differ only in the way in which they are produced: gamma rays arc produced intranuclearly and roentgen rays are produced extra nuclearly. In practice, this means that gamma rays used in radiation therapy are produced by decay of radioactive isotopes where as the roentgen rays used in radiation therapy are produced by electrical machine, like linear accelerator (Fig. 29.2).

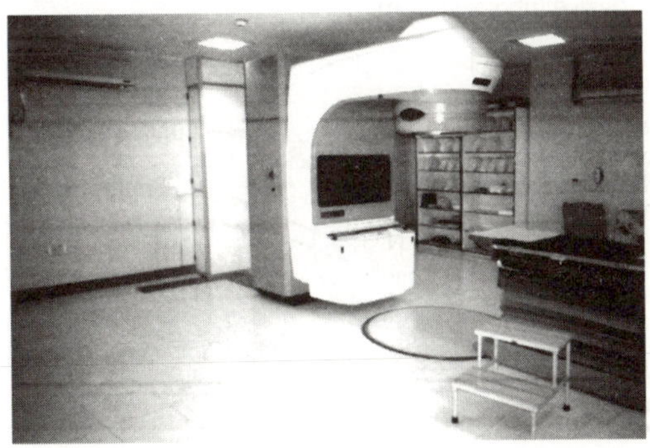

Fig. 29.2: Linear accelerator

The intensity of electromagnetic radiation dissipates as the inverse square of the distance from the source. The dose of radiation 2 cm from a point source is 25 percent of the dose of 1 cm.

Absorption mechanism of electromagnetic radiation.

The relative prevalence of the three dominant absorption mechanisms of electromagnetic radiation depends on the energy of radiation.

Photoelectric Absorption

Photoelectric is a phenomenon in which a photon interacts with an atom and ejects on of the orbital electrons from the atom (Figs 29.3A and B). The vacancy left in the atomic shell is then filled by another electron falling from an outer shell of the same atom. Thus, leaving the atom in an excited state. Photoelectric absorption varies with the cube of the atomic number (Z3). This has significant practical implications because it explains why materials with high atomic numbers, such as lead are such effective shielding material.

Compton Effect

In this process, the photon interaction is with a distant orbital electron that has a low binding energy and the electron is termed as free. In this type of absorption, the photon does not give up all its energy to a single electron; an appreciable portion reappears as a secondary photon, which is created in the interaction. Since, the Compton effect involves essentially free electrons in the absorbing material, it is independent of atomic number Z, unlike photoelectric absorption.

Pair Production

This type of absorption requires incident photon energy greater than 1.02 MeV. In this process, the photon interacts strongly with the electromagnetic field of an atomic nucleus and

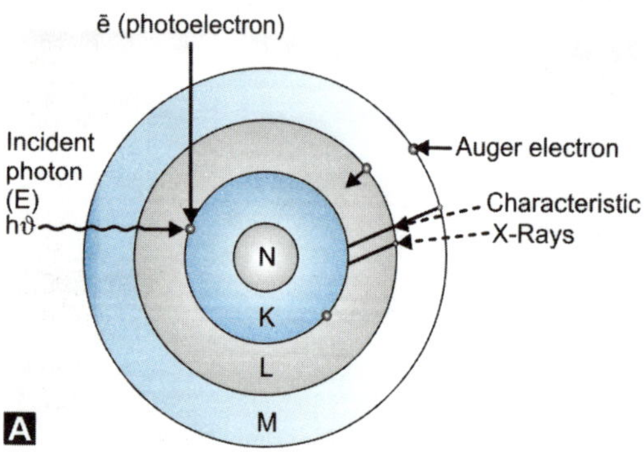

Fig. 29.3A: Photoelectric effect

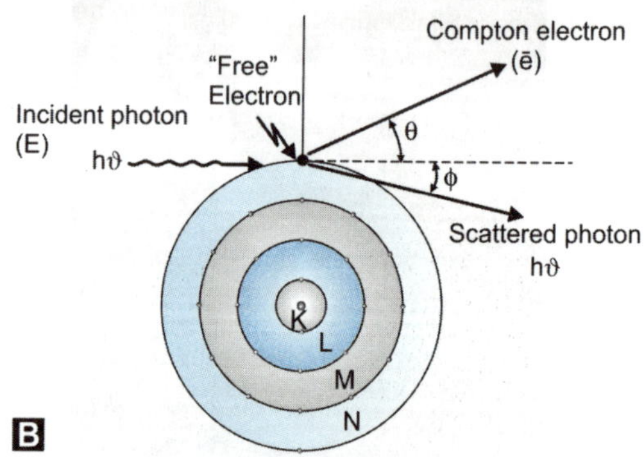

Fig. 29.3B: Compton effect

gives up all its energy in the process of creating a pair consisting of a negative electron (e–) and a positive electron (e+). Since, the rest mass energy of the electron is equivalent to 0.51 MeV. A minimum energy of the 1.02 MeV is required in order to create the pair of electron (Fig. 29.4).

The Fundamental Quantity

Necessary to describe the interaction of radiation with matter is the amount of energy absorbed per unit mass. This quantity is called absorbed dose and the rad was the most commonly used unit. Absorbed dose is measured in joules per kilogram; another name for 1 joule/kg is the Gray (1 Gray = 100 rad), which is now the recommended unit the roentgen (R) is a unit of roentgen rays or gamma rays-based on the ability of radiation to ionize air. At the energies used in radiation therapy, 1 R of roentgen rays or gamma rays results in a dose of somewhat less than 1 rad (0.01 Gy) in soft tissue on the energy increases depth of penetration of radiation increases (Figs 29.5 and 29.6) after entering into radiation causes DNA damage into cell nucleus which is the prime target for radiation induce cell killing (Fig. 29.7).

Spectrum of Electromagnetic Radiations

The different ranges of electromagnetic radiations used in clinical practice are super voltage radiation or roentgen from about 10 to 125 keV; orthovoltage radiation or electromagnetic radiation between 125 and 400 keV; and super voltage or mega voltage radiation for energies above 400 keV. As energy increases, the penetration of the roentgen rays increases, and at super voltage energies, absorption in bone is not higher than that in surrounding soft tissues as is the case with lower energies. This is because at super voltage energies, Compton absorption predominates.

MOVEMENT OF COBALT MACHINE

Compared with the orthovoltage, supervoltage radiation is skin sparing, meaning that the maximum dose is not reached in the skin, but instead occurs below the surface. The electrons

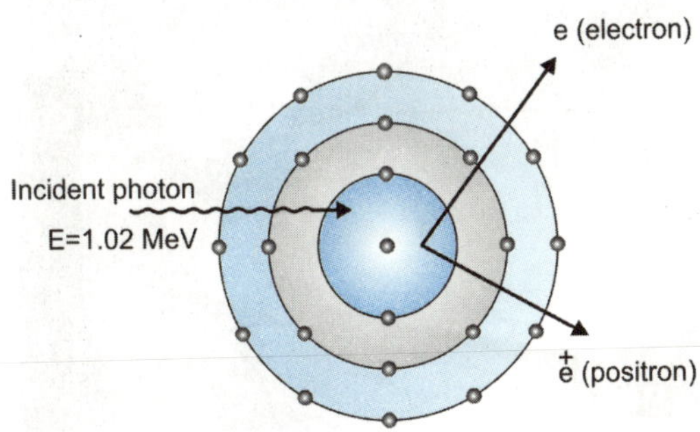

Fig. 29.4: Pair production

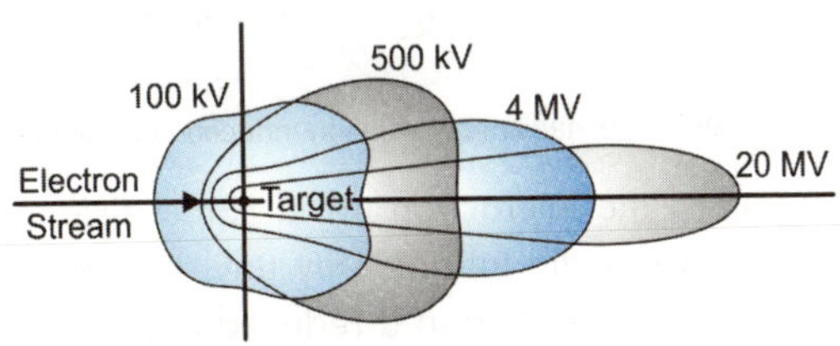

Fig. 29.5

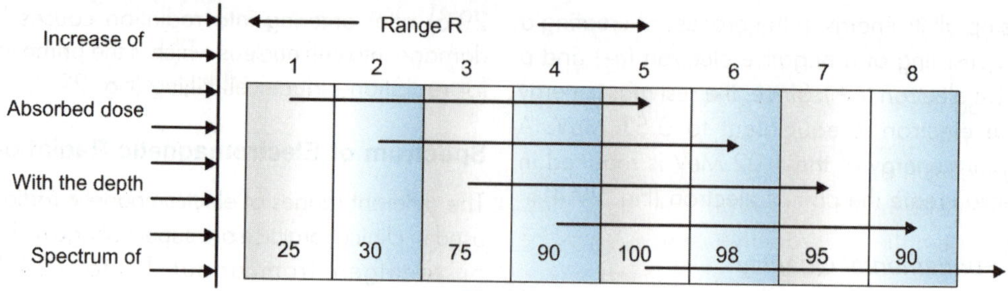

Fig. 29.6

Fig. 29.5 and 29.6: Increase in energy will lead increase in depth

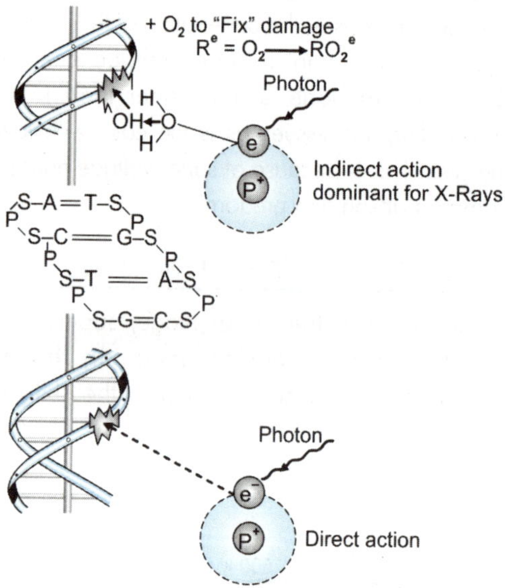

Fig. 29.7: Mechanism of radiation induced cell killing

created in the interaction travel some distance and do not attain full intensity until they reach some depth, resulting in a reduced dose to the skin.

Radiation Techniques

Two general type of radiation techniques are used clinically, teletherapy and brachytherapy.

Teletherapy

Mainly two type of teletherapy are in use for cancer treatment purpose cobalt machine (Fig. 29.8) and linear accelerator, cobalt machine are very common in India. It can move in various

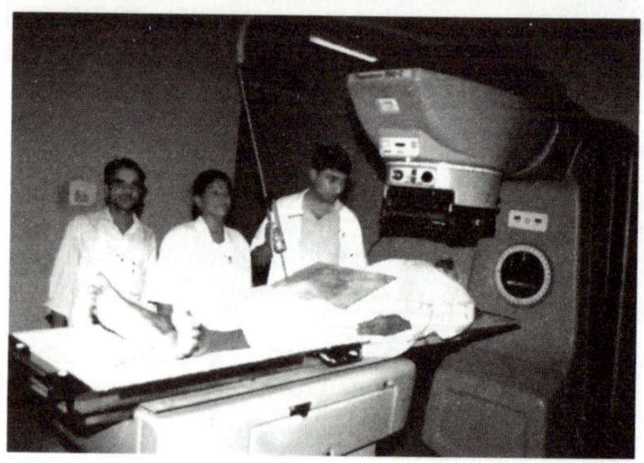

Fig. 29.8: Teletherapy unit cobalt 60

direction to treat cancer patients (Fig. 29.9) main part of cobalt machine is its head which accomodates its source (Figs 29.10 to 29.12).

Teletherapy uses a device located at a distance from the patient, as in the case in most ortho- voltage or supervoltage machines. Gamma emitting radioactive isotopes may be

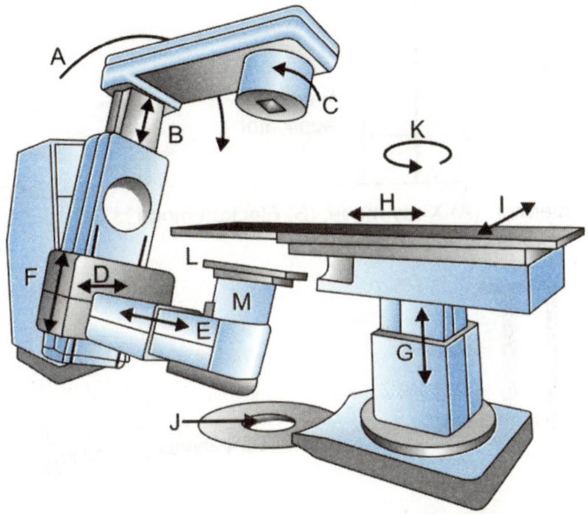

Fig. 29.9: Movement of cobalt machine

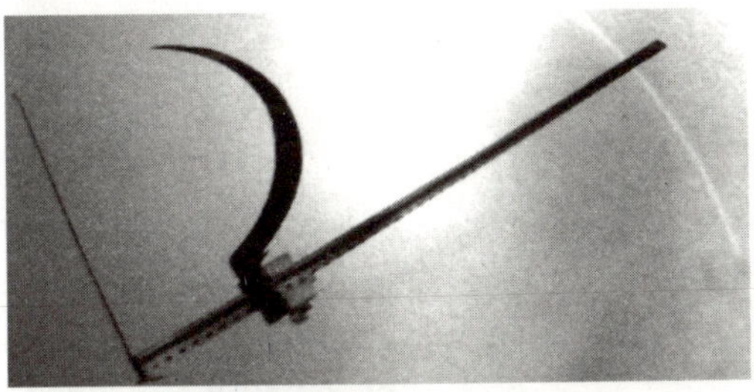

Fig. 29.10: The 45 cm curved caliper

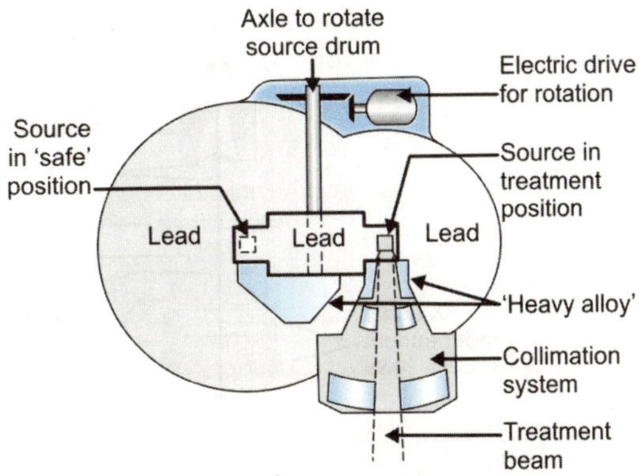

Fig. 29.11: Treatment head of cobalt 60

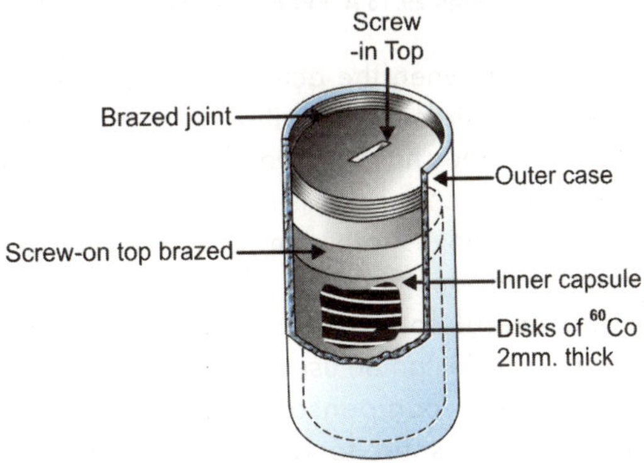

Fig. 29.12: Cobalt source

used to produce a useful gamma ray beam for radiotherapy. It must be remembered that owing to the decay of activity, the source will need replacement from time-to-time. Any one source is normally, used for a period a little longer than one-half of the half-life of the

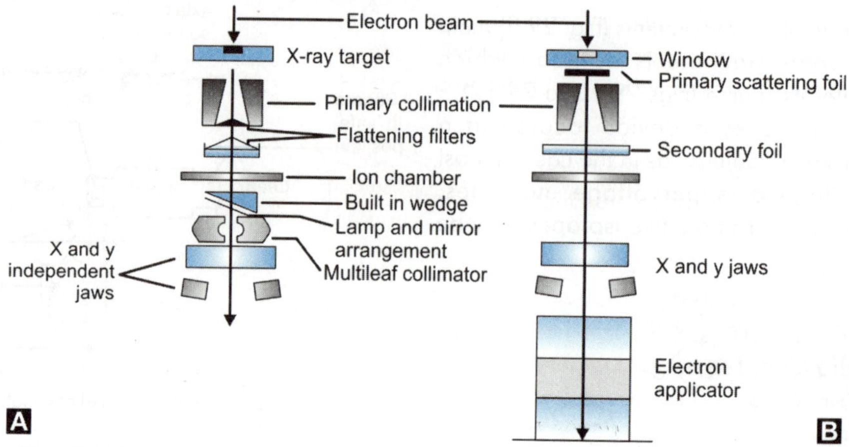

Figs 29.13 A and B: Treatment head of linear accelerator: (A) X-ray mode; (B) Electron mode

isotope, i.e. when the activity has decayed to about two-thirds of the initial activity and the treatment times have increased by about one-half. Linear accelerator is another teletherapy unit which have both componant X-ray and electron mode (Figs 29.13A and B). X-ray mode useful for deep seated tumor and electron mode can be use for superficial tumor sliding scale compensator system are the equipments useful to assist radiotherapist inorder to avoid unnecessary radiation reaction and proper dose delivery to tumor tissue (Figs 29.14A and B).

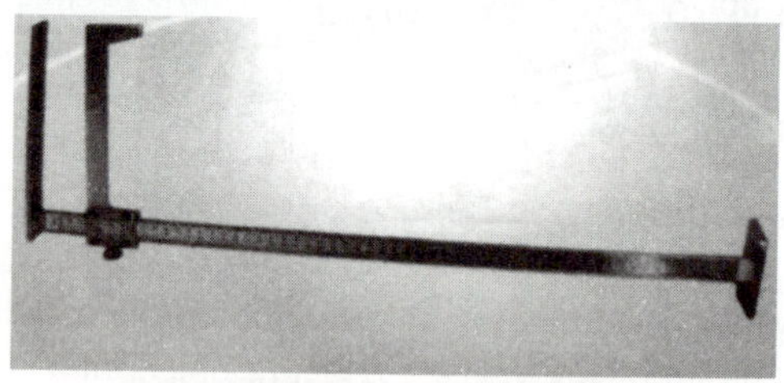

Fig. 29.14A: Sliding scale

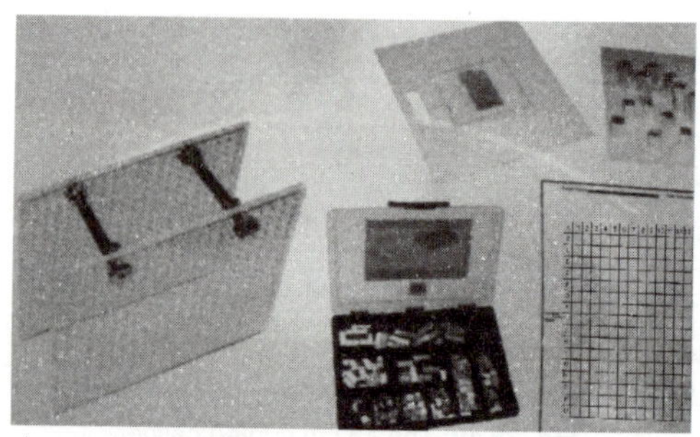

Fig. 29.14B: Compensator system used during radiation

Early units using radium had the advantage of a long half-life (1620 years) and an effectively constant output dose rate. There were however, three major disadvantages of radium:

- 1-Potential leakage of radon gas
- 2-Low specific activity

- 3-Very high photon energy making the protection on the source housing difficult. These radium sources have been replaced with either cesium-137 or cobalt–60.

Cesium-137: Cesium-137 has a long half-life (30 years) and is an attractive alternative to radium. Unfortunately, it has a low specific activity (like radium) as well as a low gamma ray constant. The advantages of cesium over radium are that it requires less shielding and is less hazardous in microsphere form. The disadvantages of cesium, however, outweigh its advantages and it is now rarely found in teletherapy units. It is widely used as a radium substitute in brachytherapy.

Cobalt-60: The effective photon energy of cobalt-60 is only slightly lower than that of radium and its half-life is relatively short (5.26 yr), but despite this, cobalt-60 is the most widely used isotope in gamma ray beam units. The main advantage of cobalt-60 is its high specific activity. Cobalt-60 is produced by neutron bombardment of cobalt-59 and decays to nickel-60 by emitting a beta particle and two gamma rays of 1.17 and 1.33 MeV.

CONCEPTS OF BRACHYTHERAPY

Bell-1903, first suggested implanting the radioactive source directly into tumor.

Forshell-1931, coined term brachytherapy initially radium was used as brachytherapy source.

Nowadays radium is not used because:

- By product of radium is radiotoxic.
- Radon gas emission is always a threat. Contamination can cause great problem.

Low specific activity therefore requires large source size.

- High-cost
- Disposal problem.

Above problem with radium as a brachytherapy source leads to discovery of many other radioactive isotopes.

IDEAL BRACHYTHERAPY SOURCE

Should be β emitter with energy 200 keV preferably monoenergetic.

Should have large half-life for temporary implant and short half-life for permanent implant.

- No gaseous by product
- High specific activity
- Insoluble and chemically nontoxic
- Should be molded in various size and shape
- Low-cost.

Isotope	*Half-life*	*Av photon energy (Mev)*	*Exp. rate constant (R Cm²/Mci-R)*
Ra 226	1622 years	0.832	8.25
Co 60	5.26 years	1.25 (Av)	13.07
Cs 137	30 years	0.662	3.226
Ir 192	74.2 days	.38 (Av)	4.62
Au 198	2.7 days	0.412	2.327
I 125	60 days	.028 (Av)	1.208
Pd 105	17 days	.21 (Av)	
Samarium145	340 days	.41 (Av)	

FORMS OF APPLICATIONS

- Intracavitary
- Interstitial brachytherapy templet system use in (Figs 29.15 and 29.16A and B)

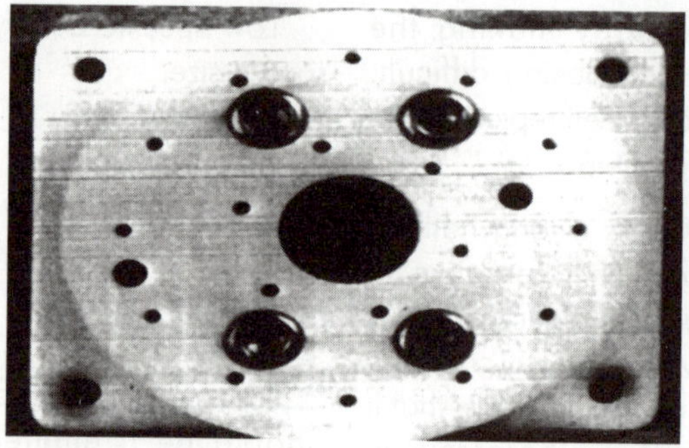

Fig. 29.15: Syed/neblett prostate template

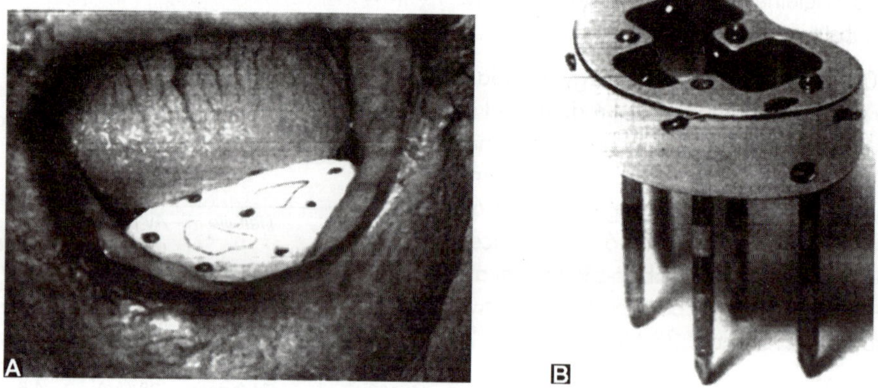

Figs 29.16 A and B: Cardboard template

- Intraluminal
- Surface molds.

Sources

Co-60 → Source available needle, tube, pellets for HDR after loading.

Cs-37 → Needle, tube, beads for after loading.

Ir-192 → As wire, pins for manual after loading.
As pellets for remote after loading.

I-125 → Seeds for permanent implant for surface applicator.

Cs-137 → Largely replaced radium as nuclide of choice.

Alkaline material, compound of cesium chloride/sulfate is chemically stable.

Recommended working half-life is 10 years.

**All sources have recommended working life beyond which manufacture will not guarantee the integrity of sources.

Cs is available in needle form or tube or small pellet for remote after loading machine.

- Ir^{192}
- Currently widely use
- High specific activity
- Flexibility—Acquire the shape of tumor
- Available in 0.8 mm diameter, 4.5 mm length
- Au^{198}/I^{125} can be used for permanent implantation short half-life
- Gurface/mold application
- Now replaced by electron treatment of linac
- Co-60-high specific activity and specific (Glastron) β-ray constant
- Make it attractive use for HDR
- Au198 Available in grains/seeds/wires
- With the help of implantation guns directly fit in tumor area
- Use as permanent implantation purpose also in malignant plural effusion and malignant ascitis
- I^{125} available in seeds form
- As permanent implant or plaque.

**Brachytherapy source is available in various physical forms such as needle, tube pellets, seeds wire which facilitates their application in the patient during interstitial implant needle placed directly into tumor tissue (Fig. 29.17). How implantation is covered is given (Fig. 29.18).

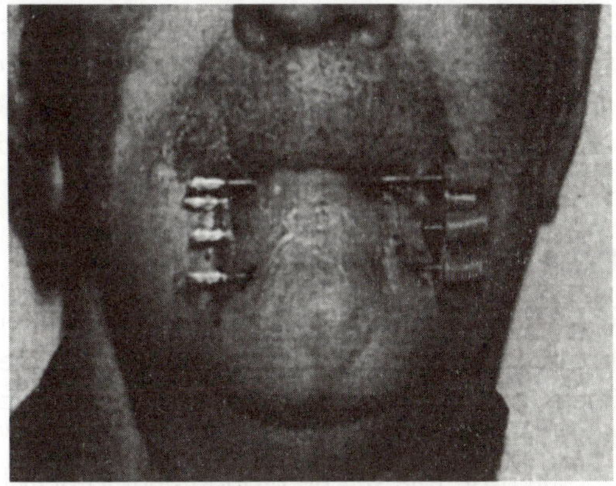

Fig. 29.17: Interstitial brachytherapy in lip cancer

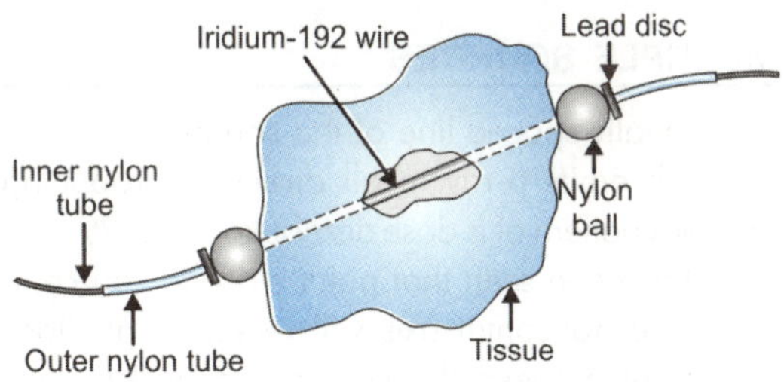

Fig. 29.18: Source train manual after loading

Directly applied in tumor area as in case of treatment of: single solitary retinoblastoma.

PRACTICAL ASPECTS IN BRACHYTHERAPY

Activity of a source is the apparent activity because real activity of source is attenuated because of source encapsulation thus true activity is always greater than this activity.

Exposure rate constant (β-rays constant of source) is defined as dose rate cGy/hr at a distance of 1 cm from millicurie activity of point source; this is however redefined because of source encapsulation (attenuation effect).

Point Source

From a single point source, X-ray is emitted isotropically. It follows inverse square law therefore, intensity of radiation will decrease with square of the distance from the source.

The dose rate will be proportional to activity of source as well as inverse square of the distance (d) from source.

MULTIPLE SOURCES

Five equally spaced line of the source.

Each emits β-ray in all direction producing complex pattern of is dose distribution (Fig. 29.19).

It has been seen that point close to source in the same horizontal axis will receive high dose and point between the two sources will receive low dose.

Uniformity of the dose further improved by increasing the activity of source at the end of the line.

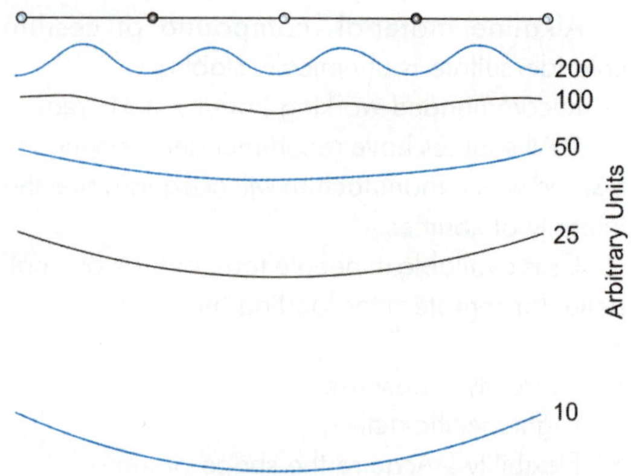

Fig. 29.19: Inference from above figure uniformity of dose achieved depends on both distance from source and spacing between the sources

Methods of Application of Brachytherapy

- Preloading method
- Manual after loading
- Remote after loading.

Preloading—Source are loaded in applicator before they are inserted into patient. Because of radiation exposure to medical and paramedical staff leads invention after loading method.

Manual after loading—First applicator are in patient then sources are manually inserted into applicators.

Remote after loading—Each applicator is fixed in the patient and check X-ray carried out to localize dummy source in applicator, many remote after loading machine life selectron (Figs 29.20 to 29.22) and micro selectron (HDR) now avialable for the purpose of remote after loading treatment.

Source Movement

Combination of various source trains with option to choose.

Small miniature source with spacer enabling the operator to create his own source configuration.

By single source with option of different (dwell times) → (How much dose to be delivered at

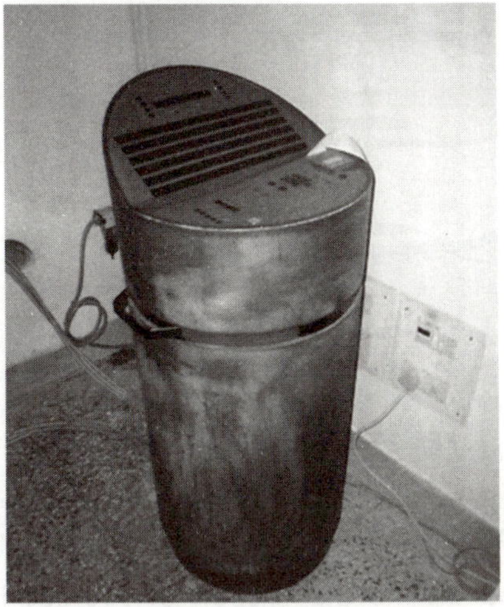

Fig. 29.20: Selectron now less in use

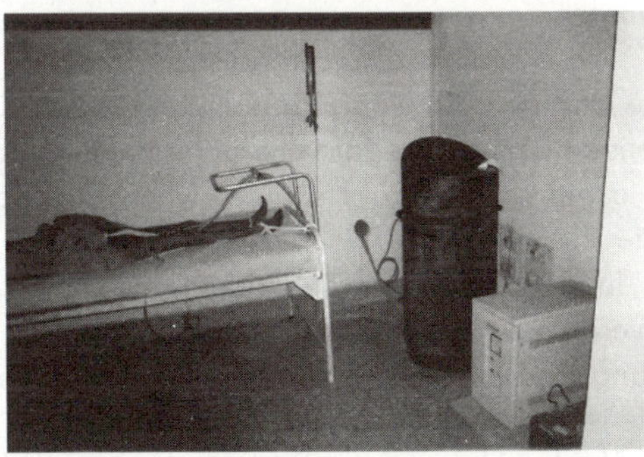

Fig. 29.21: Cancer cervix patient taking selectron treatment LDR

different site) at various position simulating either as many point.

Optimization of dose distribution—Adjusting the dwell times of the source.

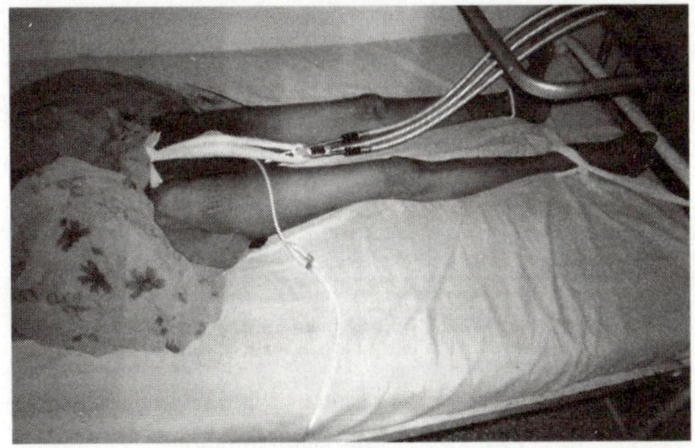

Fig. 29.22: Cancer cervix patients during brachytherapy

INTERSTITIAL IMPLANT

It is important to clearly define target volume and to have preplanned number and distribution of radioactive sources to be used.

Homogeneous dose distribution is very important because high dose around each source can cause neurosis low dose between the sources could result in recurrence (Fig. 29.23).

Rules of interstitial implant:

Active source should be parallel and straight.

Line should be equidistant.

Line or plane on which the mid-point of the source lies should be at right angle to axis of the source (Figs 29.24A to D) shown how implant used in tongue cancer see also (Figs 29.25A and B).

Linear activity of the source should be uniform along the length of each line.

Separation between sources may vary from one implant to other implant. But minimum 8 mm separation is acceptable for smallest volume rising to 20 mm largest.

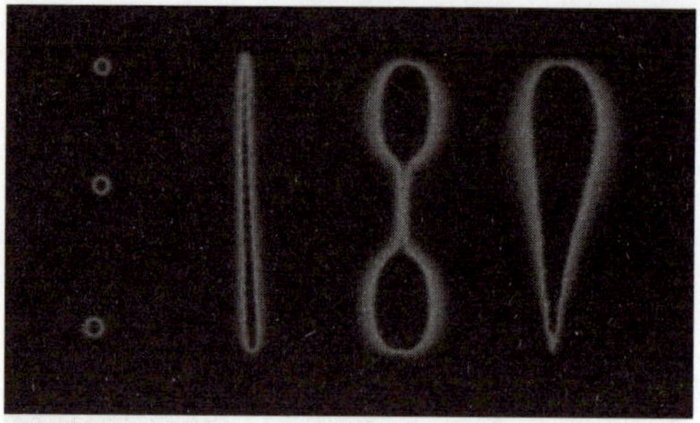

Fig. 29.23: Interstitial implant

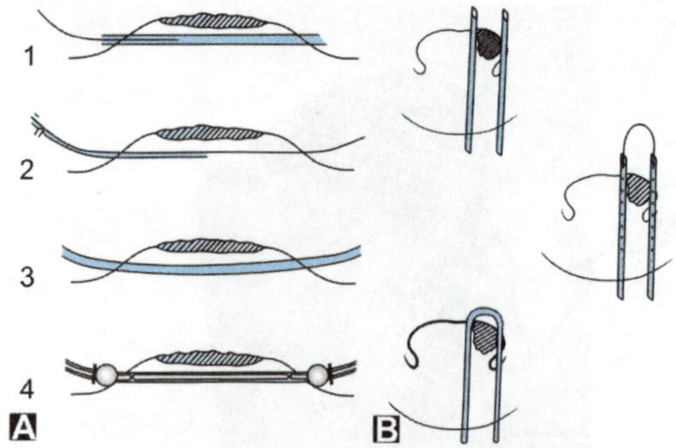

Figs 29.25 A and B: Methods of implant

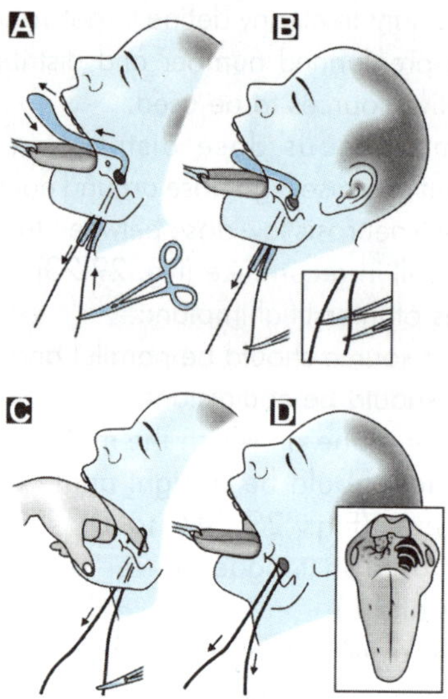

Figs 29.24A to D: Loop technique of implant

Average length of active wire should be larger than target volume by 25 to 30 percent.

Pairs System of Dose Calculation

Based on the distribution of sources in the central plane—that is, the plane which is at right angles to the axis of the mid-point of the sources.

The basal dose rate represents the dose in the center of the implanted volume, and is defined as the dose rate at a point in the middle of a pair or group of sources where the dose rate is lowest.

In the case of a large implant, there may be several pairs of groups of sources arranged in triangle or squares. For these, a mean basal dose rate is taken for the implant as a whole.

The basal dose rate a point is the summation of dose contributions from each source obtained from graphs of dose rate variations with distance from the source.

Once the basal dose rate in the center of the implant has been defined, the reference dose rate is taken as 85 percent of the BDR. This serves

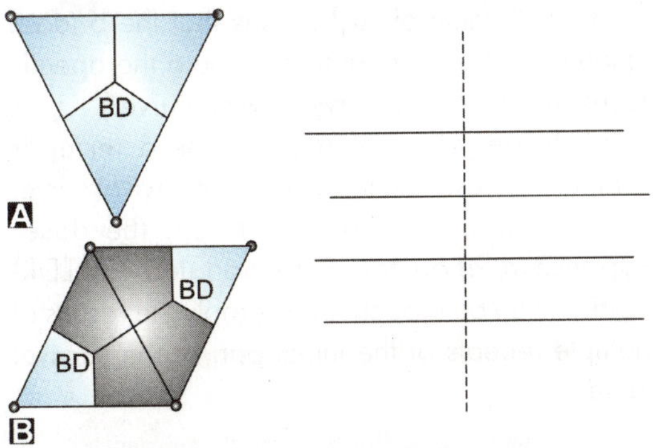

Figs 29.26 A and B: Basal dose rate

to calculate the duration of the implant, and the 85 percent is dose defines the treated volume.

A value of 85 percent has been chosen to provide the dose contour that reasonably covers the target volume with an acceptable variation between the dose at the center and that at the periphery of the target volume. The time for which at implant must be left in place is derived by dividing the prescribed dose by the reference dose rate (Figs 29.26 and 29.27).

Two Plane Implant to Deliver 25 Gy

Superficial plane = 5 cm wires × 2
Deep plane = 7 cm wires × 3

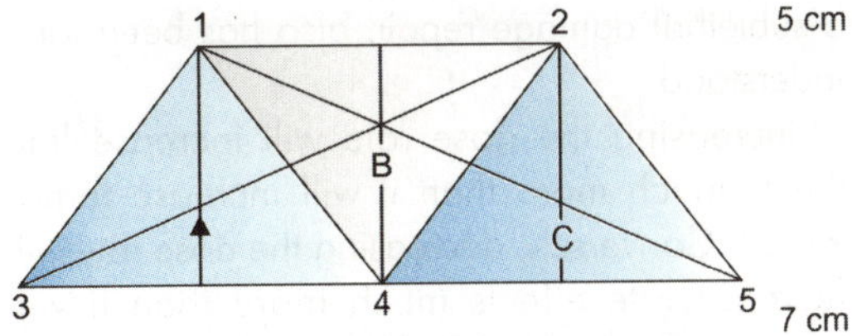

Fig. 29.27: Dose calculation

Separation between sources = 18 mm
Activity of wire (midway through treatment) =air kerma rate 0.5 μGy/hr/mm at 1 m (0.1193 μGy/hr/mm)
Mean basal dose rate

$$= \frac{0.4755 + 0.4940 + 0.4755}{3} \text{ Gy/hr}$$

= 0.4817 Gy/hr

Reference dose rate (85%) = 0.4817 × 0.85
= 0.4095 Gy/hr

$$\text{Treatment time} = \frac{25.00}{0.4095}$$

= 61.05 hr
= 2 days 13hr

It has been known for many decades that lowering the dose rate generally reduces radiobiologic damage. The explanation of this effect, relating

Wire	A Distance (mm)	A Dose rate (Gy/hr)	B Distance (mm)	B Dose rate (Gy/hr)	C Distance (mm)	C Dose rate (Gy/hr)
1	10.4	0.1245	10.4	0.1245	20.8	0.0465
2	20.8	0.0465	10.4	0.1245	10.4	0.1245
3	10.4	0.1340	20.8	0.0555	27.5	0.0365
4	10.4	0.1340	10.4	0.1340	10.4	0.1340
5	27.5	0.0365	20.8	0.0555	10.4	0.1340

to sublethal damage repair, also has been long understood.

Increasing the dose rate will increase late effects much more than it will increase tumor control. Conversely, decreasing the dose rate will decrease late effects much more than it will decrease tumor control. Thus, the "therapeutic ratio" (ratio of tumor control to complications) increase as the dose rate decreases.

Rationale for LDR brachytherapy-LQ model.

These observations can be interpreted in terms of the α/β ratio. In terms of survival curves, the α/β ratio essentially describes the degree of "curviness" of the acute survival curve (Fig. 29.28).

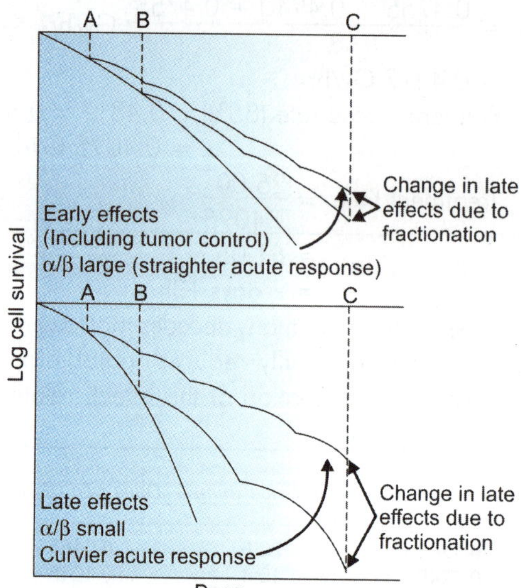

Fig. 29.28: Rationale of LDR brachytherapy—LQ model

A small value of α/β means that the b (dose squared) term is dominating at radio therapeutic doses, resulting in a curvy survival curve.

A large value of α/β means a terms is dominating, resulting in a straighter survival curve.

Now, as a first approximation, the dose-response relation for a fractionated (or LDR) regimen can be thought of as simply the results of multiple repeats of the initial part of the survival curve.

DOSE RATE AND ICRU-38 RECOMMENDATIONS

ICRU	38 defines
LDR	.4 to 2 Gy/hr
MDR	2 to 12 Gy/hr
HDR	>12 Gy/hr

Most of the LDR and MDR—CS-137 as a source HDR-Ir192, Co-60 as source.

ICRU-38 recommendations for Ca cervix T/T technique must be described.

Reference volume should be described in terms of height, width and thickness of the volume enclosed in 60 Gy is dose for LDR T/T in Ca cervix.

Absorbed dose at bladder reference/rectal reference/lymphatic trapezoid reference point and patient A and patient B as well dose determined on computer to avoid extra dose to the above said area.

PDR

Pulse dose brachytherapy

PDR was proposed to exploit the advantage of HDR as well as LDR.

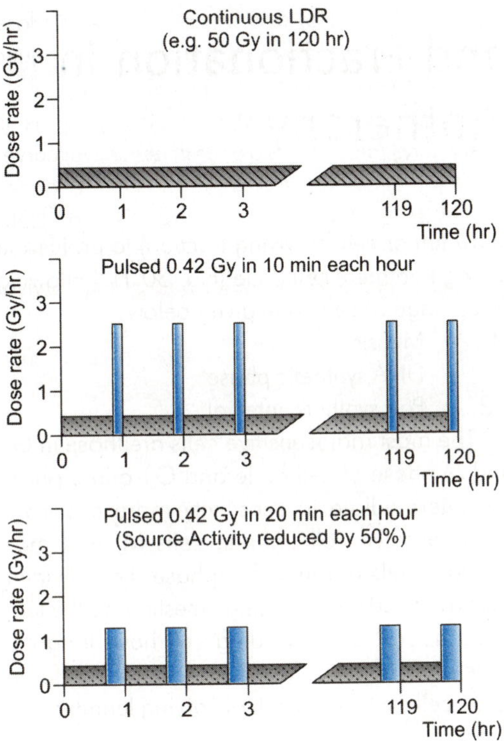

Fig. 29.29: PDR (pulse dose radiotherapy)

It was seen varying dwell time of the stepping source dose optimization could be achieved which maintain the potential benefit of LDR.

PDR

Why PDR?

In effort to replace the continuous LDR treatment lasting several days patient is hooked up for several days whereas, in PDR source of pulse 10 min/hr delivered. It offer practical advantage that patient's nursing care can be done more frequently which was not possible in LDR treatment where patient was hooked up continually for 72 hours.

Initially 0.6 Gy/10 min every hr delivered. Here single high activity source is programmed to pass all implant applicators during each pulse computer control dwell time for each position so source can deliver desired dose distribution, because of single source use, dose calculation becomes easy (Fig. 29.29).

Radiobiological advantage is that 10 min pulse every hour would produce biological effect essentially similar to continue radiation at 50 cGy/hr when the source is in safe position between the two pulses nursing care and visiting to the patient can be allowed.

DAY TIME PDR

Modification has been done in terms of day time treatment (8 am–8 pm) with no radiation in night so, It allows the patient to come out of the treatment room and to stay in the hospital ward. But this modification required an extra treatment day in compare to conventional PDR treatment.

PDR has been proposed in Europe and Asia but not in United States, Nuclear Regulatory Commission (NRC) says that during the treatment both radiation oncologist and physicist should be present which is difficult because of long treatment schedule in hospital setting. Acute reactions were similar in LDR and PDR but 2 percent raised in the late reaction observed in PDR.

Chapter 30 Time, Dose and Fractionation in Radiotherapy

Multifraction regimens mainly based on radiobiological experiments (France 1920-1930). It was found that RAM could not be sterilized by exposing its tests to a single dose of radiation without extensive skin damage to scrotum but in same case if multiple fractions, given then sterilization were possible without skin damage. So fractionation of radiation dose produces better tumor control for a given level of normal tissue toxicity than a single large dose.

The Four R of Radiobiology

The basis of fractionation-based on four R:

1. Repair of sublethal damage.
2. Reassortment of cells within cell cycle.
3. Repopulation.
4. Reoxygenation.

Dividing a dose into number of fractions spares the normal tissue because of repair of sublethal damage between dose fractions and repopulation of normal cells if over-all time is sufficient long and diving a dose in number of fraction increases damage to tumor because of reoxygenating and reassortment of tumor cells into radiosensitive phase of cell cycle however, between the fractions. Excessive prolongation allow tumor cell (surviving fraction) to proliferate during treatment cell cycle (Fig. 30.1). Following these stage of cell cycle given below:

M — Mitosis

S — DNA synthetic phase

G2 — Post synthetic interval.

The most radiosensitive cells are those in G2 and M phase of cell cycle and G1 and S phase are intermediate in sensitivity more precise is most sensitive cell (mitotic cells M) and most resistant cells are in late S phase. Fast dividing cell have short cell cycle (e.g. intestinal epithelium; 9–10 hours). Slow dividing cell have long cell cycle time. Most of the difference in the different tissue cell cycle is a result of varying length of G1 phase.

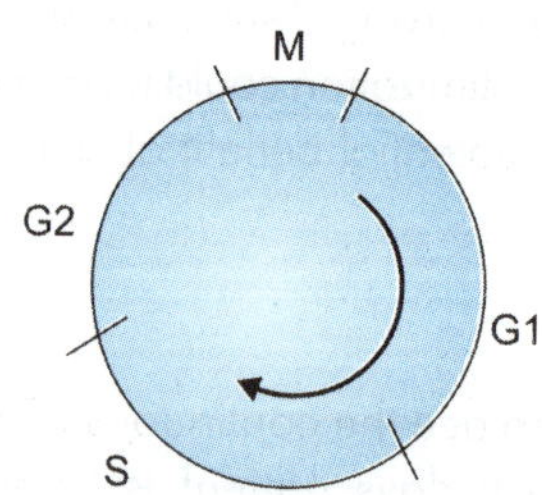

Fig. 30.1: Cell cycle

STRANDQUIST PLOT AND THE ELLIS NOMINAL STANDARD DOSE SYSTEM

Relationship between the dose of radiation delivery and the time over which dose is spread is given by Strandquist plot. Here, total dose was plotted against over all treatment time in days (Fig. 30.2).

Here, all A, B, C, D, E is parallel to each other with slope of .33 in a log scale. That means total dose for iso-effect was proportional to $T^{.33}$, here treatment given in 3 or 5 fractions/week. It is important to know overall treatment time (T) and number of fractions (N) how much contribute to total effect.

ELLIS INTRODUCED NSD SYSTEM

NSD (Nominal Standard Dose)—Because of importance of separating overall treatment time from number of fractions for skin tolerance.

Propose formulas as $TD = NSD\ (N^{.24} \times T^{.11})$

Calculation of NSD is simple but applicable on condition when

a. Uniform dose per fraction

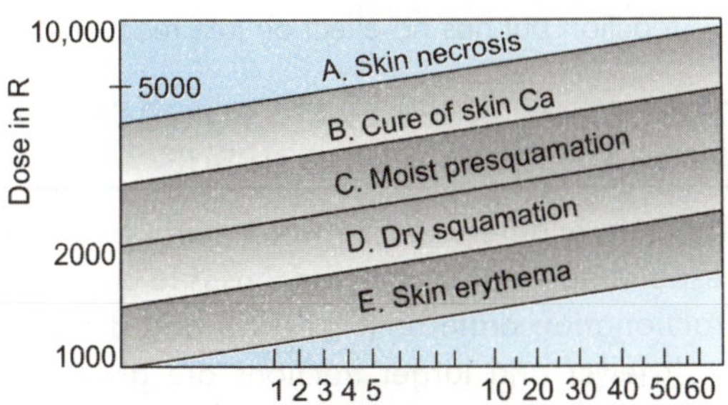

Fig. 30.2: Strandquist plot

b. Uniform number of fraction/week, for changing a treatment protocol from 5 fraction/week to 4 fraction/week. This formula can be used to calculate size of dose/fraction for same total dose.

WEAKNESS OF NSD SYSTEM

1. It was base on pure hypothesis without any direct experimental evidence.
2. NSD system is based on assumption that strand quist curve are straight lines.
3. Formula limited for 4 to 30 fraction and overall treatment<100 days.
4. Based on early skin reactions dose not predict late effects.

   Most serious criticism of NSD is T and N should not constant and should be tissue specific. Proliferation does not affect the total dose required to produce a given biological reaction. At all until some time after start of irradiation but then dependence in time is much greater than allowed by Ellis formula.

PROLIFERATION AS A FACTOR IN NORMAL TISSUE

But proliferation dose not affect the total dose required to produce a given biological reaction at all until sometime after start of irradiation but then the dependence in time is much greater than given by Ellis formula. Effects of proliferation would not be seen until longer period into fractionation regimen because of slower response of human skin and longer cell cycle of cells.

So extra dose required to counter proliferation in skin of mice as a function of time after starting daily irradiation with 300 cGy per fraction (Fig. 30.3). A delay followed by rapid rise typical of time factors in proliferating normal tissue in mouse skin the delay is about 2 weeks and in human, it is about 4 weeks. All tissues of body does not behave like skin tissue.

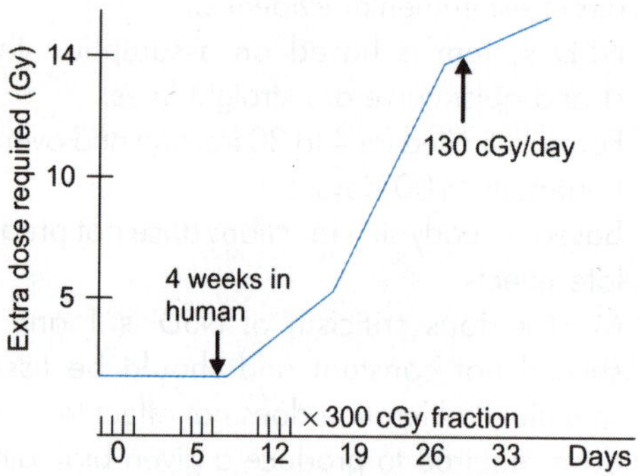

Fig. 30.3: Here we see extra dose to proliferation is sigmoidal

→ Early responding example skin epithelium (intestinal) mucosa

→ Late responding spinal cord

So, the extra dose require to counter proliferation of tissue will be different for early responding and different for late responding tissue (Fig. 30.4).

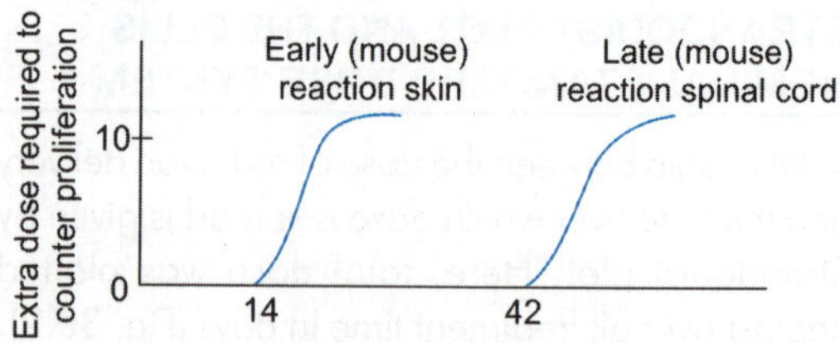

Fig. 30.4: Days after start of irradiation given delay is much longer in humans

By above experiment can converted into clinical practice that early responding tissues are triggered to proliferate with in few weeks of start of fractionated regime, so that extra dose of counter proliferation increase with time in contrast conventional radiotherapy extending 6 to 8 weeks. In never long enough to allow triggering of proliferation in late responding tissues. So important conclusion is prolonging over all treatment time with in normal radiotherapy range has little sparing effect on late reactions but large sparing effect on early reactions. So prolonging overall treatment time (within normal RT range), we can overcome early reaction but has no effect on late reactions.

DOSE RESPONSE RELATION FOR EARLY AND LATE RESPONDING TISSUE

There is a difference between early and late responding tissue in their responses to changing fractionation patterns (Figs 30.5 and 30.6).

If fewer and larger fractions are given late reaction are more severe, in dose response

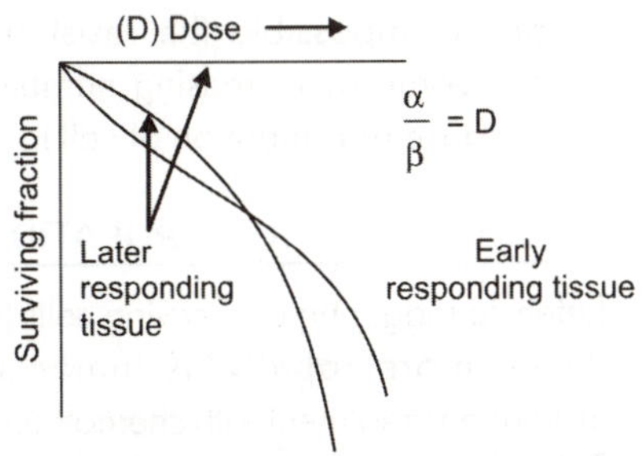

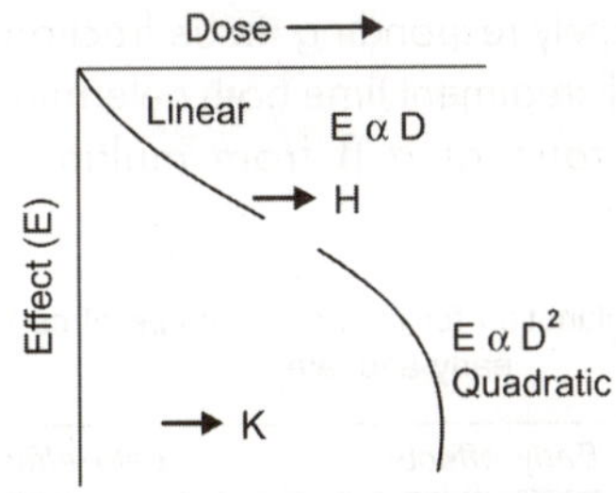

Fig. 30.5: Dose response relation for early and late responding tissue

relationship curve is more for late responding tissue (in terms of LQ relationship) than early responding tissue.

1. For early effect α/β rations larger than late effect.

   Unit α/β is $\frac{Gy}{Gy^2} = Gy^{-1}$

   a. Early effect α dominates
   b. For late effect β dominates.
2. α/β ratio is the dose at which linear and quadratic component of cell killing are equal
   a. For early effect α/β=10 Gy
   b. For late effect α/β=3 Gy

From the Shape of Curve Inference Drawn are (Fig. 30.6) and (Table 30.1)

1. If fractionation scheme is changed in clinical practice from many small doses to fewer large fraction result in more server late effects.
2. If two doses given per day for 6 to 7 weeks, appear to result in greatly reduced late effects and more sever acute effects.
3. The dose response for late effects is more curvy than early effects α/β (Dose at which single and multiple even cell killings are equal).

   10 Gy for early effects

   3 Gy for late effects

   Late responding tissue are more sensitivity to change in fractionation pattern.
4. Fraction size is dominant factor in determining late effects over all treatment time has little effects.

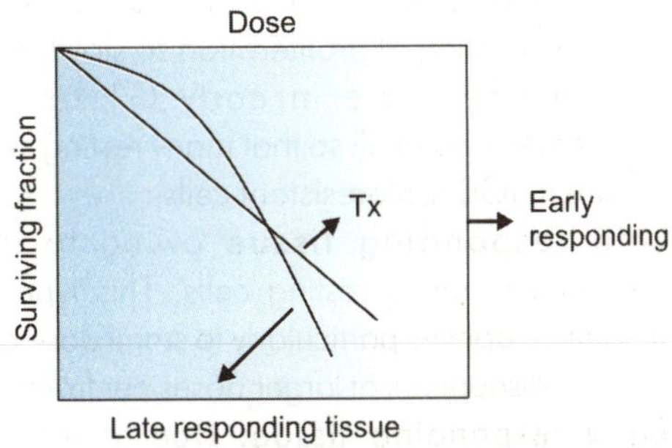

Fig. 30.6: Dose response curve for early and late responding tissues are different

5. But for acutely responding tissue fraction size and overall treatment time both determine the response ratio of α/β from multifraction experiments.

Table 30.1: Explanation for change in shape of curve for early and late

Early effects		Late effects	
	α/β Gy		α/β Gy
Skin	9–12	Spinal cord	1.7–4.9
Jejunum	6–10	Kidney	1–2.4
Colon	10–11	Lung	2–6.3
Testis	12–13	Bladder	3.1–7
Callus	9–10		

RESPONDING TISSUE

1. We know radiosensitivity of population of cells varies with distribution of cells through the cell cycle. Most resistant S phase and early G1, G0 if the cells those are out of the cell cycle. Two cell population group may be radioresistant.
   a. A population proliferating so fast that S phase occupies major portion of the cycle.
   b. A population of proliferation so slowly that many cells are in early G1 or not proliferating at all so that many resting cells are in (G0 radioresistant cells).
2. **Late responding tissue** owing to the presence of many resting cells. This type of resistance applies particularly to small dose per fraction disappears at larger doses per fraction.
3. **Early responding tissue:** Due to rapidly proliferating population, many cell are in S phase impossible the resistance it can be overcome by increasing number of fractions because redistribution of cell in cell cycle.

ACCELERATED REPOPULATION

Refers to triggering of surviving cells (clonogens) to divide more rapidly as tumor shrinks after irradiation/treatment with chemotherapeutic agent. This phenomena explained by Withers and his colleagues in head and neck cancer clonogen repopulation in this human cancer accelerates at about 28 days after start of fractionated regimen. A dose increment of about .6 Gy/day required to compensate for this population (Fig. 30.7). Conclusion drwon from fig. 30.7 are given below:

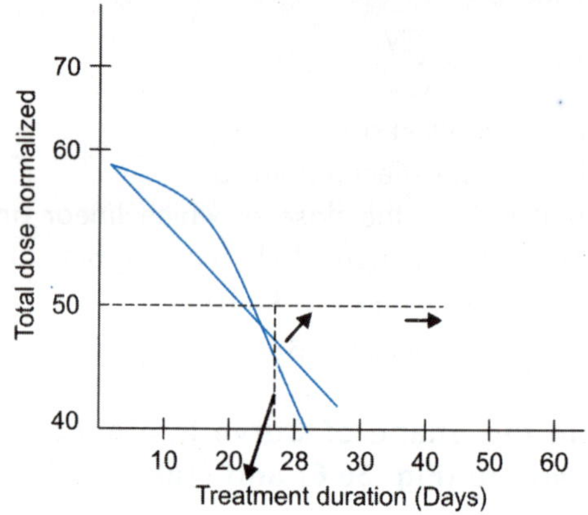

Fig. 30.7: Accelerated repopulation

1. It is better to delay initiation of treatment than to introduce delay during treatment.
2. If over all treatment is too long the effectiveness of later dose fractions is compromise because

surviving clonogens may be triggered into rapid repopulation.

3. Same is applicable for chemotherapy.
4. There is evidence that some human malignancies RT produces poor result, if preceded by NACT due accelerated repopulation.

MULTIPLE FRACTIONS PER DAY

1. Advantage of prolongation of treatment is to spare early reactions and allow reoxygenation in tumors.
2. However, excessive prolongation
   a. Do not spare late injury
   b. Allows surviving tumor cells to proliferate during treatment.

→ Hyperfractionation
→ Accelerated Treatment

HYPERFRACTIONATION

This modality of treatment to spare late responding tissue due to their capacity for repair of sublethal injury and with standing relatively higher dose of radiation.

PURE HYPERFRACTIONATION

Same total dose same overall time but by increasing number of fractions/day by increasing dose/fraction, not satisfactory because if dose/fraction decrease then total dose has to be increase.

Thus, practical is impure hyperfractionation mean increase in total dose sometimes longer over all time multiple fractions/day intent is to increase tumor control and decrease late effect but little increase in early reactions.

Trial of European Organisation of Research Treatment of Cancer (EORTC) Group

1. In head and neck cancer compare 80.5 Gy in 70 fractions (1.15 Gy twice/day). 7 weeks 70 Gy in 35 fractions, 7 weeks.
2. Local tumor control 5 years ↑–40→59 percent reflected in improved survival no increase inside effects.

FLEXURE DOSE (FD)

Two fractions/day is not limit of hyperfractionation, further ↓↓ sparing of late effect by splitting dose into more ↑↑ and more fractions of smaller size.

Wither's introduced concept of FD defined as the point at which dose response curve starts to bent significantly. In practice, it occurs at a dose of .1 a/b that is the curve bevels at the dose 1/10th of that at which lines and quadrate components are equal 1a/b for early responding tissue 6 to 12 Gy.

So FD is for early responding tissue .6 to 1.2 Gy a/b for late responding tissue 1 to 5 Gy

So FD for late responding .1 to .5 Gy (Spinal lung kidney late reactions of skin). So for hyperfractionation regimen dose/fraction can not be decrease less than [FD] because surviving fractional cell increase if total dose is less than flexure dose (FD).

ACCELERATED TREATMENT

Use in fast growing tumors. AIM is to give total dose in short overall time with in tolerable acute toxicity. Increasing overall time is to treat twice/ thrice/day in split course a break of 10 to 14 days after a dose of 30 to 36 Gy is allowed to permit the mucositis to resolve. Head and neck cancer except or pharynx test arm 72 Gy in 45 fractions (1.6 Gy 3 fractions/day) 5 weeks. Control arm 70 Gy/35 fractions, 7 weeks. 15 percent increase in local control without survival advantage. Increase acute effect, severe late effect (due to higher dose/ fractions).

CHART

Continuous Hyperfractionation Accelerated Radiation Therapy (CHART). Study carried out at Mount Vernon hospital (UK) protocol was based on 36 fractions over 12 days with 3 fractions/day without 6 hours interval no gap in treatment dose/fractions was 1.4 to 1.5 Gy to a total dose of 54 Gy. Here total dose is very low but given in very short time. The strategy was based on the low dose/fractions to minimize the late effects very short overall treatment time to decrease tumor proliferation, late effects decrease except myelopathy (spinal cord) occurred in several cases because time between two fractions was not sufficient to repair sublethal damage in spinal cord. Acute reaction are brisk but peak occur after treatment is completed.

Standard

||||| ||||| ||||| — 2 Gy × 5FR

5FR/Wk — × 7 weeks = 70 Gy

Hyperfractionation

|||||||||| |||||||||| |||||||||| — 1.2 Gy × 10 FR

× 6 weeks = 72 Gy

Chart

|||||||||||||||||||||||||||||||||||| — 1.5 Gy × 36 fraction

in 12 days = 54 Gy

TIME INTERVAL BETWEEN MULTIPLE DAILY FRACTIONS

We should ensure repair of sublethal damage should be completed before the next dose is delivered clinically 6 hours gap is kept between two fractions because late effect was worse for interfraction interval less than 4 hours.

T POT AND ACCELERATED TREATMENT

T pot (potential tumor doubling time) Patient were given intravenus tracer dose of thyamidine analogue (iododeoxyuridine) Accelerated fractionate for study of patient vs conventional fractionation tracer is given to estimate T pot A. Fast growing tumor T pot <4 days. Patient divided B, slow growing tumor T pot >4 days, study indicates there was no difference accelerated vs conventional regime for slow growing tumor but in accelerated fractionation regime in fast growing tumor show better local control. Local control of tumor (rapidly glowing) lost if overall treatment time is prolonged since rapid growth does not occur for CA breast/prostate (T pot 28 days for prostate/ 14 days for breast/4 days for H/N cancer cells) thus in both the cases overall treatment is not critical except in head and neck cancer.

LINEAR QUADRATIC CONCEPT TO CALCULATE EFFECTIVE DOSE IN RADIOTHERAPY

- Because limitation in NSD system LQ model used by Jack Fowler
- N = Number of fractions
- d = dose
- For single dose biological effect is E= ad+bd^2
- E=n (ad+bd^2)
- E=nd (a+b)

$$E = \alpha \text{ and } d\left(1+\frac{d}{\alpha/\beta}\right)$$

- n × d = Total Dose
- d = Dose/fractions
- n = Number of fractions
- E/a = nd (1+d/$_{a/b}$)
- (1+d/$_{a/b}$) is called relative effectiveness
- E/a = BED (Biologically Effective Dose) is a parameter by which different fractionation protocol can be compared. We know a/b=3 Gy for late responding tissue a/b= 10 Gy for early responding tissue, **Example:** If 30 fractions of 2 Gy/fractions, 1 fractions/ day (Fig. 30.8) 5 days/week.

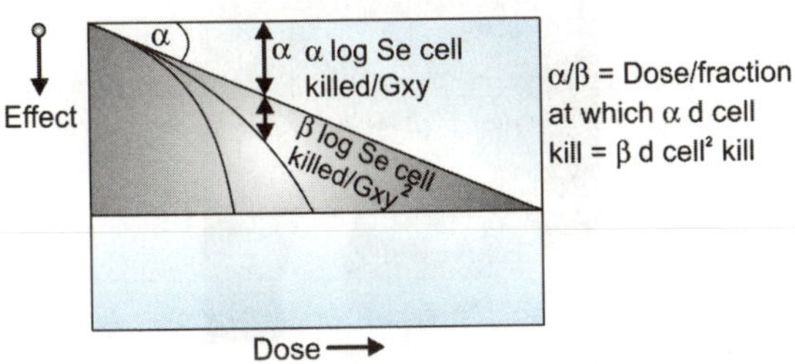

Fig. 30.8: LQ model of cell killing in radiotherapy

1. For overall treatment effect E/a=nd (1+d/$_{a/b}$)

$$\frac{E}{\alpha} = 30\times 2\left(1\pm\frac{2}{10}\right)$$

Early=72 Gy 10
late effect = E/a =30 × 2/100 Gy 3

2. Thus, we can compare early effects and late effects of one fractionation schedule to another schedule along with the biological effectiveness of various radiotherapy protocols. Few other examples. Hyperfractionation 70 fractions of 1.15 Gy given twice daily 6 hours. apart 5 day/ week. For overall treatment for 7 weeks. than BED = E/a = (nd)(1 + d/$_{a/b}$). Early effects 70 × 1.15 (1 + 1.15/10) = 89.8 Gy 10 for late effect BED=E/a=80.5(1 + 1.15/3) = 111.4 Gy 3 compare of example 1 and 2.

Explanation treatment is much hotter that is more effective than conventional for both early and late effects.

Example 3 (Control schedule) 1 fractions/day use here to compare with hyperfractionation schedule (example 2) 35 fractions of 2 Gy 1 fractions DA 5

5 fractions/week for 7 week. Early effect is BED E/a = nd (1 + d$_{/a/b}$) = 2 × 23 (1 + 2/3) = 84 Gy 10 late effects BED = 2 × 35 (1 + 2/ 3) =116.7 Gy 3 example 3 (Control schedule) is not comparable with example 2 (Hyperfractionation) because it is less effective (example 3) by 7 percent for early effect which include tumor control but hotter for latter effect b x 5 percent (116.7 vs 111.4 Gy 3) .

Chapter 31

Effects of Radiation on Normal Human Tissue

- When ionizing radiation passes through tissues result in damage to DNA mainly through the effects of free radicals. Damage to DNA results in immediate cell death or at next mitosis or result in permanent changes in genotype (mutation) which transmitted to future generation cells. Low dose radiation is more likely to cause changes in genotype since it will be below the level of cell death. Radiation exposure can be under following heads:
  a. Radiation accident
     i. Atomic bomb explosion severe radiation reaction nuclear reactor.
     ii. Radiation devices (X-rays).
     iii. Radiation isotope.
  b. Radiation as a part of treatment
     i. To feel body irradiation called magnified irradiation.
     ii. HBI (Hemi Body Irradiation).
  c. Human body exposure by radiation sources
     i. From background sources radioactive material present in earth such as uranium/radium/thorium.
     ii. Cosmic radiation—Dose Se with height from surface.
     iii. Human body itself contains radioactive elements like $P^{40}/C^{14}/Sr^{90}$. They can be grouped under source of internal exposure.

ACUTE EFFECTS

Symptoms which appears early and last for a limited period of time called prodroma and radiation syndrome. It may occur even at very low dose (e.g. 5 Gy within 5–15 minutes of exposure) (Fig. 31.1).

Prodromal Symptom

- LD_{50} is the radiation dose that is equal to the dose that would be fatal to 50 percent of the

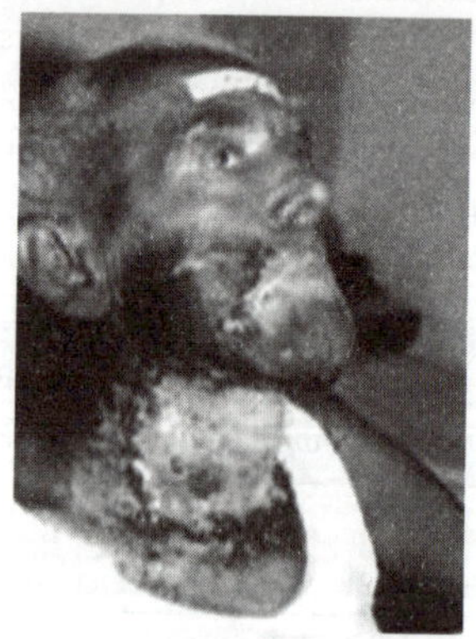

Fig. 31.1: Severe skin reaction
(For color version, see Plate 2)

population within specified period of time. Human prodromal syndrome vary with:

- Time of onset
- Maximum severity
- Duration
- Size of dose.

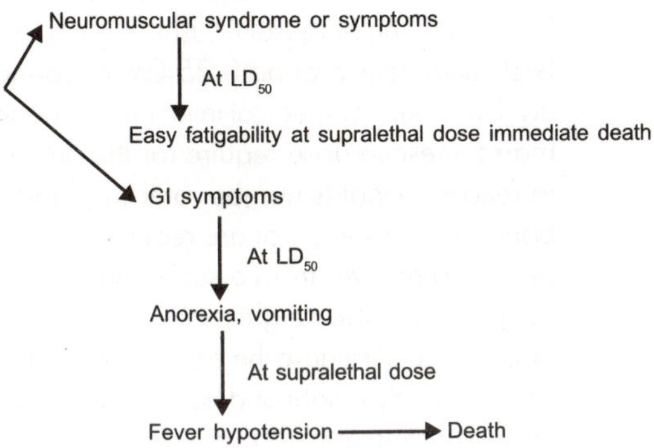

EARLY LETHAL EFFECTS

A. Acute cerebrovascular syndrome
B. Gastrointestinal syndrome
C. Hemopoietic syndrome (Bone marrow toxicity). Cerebrovascular syndrome occurs about 100 Gy. Death occurs 24 to 48 hours after exposure.

Acute Cerebrovascular Syndrome

Symptoms: Nausea, vomiting, diarrhea, loss of coordination of muscular movement, disorientation seizures, coma, death. Cause of death increase leakage from small blood vessels of brain resulting increase ICP, it has been found much higher doses are required to produce death, if head alone irradiated rather than entire body thus, radiation effects on the rest of the body, do have some effect as well.

Gastrointestinal Syndrome

- Nausea, vomiting, prolonged diarrhea, loss of appetite appears sluggish and lethargic. Death symptoms that appear and deaths that follow are attributed to depopulation of epithelial lining of gastrointestinal (GI) tract. Lining of GI tract compose of:
  - Stem cell compartment
  - Differentiating compartment
  - Mature functioning cell
  - Dividing cell confined to crypts which produces (stem cell)
  - Continuous supply of new cells
- These cells move up to villi, differentiate and become functioning cells. Cells at the top of the fold of villi are slough off slowly but replaced by new cells which originate from mitosis in the crypts. Intestinal villi, mature functioning cell, stem cell.

RADIATION

Sterilizes a large proportion of dividing cell in the crypts thus, as the surface of the villi slough off there are no replacement of cells from crypts, thus villi began to shorten and shrink (villus atropy) on the worst stage of radiation enteritis villi are flat and completely free of cells. Most severe effects—noted in intestine, large intestine some what have better tolerance. Delay between time of radiation and onset of GI (radiation syndrome) depends upon life span (14 days) of mature functioning cells at the top of villi.

Hemopoietic Syndrome (Bone Marrow Toxicity)

At the dose of 3 to 8 Gy death occurs. At about 30 days after exposure and continue up to 60 days thus, LD expressed for human as $LD_{50/60}$. Cause: Mitotically active cell (precursor cell) sterilized by radiation, thus supply of WBC, platelet, RBCs thereby diminished. Most marked effect fall on lymphocytes (half-life 24 hour) than platelet (half-life 7 days) than RBC (half-life 120 days). Crisis occurs at which point of time when circulating cells in blood reaches a minimum level. It is only when mature circulating cells began to die off and supply of new cell is inadequate.

INDIVIDUAL VARIATION

Do have role to play like—very young and very old. Old persons are more radiation sensitive than young adult. Female have greater degree tolerance than male.

$LD_{50/30}$ at 5.3 Gy in rhesus monkey $LD_{50/30}$ 30 denotes death continue up to 30 days after exposure.

SYMPTOMS

Three weeks after exposure onset of chills, fatigue, patechial hemorrhage, ulceration of mouth, epilation decrease granulocyte counts causes fever, infection impairment of immune status, bleeding due to low platelet count. Usually-anemia due to hemorrhage (normally) not due to decrease RBC count (life span 120 days). Important cause of death (Fig. 31.2)—that is infection can be controlled by antibiotic treatment mean lethal dose and **bone marrow transplantation TBI** has been of interest from the point of view of bone marrow transplantation or in the case of rescue of patient receiving chemotherapy or radiotherapy.

1. TBI (Total body irradiation)
2. Radiolabelled antibodies
   - $LD_{50/60}$ for human-based on experiments at Hiroshima and Nagasaki. Lushbaugh claims best estimate is around 3.25 Gy for young adult without any medical intervention. Bone marrow rescue dose require for the person to recover—that is number of transplanted bone marrow cells that are required for the person to recover from a supralethal dose. Larger the height, weight more hemopoietic toxicity occurs because there is inverse relation between body weight and hemopoietic stem cell concentration (that is number of hemopoietic stem cell). Human require 10 times more bone marrow cell per kg body weight as mouse for successful bone marrow rescue. After supralethal dose because of lower concentration of hemopoietic stem cell (Table 31.1).

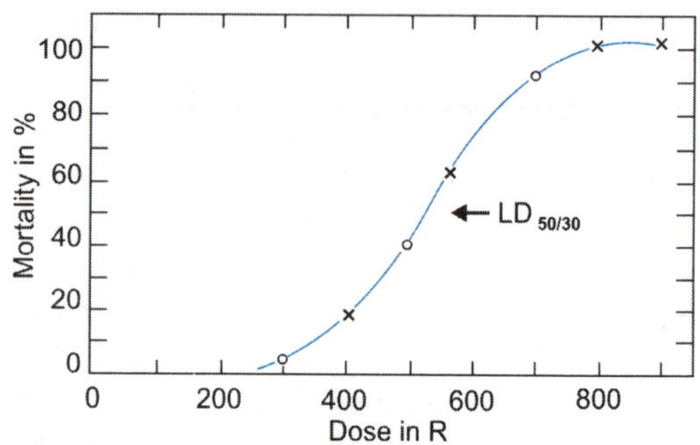

Fig. 31.2: Radiation effect

Table 31.1: Radiation effect of mouse and dog

Species	*Per body unit Average body wt.*	*LD_{50} Gy*	*Rescue dose per kg × 10^{-8}*	*Relative hemopoietic stem cell concentration*
Mouse	0.05 kg	7 Gy	2	10
Dog	12 kg	3.7 Gy	17.5	1.1

- Delay between the time of irradiation and the onset of subsequent radiation syndrome is dictated by the "normal life span of the mature functioning cell."

ACUTE RADIATION INDUCE TOXICITY PROFILE

Result from total body exposure to about 100 Gy result in death between 30 – 50 hours. The cause of cerebrovascular syndrome is due to permeability of small blood vessels in brain. GIT syndrome do occur from TBI to about 10 Gy dose, death occur in 9 days in human population due to depopulation of epithelial lining of GI tract. Emopoietic syndrome—It results from total body exposure to 3 to 8 Gy since radiation sterilizes some or all mitotically active precursor cell symptoms occur after 3 week. LD_{50} for human is about 3 to 4 Gy for youth, adults without medical intervention dose will be little less to very young or very old. The dose window over which bone marrow transplantation is useful is very narrow 8 to 10 Gy.

MANAGEMENT OF ACUTE RADIATION EXPOSURE AT THE DOSE CLOSE TO LD_{50}

- Patient should be taken out from the place of exposure and isolated in a barrier (nursing room)
- Blood count: Should be done 6 hourly interval up to 72 hours, since TLC may fall to less than 1000 cell/mm^3 with in 24 hours
- To know the amount of dose count should be sent before 24 hours of exposure because peripheral lymphocytes (in which chromosomal abberation occurs provide clue that how much dose patient has been exposed) disappear from peripheral blood before 24 hours, so we can do cytogenetic study
- LFT, KFT, electrolytes should be done
- Blood culture in order to start appropriate antibiotic
- ECG to be done
- Patient should be given antiseptic bath (with diluted savlon)
- A part from IV antibiotic, oral antifungal to be given, (e.g. fluconazole, ketoconazole) to combat fungal infection in upper aerodigestive tract
- For gut sterilization oral antibiotic (cotrimoxazole) should be given
- IV fluid and electrolytes according to need should be given
- Gramulocyle macrophage colony stimulating factor (GM-CSF) can be given subcutaneously to promote hemopoiesis
- Blood component can be given (fresh blood, packed cell, fresh platelets)
- In blood component—we should prefer (platelet, packed cell, RBC) because whole blood itself causes bone marrow suppression
- In bone marrow failure cases, BMT can be done with appropriate HLA matched donor/autologous BMT window period within which BMT is use for 8 to 10 Gy up to dose of

8 Gy. Most persons would survive with proper antibiotic and careful nursing
- Above 10 Gy most of the patient dies due to radiation induced GI syndrome and dose up to 2 Gy no treatment is required (Fig. 31.3)
- Overall LD_{50} for human is 3 to 4 Gy for young adult without medical intervention, it may be less for young and old age group.

BONE MARROW TRANSPLANTATION (BMT)

- Allogenic BMT (taking other marrow done by matching with HLA typing (human leukocyte antigen).

Just to abate recipient hemopoietic and immunological tissue now, injected cell home to bone marrow and produces erythrocytes/ granulocytes/ platelets in about 3 to 4 weeks period is important. We should give antibiotic/antifungal in the patient. Best result from BMT seen in young age. Old age BMT results are not so good.

COMPLICATION DUE TO BMT

- Complication occurs in 30 percent cases of BMT more in allogenic type.
  - GVHR (Graft versus host disease)
  - Interstitial pneumonitis.

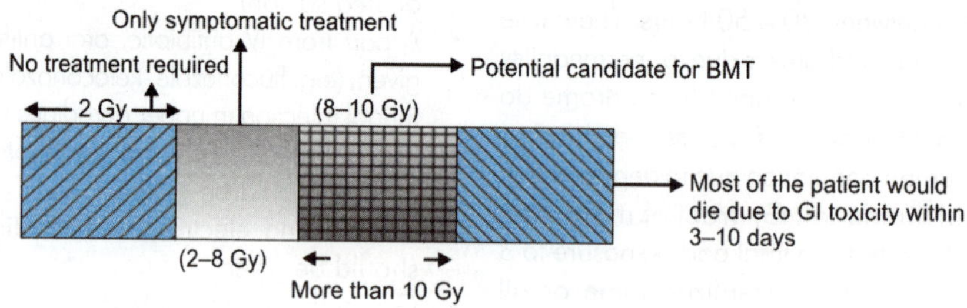

Fig. 31.3: Bone marrow transplant treatment window

- Autologous—Patient's own marrow taken for BMT no HLA typing test is required
- In allogenic bone marrow transplantation, marrow injected intravenously into recipient who is suitably undergone conditioning
- What is conditioning therapy before allogenic BMT require?
  i. High dose of cyclophosphamide
  ii. Give total body irradiation

- GVHR: Mainly because of donor T-lymphocytes and its cytotoxic activity due to lymphocyte sensitization to new host. It can attack liver, skin, gut, decrease immune status leads to infection. Treatment is antibiotic/antifungal, cyclosporine, steroids, methotrexate intestinal pneumonitis—Immunological injury occur to lung for this treatment is steroid.

Chapter 32

Latest Radiotherapy Technique

IMAGE-GUIDED RADIATION THERAPY (IGRT)

Using IMRT does not necessarily mean that margins can be reduced. Remember that margins are based on immobilization and repositioning techniques, not dose delivery techniques. One patient immobilization techniques are mastered, new techniques may then be introduced with the expectation of reducing margins. Practitioners are using new image—guided techniques to verify the tumor location each day. Ultrasound systems have begun to find their way into the clinic but they only work well in the abdomen where there are no air cavities or significant amounts of bone. An alternative approach is electronic portal imaging, which requires the placement of small, inert marker seeds in the soft-tissue tumor as an aid to visualization. Yet, another technique is to produce a computed tomography (CT) image of the patient using the "cone beam" technique. The linear accelerators larger conical beam is used and the entire 3-D volume can be imaged with just one linac rotation. The cone-beam approach works for either kV or mv X-ray beams but a kV beam produces the highest image using the least amount of dose.

Treating cancer in the lung, liver, or pancreas can be problematic since these organs move with respiration. Practitioners have tried to manage tumor motion by asking patients to hold their breath at a specific point in the respiratory cycle ("deep inspiration breath hold"), allowing them to breathe only when the linac allows (active breath control) or using physical restraints that limit the distance the chest can move. Since most patients with thoracic malignancies have limited respiratory capacity and cannot tolerate further reductions in oxygen, patient compliance has sometimes been an issue.

An alternative solution is an automated respiratory gating system that uses an infrared camera to track a passive marker block placed on a patient's chest or abdomen. The system processes the tracked motion to characterize the patient's normal breathing pattern in the form of respiratory waveform. The data are typically gathered during CT simulation so that the respiratory motion can be synchronized with the CT image acquisition, i.e. "4 D" CT, the fourth dimension being time. During treatment, the system automatically gates the radiation beam on only when the tumor falls within the planned treatment field. Throughout the simulation and treatment processes, the patient can breathe naturally and remain comfortable.

INTENSITY-MODULATED RADIATION THERAPY (IMRT)

The aim of radiation therapy is to give high dose confined to tumor area and avoiding dose to normal critical structures. Three dimensional conformal radiation therapies (3D-CRT) was the first technological advancement for this approach which improved the tumor control and decreased the normal tissue damage. Intensity-modulated radiation therapy (IMRT) is the latest step to achieve this goal. IMRT has clear theoretical advantage over conventional radiation in tumors of various sites (Figs 32.1A and B). Excellent target coverage and normal tissue sparing are the two main features of IMRT. Avoidance of permanent xerostomia is the hallmark of health related quality of life benefit for head and neck cancer patients

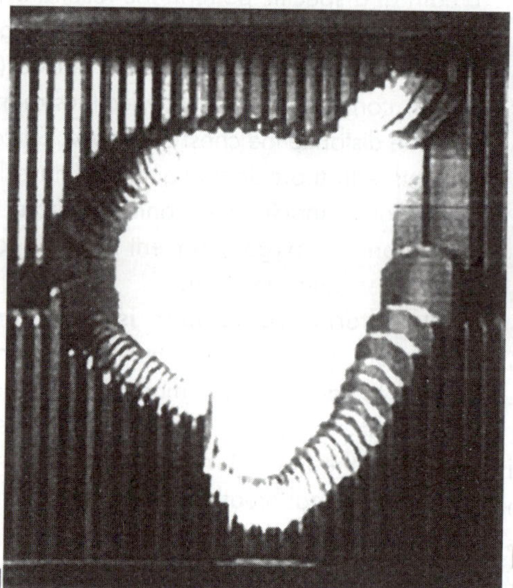

A

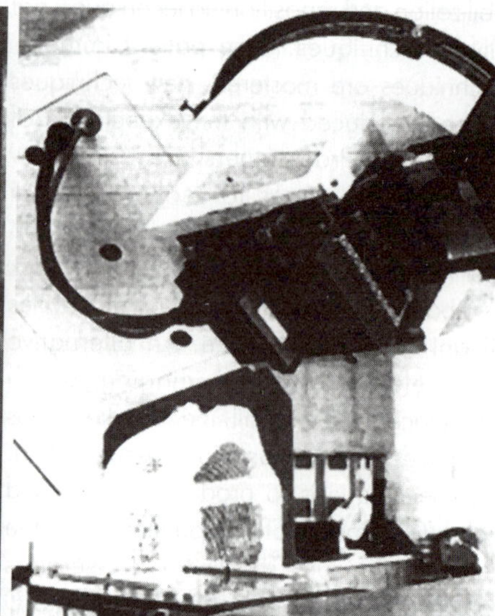

B

Figs 32.1A and B: A typical multileaf collimator used for delivery of intensity-modulated radiation therapy (IMRT) looking toward the radiation source. In the dynamic mode, the leaves move back and forth or sweep across the field continuously to form the sequence of enquired field shapes while the beam is on. In the static or step and shoot mode, the beam is turned off when the leaves move to form the required field shapes. (*Courtesy:* Varian Medical System)

undergoing IMRT. The shape, location and extant of head and neck tumors make them well-suited for IMRT, as maintenance of baseline salivary flow through preservation of parotid glands is of utmost importance.

Physics of IMRT

IMRT is the delivery of uniform radiation to the tumor area via multiple fields which have non-uniform radiation fluence. The fluence not the intensity of radiation is modulated by collimators/ compensators. A number of beams are brought together around an isocenter and fluence of each beam is modulated in such a way across the field, so high dose volume of any shape and size is created by superimposition of beams in IMRT dose delivery. Mechanical parameters as gantry position and multileaf collimator (MLC) configuration are continuously varied during IMRT dose delivery. IMRT dose delivery is of two types:

1. Dynamic IMRT: When beam is turned on, the MLC leaves along with the gantry moves.
2. Step and shoot IMRT: When beam is off between the control points, the MLC leaves along with the gantry moves and dose delivery in stepwise fashion.

Requirements for IMRT Dose Delivery

IMRT is multistep delivery process requires various steps such as positioning and immobilization, image acquisition (CT, MRI), transfer of data to planning system, segmentation (contouring of tumor and critical structures), IMRT treatment planning and plan evaluation, position (initial set-up and daily set-up) and finally IMRT dose delivery.

Why IMRT in head and neck cancers?

The potential benefit of IMRT is ability to treat the target volume which partially or completely surrounds the organ at risk of radiation injury or the target volume is irregularly shaped and is close proximity to critical structures. The long-term morbidity or sequel of conventionally treated head and neck cancers is xerostomia (dryness of mouth) which is major concern of poor quality of life. It also affects speech, taste, mastication and deglutition. By IMRT higher dose can be delivered to tumor with sharp decrease in dose to normal and critical structures such as parotid, spinal cord, brain stem, optic nerve and chiasma.

Treatment Planning and Delivery

All patients are immobilized in the supine position with custom aquaplast marks and target localization is accomplished using CT simulation. Computed tomography images indexed every 3 to 5 mm is obtained, extending from the vertex to 5 cm inferior to the clavicle heads. Treatment planning is performed using the inverse planning software, which is integrated with the treatment planning system. Patients are treated with IMRT delivered with dynamic multileaf collimation (DMLC) on an accelerator. The IMRT beam arrangement consisted of equispaced coplanar beams.

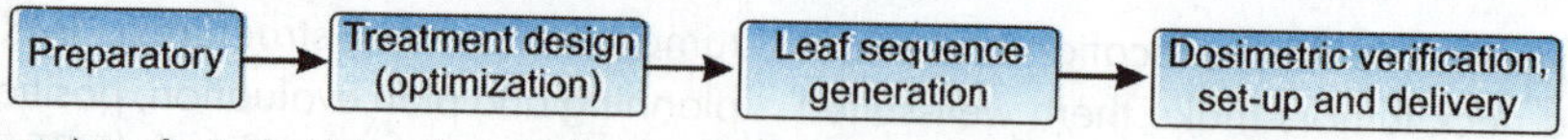
Preparatory
Treatment design (optimization)
Leaf sequence generation
Dosimetric verification, set-up and delivery

Overview of a typical intensity-modulated radiation therapy (IMRT) planning and delivery process.

CONCLUSION

In terms of effectiveness and tolerability, IMRT is an ideal choice for head and neck cancers various sites. With a short follow-up of patients had their disease controlled locally, acute toxicities were manageable and the focused sparing of critical organs such as the parotids enabled a better quality of life for patients both during and after treatment. Longer follow-up will be necessary to validate the early clinical results and elucidate long-term side effects. However, the universally excellent results to date from various institutions on the use of IMRT for head and neck cancers are encouraging.

Chapter

33 Imaging in Oncology

INTRODUCTION

Radiation oncology is an art of treating an invisible target by an invisible radiation, knowledge of tumor morphology, tumor biology and body movements which are one of the important applications of various imaging modalities with newer radiotherapy machines. Accurate, patient-specific anatomical information is a prerequisite for planning and implementing the delivery of radiation to the entire extent of the malignancy while minimizing exposure to critical structures. For this reason, radiological and medical images are of utmost importance in radiotherapy.

Images
- Radiologic images
- Medical images

Useful for:

1. Diagnosis
2. Treatment planning
3. Treatment delivery
4. Follow-up
5. Response assessment CT scan

Images
- Cross-sectional image – MRI, PET
- Projectional image – DRR

- Radiation oncology imaging solutions fall into two categories: Those that provide more precise treatment planning images and systems that facilitate increasingly accurate dose delivery. In fact, most of the significant recent advances in radiation oncology have resulted from developments in application of imaging modalities such as computed tomography (CT) and magnetic resonance imaging (MRI).
- With information from the new imaging modalities, it is now possible to define treatment volumes and critical structures with greater precision, thus reducing marginal misses and irradiation of normal tissues.
- **Tumor morphology**: Knowledge of morphology is essential because we intend to give high dose to tumor and minimum dose to surrounding normal tissue. Various imaging modalities (e.g. USG CT, MRI, PET), are available to understand better tumor morphology so that we can give maximum radiation to the tumor bed and minimum radiation to the normal tissue.
- Like in case of glioma functional MRI, diffusion tumor imaging, MR spectroscopy, functional MRI and tactography is required to delineate the exact anatomical structure involve by the tumor.

- **CT scan:** Many aspects of medical imaging have benefited from the substantial and sustained developments in computer technology, both in hardware and in software (Figs 33.1 to 33.3).

Computed tomographic images have already gained widespread utilization in various areas of radiation oncology including:

1. The delineation of the target volume.
2. The determination of the relative geometry of critical structures.
3. The optimal placement of beams and the shaping of apertures.
4. The calculation of dose distribution.
5. Follow-up evaluation of treatment outcome.
6. **MRI:** MR images present unique anatomical information and tumor detail. Although the digital values cannot be directly used in dose calculations.
7. The MR image detail, when correlated with CT attenuation, values, can provide a powerful planning tool as it gives an 3-d imaging and better tissue contrast. MRI has been effectively utilized for the treatment

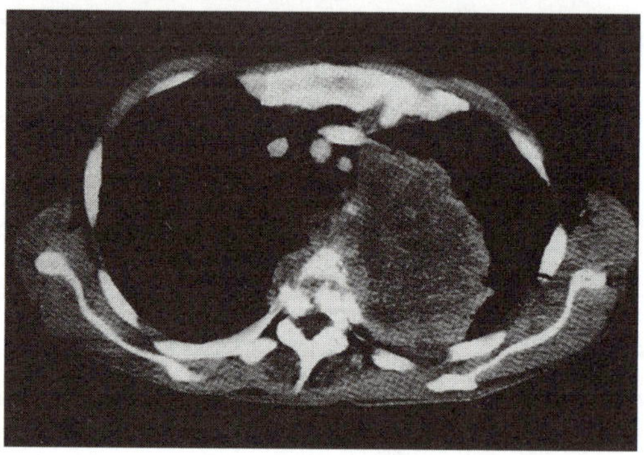

Fig. 33.1: CECT thorax showing left lung mass *(For color version, see Plate 2)*

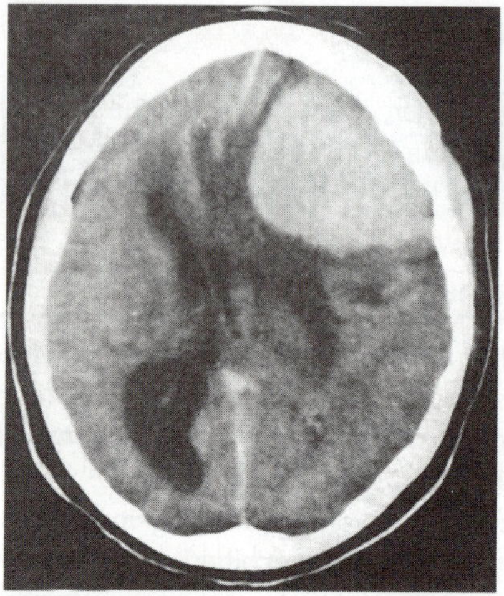

Fig. 33.2: CECT head, meningioma left frontal *(For color version, see Plate 3)*

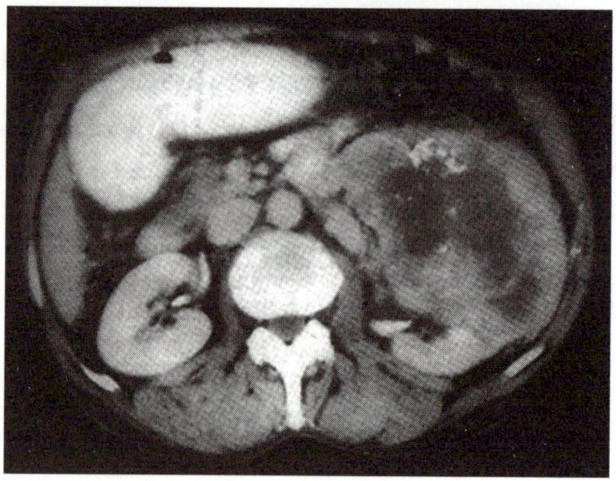

CECT shows left renal cell carcinoma

planning of brain, pelvis and prostate disease.

8. In 53 percent case MR alter the CT planning in brain tumor but MR has own limitations due to its slow speed, motion artifact, inadequate software for radiotherapy planning. The images may be distorted by variations in local magnetic field caused by the presence of metal objects in the environment and within the patient. In addition, bone does not explicitly appear in MR images.
9. **PET:** Positron emission tomography images do not provide the resolution as of CT or MR images but it do provide physiologic information that may be important for localizing certain diseases and for determining responses to radiation therapy. PET – CT fusion images are very helpful in treatment planning and follow-up.
10. **USG:** Ultrasonography is a good imaging tool for abdomen, prostate and detection of lymph node metastasis in head and neck. It helps as guidance of various implants, e.g. perineal implants in prostate and cervix. It is also an important tool for assessing the response of therapy.
11. **Simulation**: In the conventional method, 24 to 47 percent cases shows inadequate tumor coverage and it was observed that 55 percent cases need CT information and this will help to increase the overall survival by 6 to 10 percent by giving 20 percent more dose to the tumor.
12. This can be achieved only if radiation oncologist gets proper information by radiology about tumor morphology. The modern CT simulation have advantage over conventional simulation machine, in which tumor localization and verification is better and the digital date can be directly transferred to planning system. A linear array of detectors is mounted on the gantry arm and digital information on the radiation exiting from the patient is acquired by rotating the simulator gantry (with the X-ray tube). The advantages of such CT-simulators over conventional units is that, with the elimination of spacial restrictions of the CT gantry, the patient is more likely to be imaged in the exact treatment position including the use of patient support devices. The major disadvantage is the time needed to image a large number of CT planes and the poorer image quality. In tomotherapy, the CT is mounted with therapy system so online treatment planning can be rectified as and when needed, CT also very helpful for SRS/SRT radiotherapy tecnique useful for mainly small size brain tumors (Fig. 33.4).
13. **EPIDS:** Electronic portal imaging devices in radiation oncology is the recent development and may have a profound impact on the overall accuracy of radiation treatment delivery. With these devices, daily imaging for treatment localization and verification may become feasible, as the acquisition, analysis, storage and distribution of portal images can

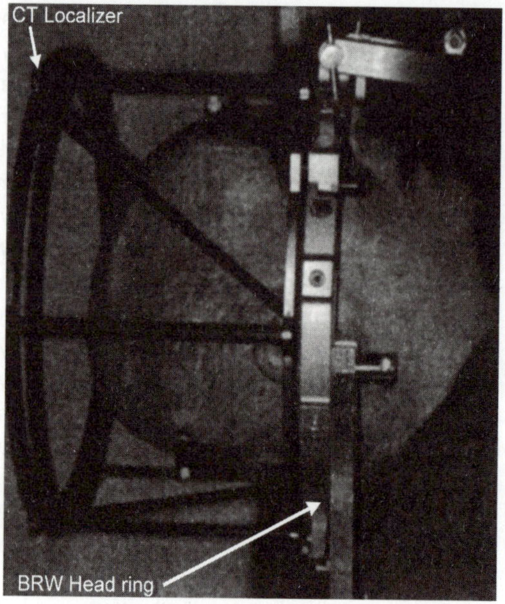

Fig. 33.4: Patient under SRT treatment

be performed with relatively easy. Besides its use as a replacement of port film, EPID can be applied to other areas of radiation oncology. These include the monitoring of patient and organ motion during treatment, the use in exit dosimetry treatment plan verification and the recording of dynamic multileaf collimator (MLC) movement for intensity modulated beams, and in accelerator quality assurance procedures.

14. In the future image acquisition, communication and storage procedures for acquiring different images (CT, MRI, PET stimulator, etc.) for planning and verification will for a part of an integrated system in the field of radiotherapy.

TREATMENT PLANNING AND RESPONSE ASSESSMENT

- Imaging can be used for the planning of the treatment and its response keeping in mind the importance of proper operational utility of the imaging modality as the assessment of response and treatment planning execution may be effected by improper knowledge about the imaging.
- For example, assessment of response in reduction of tumor size should be done by measuring the tumor volume in the largest dimension in the contrast scan images.
- Assessment may occur if patients scanned while patient is on steroids which gives a false information about the extent of response because steroid reduces the edema and vascularity (contrast enhancement), so tumor volume falsely appears to be less than the tumor.
- If patient imaged in different makes of machine and by different modalities or patient scanning done in nonidentical position than there are high chances of false assessment. Now, this can be minimize by using the CT, MRI, PET fusion. Therefore, it is necessary that diagnostic radiologist should have the basic knowledge of the radiotherapy, importance of the radiotherapy position.

- **Patient and tumor movements:** Problem of moving structure specially in the thorax and abdomen is one of the concerned in radiotherapy planning and treatment delivery. It was observed that the movements of 1 cm. size tumor is approximately 3 cm and it increases the treatment volume by the factor of 50. The movements depend how does the tumor shape and the morphology changes by day-to-day (interfractional) and during radiation (intrafractional), so it is very important to deal the problem of tumor movements. This problem is now tackled by TART (Tumor adapted radiotherapy/image guided radiotherapy). IGRT and tomotherapy is the latest advancement. IGRT and tomotherapy in the field of radiation oncology imaging has come of age. New imaging modalities like CT, 4D CT, PET-CT now, integrated with treatment planning and delivery realms, enabling radiation oncologists to plan deliver razor-sharp treatment especially for lung and abdominal cancer are benefiting form ultra-precise respiratory gating and image-guided adaptive radiation therapy (IGART).

CONCLUSION

The radiation oncologist should have a knowledge of various imaging modalities and their application in the field of radiotherapy this should be an integral part of the postgraduate training program. There is need of future research for improvement in the accurate diagnosis and better understanding of tumor biology and the problem of hypoxia and radio-resistance. Targeted treatment delivery is the key issue in the future which can be solved with the help of various imaging modalities.

Improvement in image fusion and the portal imaging related to organ movement during treatment and evaluation of treatment response is being tackled in better way.

Organ movements and dose delivery to the biologically sensitive biologically resistant tumor will be another area of research. In future time, adapted radiotherapy and biological adapted RT will be the major area of research.

Chapter 34

Radiation Oncologist with Benign Tumors

Regarding the radiation treatment of benign disease bureau of radiological health recommends that:

1. Before start of treatment ensure, quality of radiation/total dose/overall treatment time/ underlying organ at risk.
2. Infant and children should be treated under-exceptional circumstances.
3. Underlying organ must be appropriately protected by the help of lead shield/cones. For example, thyroid/eye/gonads/breast/ bone marrow.
4. Appropriate energy must be chosen according to the depth of tumor.

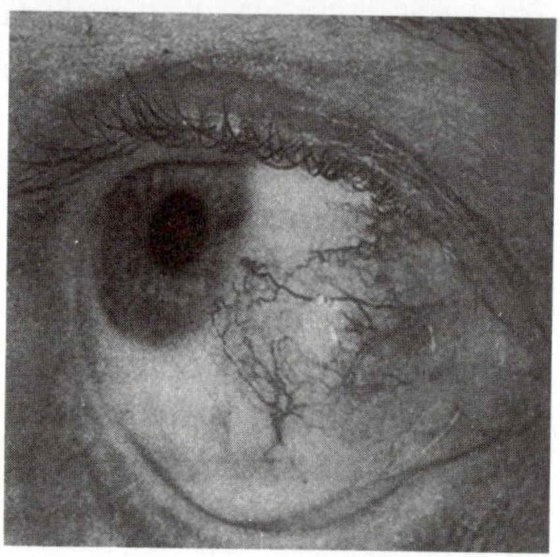

Fig. 34.1: Pterygium
(For color version, see Plate 3)

OCULAR DISORDER

Pterygium (Fig. 34.1) postoperative recurrence is 20 to 30 percent with use of post of RT recurrence decreases up to 1.4 percent.

Commonly use Sr^{90} (8×10 Gy) applicators. Dose given in 3 sittings at 0, 7, 14 days after surgery.

EXOPHTHALMOS

Grave's ophthalmopathy (Fig. 34.2) clinically presents

a. Extraocular muscle dysfunction
b. Diplopic
c. Periorbital edema
d. Chemosis
e. Lid lag proposes occurs because of T-lymphocytes and fibroblast infiltration in the

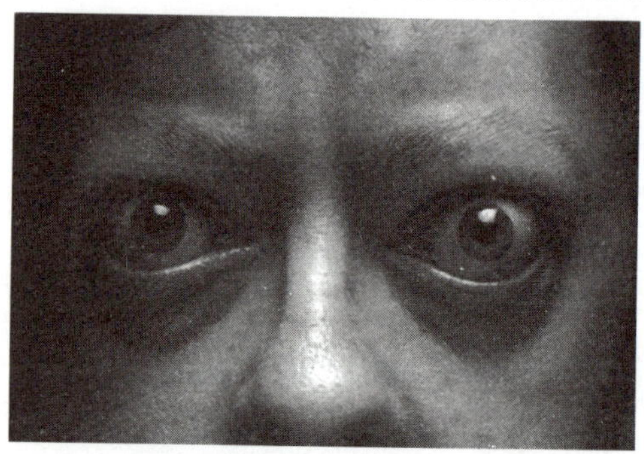

Fig. 34.2: Grave's ophthalmopathy
(For color version, see Plate 3)

retro-orbital region both T-lymphocysts/ fibroblast highly sensitive to radiation thus 20 Gy/10 fraction RT given while protecting lens by giving 15 percent posterior angulation in beam by single lateral field.

ORBITAL PSEUDOTUMOR

Cause by
- Orbital lymphoma
- Atypical lymphoid

Hyperplasia of orbit

Dose 20 Gy/10 fraction in 2 weeks.

Macular degeneration age related and is most common and leading – cause of blindness

In USA treatment given by
- Laser photocoagulation
- External beam radiation 10 Gy/ 5 fraction By 6 MV photon

Skin Disorders

Keloid skin tissue have tendency to react trauma with excessive production of fibrous tissue leading to keloids.

Cause of keloid
- Infection
- Trauma
- Burn
- Surgery

Recurrent keloid (after surgery) required T/T kilovoltage

T/T 10 Gy/2 fraction

PLANTAR WARTS

1. Salicylic ointment T/T very effective 70 percent.
2. Liquid nitrogen (Cryosurgery) very effective 80 percent cure rate.
3. Intralesional injection of bleomycin effective in resistant cases with 77 percent cure rate. But radiation T/T with kilovoltage has been got cure rate 87 percent. Dose 10 Gy of KV T/T warts usually fall off in 3 weeks after RT treatment.

Hemangiomas (Fig. 34.3)

A. Skin hemangioma RT recommended for those having life-threatening situation that failed all other methods.

Dose 10 Gy/5 fraction

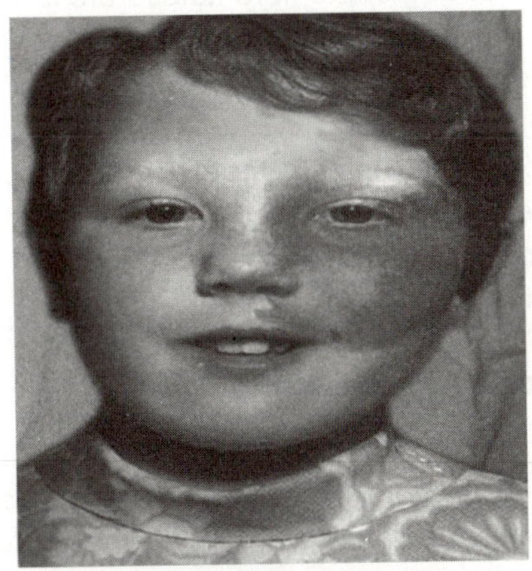

Fig. 34.3: Hemangioma

(For color version, see Plate 3)

B. **Cavernous hemangioma of liver:** It is a congenital anomaly—most people remain asymptomatic unless until lesion bleeds.
Present in 50 percent cases.

Radiation use when hemangioma is large diffuse not fit for surgical intervention dose 20 Gy/10 fraction. If partial response dose—to 10 Gy/5 fraction.

AV malformation of brain: It fall underlate responding tissue under RT (have low α/β ratio) thus, fit case to be treated large dose in single fraction by radiosurgery/cyber knife response rate 70 to 89 percent.

Trigeminal nuralgia: Radiotherapy given at the point of nerve root entry one 70 Gy dose have response rate around 90 percent complete pain relief.

DESMOID TUMOR

Known as aggressive fibromatosis are low grade locally invasive nonmetastatic tumor surgery is main treatment but recurrence occurs in a range of 10 to100 percent.

Recurrence after surgery require resurgical excision plus adjuvant radiotherapy.

Dose 50 Gy/25 fraction 5 cm along 2 cm margin.

Peyronie's Disease (Fig. 34.4)

Inflamatory lesion of corpora cavernosa of penis.

Leads to hard plaque nodule or bands pain and tenderness commonest site on the dorsum of the penis.

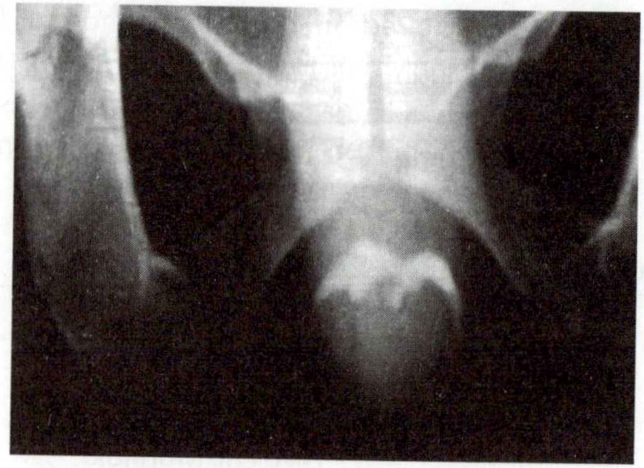

Fig. 34.4: Peyronie's disease of penis
(For color version, see Plate 4)

Treatment with radiation dose 25 Gy/10 fraction @ 2.5 Gy/fraction response rate and pain relief occurs in 75 percent cases.

PREVENTION OF RESTENOSIS AFTER PTCA (PERCUTANEOUS TRANSLUMINAL CORONARY ANGIOPLASTY)

Since, balloon dilatation done in PTCA causes injury to smooth muscle of coronary vessels leading the restenosis of coronary vessel at the upper and lower edge of angioplasty site drugs use to prevent restenosis are trapidil and protocol (antioxidant), trapidil is a platlet derived growth factor inhibitor after angioplasty percent of restenosis is as high as 30 percent but by adding postangioplasty. endovascular brachytherapy (Sr^{90} β-emitter). via catheter based hydrolic delivery system decreases the percent of restenosis up to 8 percent.

AMELOBLASTOMA OF JAW (FIG. 34.5)

Treatment after surgical curattage recurrence is very common but adjuvant RT 50 Gy/25 fraction after surgery decrease recurrence in 90 percent cases.

ANEURYSMAL BONE CYST

Recurrence after curettage is as high as 30 to 60 percent cases but adding postoperative RT ↓↓ recurrence in 80 percent cases (dose of RT 20 Gy/10 fraction).

VERTEBRAL HEMANGIOMA

Surgery usually not possible or difficult require 30 Gy/15 fraction glandular disease.

A. **Gynecomastia:** Patient on flutamide T/T for prostatic cancer patients 90 percent develops gynecomastia, after orchidectomy in 8 percent cases patient develops gynecomastia.
   RT Dose 1500 cGy/3 fraction
B. **Ovarian Ablation**
   Not done nowadays
   In breast cancer used in early years 20 Gy/10 fraction as ovarian ablation dose.

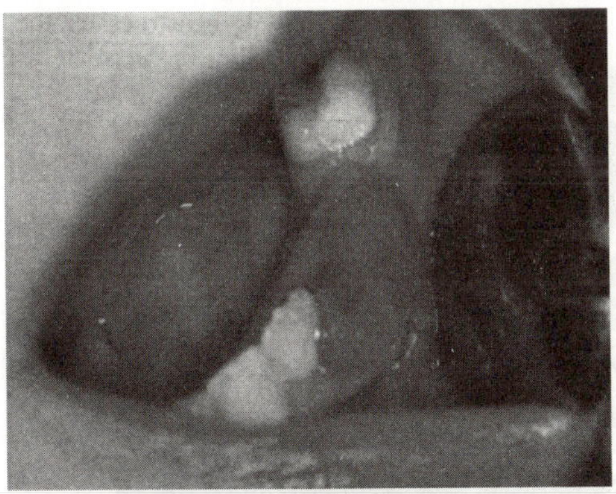

Fig. 34.5: Ameloblastoma of jaw
(For color version, see Plate 3)

RHEUMATOID ARTHRITIS

Response to methotrexate/azathioprine T/T/cyclophosfamide.

Response

i. 60 percent get complete pain relief
ii. 50 percent cases ↓↓ joint swelling
iii. 72 percent ↓↓ morning stiffness of joint.

We give TBI <
- 20 Gy/10 fraction by mental field
- 20 Gy/13 fraction by inverted Y field technique

JUVENILE NASOPHARYNGEAL ANGIOFIBROMA

- Seen in adolescent male
- Epistaxis, nasal obstruction on and off
- T/T SX is gold standard
- RT advised in recurrent tumor or in anticipation of excessive bleeding 30 Gy/15 fraction by anterior/lateral wedge pair cure rate with RT alone in 80 percent cases.

INVERTED PAPILLOMA (FIG. 34.6)

- Common in male
- Unilateral
- Clinically present firm red and gray mass
- Invasion of squamous epithelium under stroma unlike papilloma which grows outwards.

EOSINOPHILIC GRANULOMA LCH (FIGS 34.7A AND B)

Single solitary lesion presence of langerhans-gaint cells is hallmark thus called as langerhans cell histocytosis male female ratio 2:1 usually occurs 1 to 3 years of age treatment is:

i. Surgery curettage cure rate 50 percent intralesional steroid (methylprednisolone) surgical failure—option is radiotherapy 6 Gy/ 3 fraction.

RADIOTHERAPY STRONGLY ADVISED

If lesion is at vertebra/base of skull response rate with radiotherapy 90 to 100 percent.

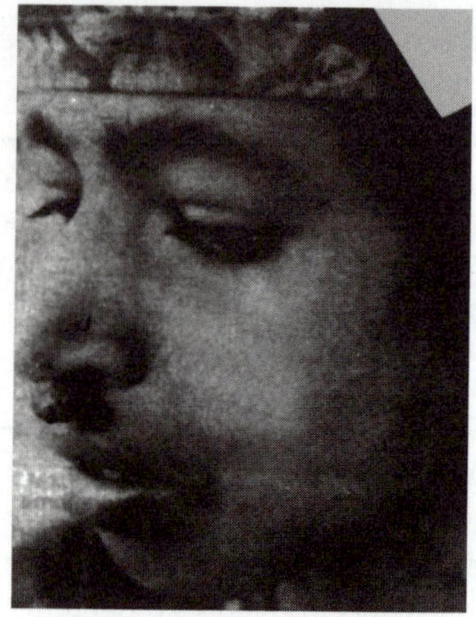

Fig. 34.6: Inverted papilloma

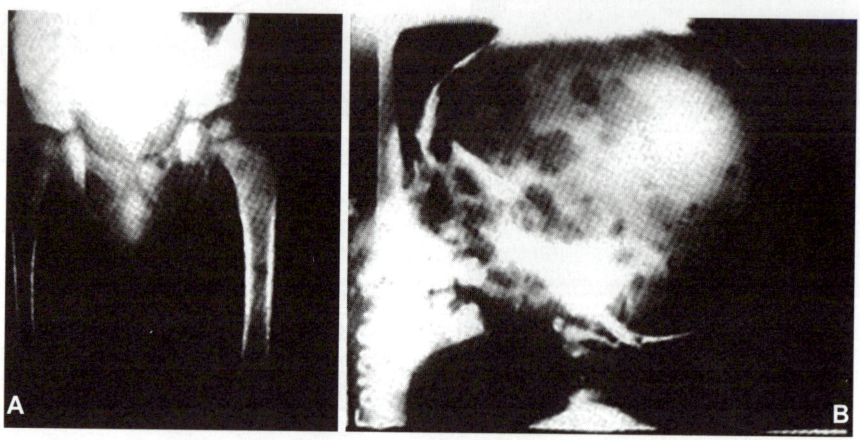

Figs 34.7A and B: Eosinophilic granuloma

Bibliography

1. Alexander MC, Yankaskas BC, Biesemier KW. Association of stellate mammographic pattern with survival in small invasive breast tumors. Am J Roentgenol 2006;187:29-37.
2. American Pain Society Quality of Care Committee. Quality improvement guidelines for the treatment of acute pain and cancer pain. JAMA 1995;274:1874-80.
3. Anderson SJ, Wapnir I, Dignam JJ, Fisher B, Mamounas EP, Jeong JH, Geyer CE, Wickerham DL, Costantino JP, Wolmark N. Prognosis after ipsilateral breast tumor recurrence and locoregional recurrences in patients treated by breast-conserving therapy in five national surgical adjuvant breast and bowel project protocols of Node-Negative Breast Cancer. JCO 2009;27:2466-73.
4. Ansuategui M, Naharro L, Feria M. Noradrenergic and opioidergic influences on the antinociceptive effect of clomipramine in the formalin test in rats. Psychopharmacology 1989;98:93-6.
5. Areta KV, Bryan KC. Burn scar neoplasms: A literature review and statistical analysis. Burns 2005; 31(4):403-13.
6. Arons MS, Rodin AE, Lynch JB, Lewis SR, Blocker TG. Scar tissue carcinoma: II An experimental study with special reference to burn scar carcinoma. Ann Surg1966;163:445-60.
7. Arthur DW, Vicini FA. Accelerated partial breast irradiation as a part of breast conservation therapy. JCO 2005;23:1726-35.
8. Bartelink H, Horiot JC, Poortmans PM, Struikmans H, Van den BW, Fourquet A, Jager JJ, Hoogenraad WJ, Oei SB, Warlam-Rodenhuis CC, Pierart M, Collette L. Impact of a higher radiation dose on local control and survival in breast-conserving therapy of early breast cancer: 10-year results of the randomized boost versus no boost EORTC 22881-10882 Trial. JCO 2007;25:3259-65.
9. Bergouignan M. Cures heureuses de nevralgies faciales essentielles par le diphenylhydantoinate de soude. Rev Laryngol Otol Rhinol 1942;63:34-41.
10. Bijker N, Meijnen P, Peterse JL, Bogaerts J, Van Hoorebeeck I, Julien JP, Gennaro M, Rouanet P, Avril A, Fentiman IS, Bartelink H, Rutgers EJ. The breast-conserving treatment with or without radiotherapy in ductal carcinoma *in situ*: Ten-year results of European Organisation for Research and Treatment of Cancer Randomized Phase III Trial 10853—A Study by the EORTC Breast Cancer Cooperative Group and EORTC Radiotherapy Group. JCO 2006;24:3381-87.
11. Bilimoria KY, Bentrem DJ, Hansen NM, Bethke KP, Rademaker AW, Ko CY, Winchester DP, Winchester DJ. Comparison of sentinel lymph Node biopsy alone and completion axillary lymph node dissection for node-positive Breast Cancer. JCO 2009;27:2946-53.
12. Bogart JA, Seagren SL, Glicksman A. Radiation oncology research in the cancer and leukemia group B. Clin Cancer Res 2006;12:s3628-34.

13. Botteri E, Bagnardi V, Rotmensz N, Gentilini O, Disalvatore D, Bazolli B, Luini A, Veronesi U. Analysis of local and regional recurrences in breast cancer after conservative surgery. Ann Oncol 2009;1:386.
14. Botteri E, Rotmensz N, Sangalli C, Toesca A, Peradze N, De Oliveira Filho HR, Sagona A, Intra M, Veronesi P, Galimberti V, Luini A, Veronesi U, Gentilini O. Unavoidable mastectomy for ipsilateral breast tumour recurrence after conservative surgery: Patient outcome. Ann Oncol 2009;20:1008-12.
15. Bowers RF, Young JM, Carcinoma arising in scars, osteomyelitis, and fistulae. Arch Surg1960; 80: 564-70.
16. Bowsher D. Neurogenic pain syndromes and their management. British Medical Bulletin 1991; 47:644-66.
17. Brachtel EF, Rusby JE, Michaelson JS, Chen LL, Muzikansky A, Smith BL, Koerner FC. Occult nipple involvement in breast cancer: Clinicopathologic findings in 316 consecutive mastectomy specimens. JCO 2009;27:4948-54.
18. Brenner DJ, Shuryak I, Russo S, Sachs RK. Reducing second breast cancers: A potential role for prophylactic mammary irradiation. JCO 2007;25: 4868-72.
19. Brewster K, Wileyto EP, Kessler L, Collier A, Weathers B, Stopfer JE, Domchek S, Halbert CH. Sociocultural predictors of breast cancer risk perceptions in African. American breast cancer survivors. Cancer Epidemiol. Biomarkers Prev 2007;16:244-8.
20. Brown JM. Hypoxic cell radiosensitisers: Where next? International Journal of Radiation Oncology, Biology, Physics1989;16:987-93.
21. Brown JP, Boden P, Singh L, Gee NS. Mechanisms of action of gabapentin. Rev Contemp Pharmacother 1996;7:203-14.
22. Buchholz TA, Theriault RL, Niland JC, Hughes ME, Ottesen R, Edge SB, Bookman MA, Weeks JC. The use of radiation as a component of breast conservation therapy in National Comprehensive Cancer Network Centers. JCO 2006;24:361-9.
23. Buchholz TA: Radiation therapy for early-stage breast cancer after breast-conserving surgery. NEJM 2009;360:63-70
24. Burnet NG, Nyman J, Turesson I, Wurm R, Yarnold JR, Peacock JH. Prediction of normal-tissue tolerance to radiotherapy from *in vitro* cellular radiation sensitivity. Lancet 1992;339:1570-1.
25. Caplin ME, Buscombe JR, Hilson AJ, Jones AL, Watkinson A, Burroughs AK. Carcinoid tumour. Lancet 1998;352:799-805.
26. Cavalli F, Hansen HH, Kaye SB. Textbook of medical Oncology, 2nd Edn. Martin D (Ed). London; 2000.
27. Chabal C, Russell LC, Burchiel KJ. The effect of intravenous lidocaine, tocainide, and mexiletene on spontaneously active fibers originating in rat sciatic neuromas. Pain 1989;38:333-8.
28. Chaplin DJ, Durand RE, Olive PL. Acute hypoxia in tumors: Implications for modifiers of radiation effects. International Journal of Radiation Oncology, Biology, Physics 1986;12:1279-82.
29. Chapman V, Dickenson AH. The combination of NMDA receptor antagonism and morphine produces profound antinociception in the rat dorsal horn. Brain Res 1992;573:321-3.
30. Charney DS, Heninger GR, Sternberg DE. Serotonin function and mechanisms of action of antidepressant treatment. Arch Gen Psychiatry 1984;41:359-65.
31. Clouse ME, Chen J, Krumholz HM, Clouse ME, Chen J, Krumholz HM. Noninvasive screening for coronary artery disease with computed tomography is useful. Circulation 2006;113:125-46.

32. Cohen L. Carrier EK, Horning SJ, Radiation parameters. Thesis, University of Witwatersrand; 1960. pp66.
33. Coleman CN. Beneficial liaisons: Radiobiology meets cellular and molecular biology. Radiotherapy and Oncology 1993;28:1-15.
34. Collins ED, Moore CP, Clay KF, Kearing SA, O'Connor AM, Llewellyn-Thomas H, Barth RJ, Sepucha K. Reply to MM Mohiuddin, et al. JCO 2009; 27: e162-3.
35. Collins ED, Moore CP, Clay KF, Kearing SA, O'Connor AM, Llewellyn-Thomas HA, Barth RJ, Sepucha KR. Can women with early-stage breast cancer make an informed decision for mastectomy?. JCO 2009;27:519-25.
36. Come SE. A 62-Year-old woman with a new diagnosis of breast cancer. JAMA 2006;295:1434-42.
37. Coventry DM, Todd G. Epidural clonidine in lower limb deafferentation pain. Anesth Analg 1989;69: 407-8.
38. D' AAV, Hanks G (Eds). Radiotherapeutic management of prostate adenocarcinoma. Arnold, London;1999.
39. Dabakuyo TS, Fraisse J, Causeret S, Gouy S, Padeano MM, Loustalot C, Cuisenier J, Sauzedde JM, Smail M, Combier JP, Chevillote P, Rosburger C, Boulet S, Arveux P, Bonnetain F. A multicenter cohort study to compare quality of life in breast cancer patients according to sentinel lymph node biopsy or axillary lymph node dissection. Ann Oncol 2009;20:1352-61.
40. Dachs GU, Dougherty GJ, Stratford IJ, Chaplin DJ. Targeting gene therapy to cancer: A review. Oncology Research 1997;9:313-25.
41. Davidson NE, Morrow M, Kopans DB, Koerner FC. Case 35—A 56-year-old woman with breast cancer and isolated tumor cells in a sentinel lymph node. NEJM 2005;353:2177-85.
42. Deacon J, Peckham MJ, Steel GG. The radiores-ponsiveness of human tumours and the initial slope of the cell survival curve. Radiotherapy and Oncology 1984;2:317-23.
43. Desch CE, McNiff KK, Schneider EC, Schrag D, McClure J, Lepisto E, Donaldson MS, Kahn KL, Weeks JC, Ko CY, Stewart AK, Edge SB. American Society of Clinical Oncology/National Comprehensive Cancer Network Quality Measures. JCO 2008;26:3631-7.
44. Devor M, Govrin-Lippmann R, Raber P. Corticosteroids suppress ectopic neural discharge originating in experimental neuromas. Pain 1985;22:127-37.
45. Devor M, Wall PD, Catalan N. Systemic lidocaine silences ectopic neuroma and DRG discharge without blocking nerve conduction. Pain 1992;48: 261-8.
46. DiFronzo LA, Tsai PI, Hwang JM, Lee JJ, Ryoo MC, Rahimian J, Tome M, Takasugi JK, Haigh PI. Breast conserving surgery and accelerated partial breast irradiation using the mammo site system: Initial clinical experience. Arch surg 2005;140:787-94.
47. Dixon JM. ABC of Breast Diseases, 2nd Edn. BMJ Publishing Group, London; 2000.
48. Dobbs J, Barrett A, Ash D. Practical Radiotherapy Planning, 3rd Edn. Arnold, London; 1999.
49. Eide PK, Jorum E, Stubhaug A, Bremnes J, Breivik H. Relief of post-herpetic neuralgia with the N-met-hyl-D-aspartic acid receptor antagonist ketamine: A double-blind, cross-over comparison with morphine and placebo. Pain 1994;58:347-54.
50. Eisenach JC, Rauck RL, Buzzanell C, Lysak SZ. Epidural clonidine analgesia for intractable cancer pain: Phase I. Anesthesiology 1989;71:647-52.
51. Fisher B, Anderson SJ. The breast cancer alternative hypothesis: Is there evidence to justify replacing it?. JCO 2010;28:366-74.

52. Fisher B. Biological research in the evolution of cancer surgery: A personal perspective. Cancer Res 2008;68:10007-20.
53. Fitzgerald M. Capsaicin and sensory neurones: A review. Pain 1983;15:109-30.
54. Ford HT, Coombes RC, Gazet JC, Gray R, McConkey CC, Sutcliffe R, Quilliam J, Lowndes S. Long-term follow-up of a randomised trial designed to determine the need for irradiation following conservative surgery for the treatment of invasive breast cancer. Ann Oncol 2006;17:401-08.
55. Fowler JF. Intercomparison of now and old schedules in fractionated radiotherapy. Sem Radiat Oncol 1992;2:67-72.
56. Freedman RA, He Y, Winer EP, Keating NL. Trends in racial and age disparities in definitive local therapy of early-stage breast cancer. JCO 2009;27:713-9.
57. Freund H, Biran S, Laufer N, Eyal Z. Breast cancer arising in surgical scars. J Surg Oncol 1976; 8(6):477-80.
58. Gee NS, Brown JP, Dissanayake VUK, Offord J, Thurlow R, Woodruff GN. The novel anticonvulsant drug, gabapentin (Neurontin), binds to the alpha delta 2 subunit of a calcium channel. The Journal of Biological Chemistry 1996;271:5768-76.
59. Gentilini O, Botteri E, Rotmensz N, Santillo B, Peradze N, Saihum R, Intra M, Luini A, Galimberti V, Goldhirsch A, Veronesi U. When can a second conservative approach be considered for ipsilateral breast tumour recurrence. Ann Oncol 2007;18:468-72.
60. Gilron I. The role of anticonvulsant drugs in postoperative pain management: a bench-to-bedside perspective. Canadian Journal of Anesthesia 2006;53:562-71.
61. Gimlin D. Accounting for cosmetic Surgery in the USA and Great Britain: A cross-cultural analysis of women's Narratives. Body Society 2007;13: 41-60.
62. Godinez J, Gombos E. C, Chikarmane SA, Griffin GK, Birdwell RL. Breast MRI in the evaluation of eligibility for accelerated partial breast irradiation. Am J Roentgenol 2008;191:272-77.
63. Guay DRP. Adjunctive agents in the management of chronic pain. Pharmacotherapy.
64. Haffty BG, Buchholz TA, McCormick B. should intensity-modulated radiation therapy be the standard of care in the conservatively managed breast cancer patient. JCO 2008;26: 2072-74.
65. Hall ED. Acute effects of intravenous gluco-corticosteroids on cat spinal motor neurone electrical properties. Brain Research 1982;240:186-90.
66. Halperin EC, Constine LS, Tarbell NJ, Kun LE. Pediatric Radiation Oncology, 3rd Edn. Raven Press, New York;1999.
67. Hancock BW, Selby PJ, MacLennan K, Armitage JO (Eds). Malignant lymphoma. Arnold, London, 2000.
68. Hansen NM, Grube B, Ye X, Turner RR, Brenner RJ, Sim MS, Giuliano, AE. Impact of micrometastases in the sentinel node of patients with invasive breast cancer. JCO 2009;27:4679-84.
69. Harris EER, Correa C, Hwang WT, Liao J, Litt HI, Ferrari VA, Solin LJ. Late cardiac mortality and morbidity in early-stage breast cancer patients after breast-conservation treatment. JCO 2006;24:4100-06.
70. Hawley ST, Griggs JJ, Hamilton AS, Graff JJ, Janz NK, Morrow M, Jagsi R, Salem B, Katz SJ. Decision involvement and receipt of mastectomy among racially and ethnically diverse breast cancer patients. JNCI J Natl Cancer Inst (2009);101:1337-47.
71. Helzlsouer KJ. Contralateral prophylactic mastectomy: Quantifying benefits and weighing the Harms. JCO 2005;23:4251-53.
72. Hemminki K. Variation in the risk for liver and gallbladder cancers in socioeconomic and occupational groups in Sweden with etiological

implications. Int Arch Occup Environ Health 2005; 78(8): 641-9. PMID 16001211. Retrieved on 28 May 2007.

73. Hershman DL, Buono D, McBride RB, Tsai W.Y, Joseph, KA, Grann VR, Jacobson JS. Surgeon characteristics and receipt of adjuvant radiotherapy in women with breast cancer. JNCI J Natl Cancer Inst 2008;100:199-206.

74. Hiley C, Tutt A, Torres M, Palmieri C. Adjuvant radiotherapy for breast cancer. BMJ 2008;337: a2843.

75. Hockel M, Dornhofer N. The hydra phenomenon of cancer: why tumors recur locally after microscopically complete resection. Cancer Res 2005;65:2997-3002.

76. Hoffmann V, Coppejans H, Vercauteren M, Adriaensen H. Successful treatment of postherpetic neuralgia with oral ketamine. Clin J Pain 1994;10: 240-2.

77. Holland JF, Frei E, Bast RC, Morton DL, Kufe DW, Weichelsbaum RR. Cancer medicine, 4th edn. Williams and Wilkins, Philadelphia; 1997.

78. Holli K, Hietanen P, Saaristo R, Huhtala H, Hakama M, Joensuu H. Radiotherapy after segmental resection of breast cancer with favorable prognostic features: 12-year follow-up results of a randomized trial. JCO 2009;27:927-32.

79. Horsman MR, Khalil AA, Siemann DW, Grau C, Hill SA, Lynch EM, Chaplin DJ, Overgaard J. Relationship between radiobiological hypoxia in tumors and electrode measurements of tumor oxygenation. International Journal of Radiation Oncology, Biology, Physics 1994;29:439-42.

80. Horton CE, Crawford, HH, Love HG, Loeffler HA. The malignant potential of burn scar. Plast Reconstr Surg 1958;22:348-52.

81. Houssami N, Hayes DF. Review of preoperative magnetic resonance imaging (MRI) in breast cancer: Should MRI be performed on all women with newly diagnosed, Early Stage Breast Cancer. CA Cancer. J Clin 2009;59: 290-302.

82. Houtchens MK, Richert JR, Sami A, Rose JW. Open label gabapentin treatment for pain in multiple sclerosis. Multiple Sclerosis 1997;3:250-3.

83. J Couto E, Hemminki K. Incidence differences for gallbladder cancer between occupational groups suggest an etiological role for alcohol. In: J Cancer 2005;116(3):492-3.

84. Johansson AJ, Hao J, Sjolund B. Local corticosteroid application blocks transmission in normal nociceptive C-fibres. Acta Anaesth Scand 1990; 34:335-8.

85. Jones HA, Antonini N, Hart A AM, Peterse JL, Horiot, JC, Collin F, Poortmans PM, Oei SB, Collette L, Struikmans H, Van den Bogaert WF, Fourquet A, Jager JJ, Schinagl D AX, Warlam-Rodenhuis CC, Bartelink, H. Impact of pathological characteristics on local relapse after breast-conserving therapy: A subgroup analysis of the EORTC boost versus no boost trial. JCO 2009;27:4939-47.

86. Kaisary AV, Murphy GP, Denis L, Griffiths K (Eds). Textbook of prostate cancer, pathology, diagnosis and treatment. Martin Dunitz, London, 1999.

87. Kanaar R, Hoeijmaders JHJ, van Gent DC. Molecular mechanisms of DNA double-strand break repair. Trends in Cell Biology 1998;8:483-9.

88. Kapoor VK, McMichael AJ. Gallbladder cancer – An Indian disease. National Medical Journal of India 2003;16:209-13.

89. Kapoor VK. Incidental gallbladder cancer. American Journal of Gastroenterology 2001;96:627-9.

90. Katz SJ, Hawley ST. From policy to patients and back: Surgical treatment decision making for patients with breast cancer. Health Aff (Millwood) 2007;26:761-9.

91. Kell MR, Burke JP. Management of breast cancer in women with BRCA gene mutation. BMJ 2007;334:437-8.

92. Kimmick G, Camacho F, Foley KL, Levine EA, Balkrishnan R, Anderson R. Racial differences in patterns of care among medicaid: Enrolled patients with breast cancer. J Oncol Pract 2006;2:205-13.
93. Kingery WS. A critical review of controlled trials for peripheral neuropathic pain and complex regional pain syndrome. Pain 1997;73:123-39.
94. Koga Y, Sawada Y. Basal cell carcinoma developing in burn scar. Burns 1997;23(1):75-7.
95. Kreike B, Halfwerk H, Armstrong N, Bult P, Foekens JA, Veltkamp SC, Nuyten DSA, Bartelink H, van de Vijver MJ. Local recurrence after breast-conserving therapy in relation to gene expression patterns in a large series of patients. Clin Cancer Res 2009;15:4181-90.
96. Kreike B, Halfwerk H, Kristel P, Glas A, Peterse H, Bartelink H, van de Vijver MJ. Gene expression profiles of primary breast carcinomas from patients at high risk for local recurrence after breast-conserving therapy. Clin. Cancer Res 2006; 12:5705-12.
97. Kushi LH, Kwan ML, Lee MM, Ambrosone CB. Lifestyle factors and survival in women with breast cancer J. Nutr. 2007;137:S236-42.
98. Kwan W, Al-Tourah AJ, Speers C, Woods R, Kennecke H, Olivotto IA. Does HER2 status influence locoregional failure rates in breast cancer patients treated with mastectomy for pT1-2pN0 disease?. Ann Oncol 2009; 0: mdp396v1-mdp396.
99. Lakhani SR, Dilly SA, Finlayson CJ. Basic pathology, 2nd edn. Arnold, London; 1998.
100. Lang DG, Wang CM, Cooper BR. Lamotrigine, phenytoin and carbamazepine interactions on the sodium current present in N4TG1 mouse neuroblastoma cells. J Pharmacol Exp Ther 1993; 266:829-35.
101. Lees G, Leach MJ. Studies on the mechanism of action of the novel anticonvulsant lamotrigine (Lamictal) using primary neuroglial cultures from rat cortex. Brain Research 1993;612:190-9.
102. Leijon G, Boivie J. Treatment of neurogenic pain with antidepressants. Nordic Journal of Psychiatry. 1989;43:83-7 / Nord Psykiatr Tids- skr 1989;43: p83-87.
103. Lenhard RE, Osteen RT, Gansler E. Clinical oncology. American Cancer Society, Atlanta; 2001.
104. MacDonald S, Taghian AG. Prognostic factors for local control after breast conservation: Does margin status still matter?. JCO 2009;27:4929-30.
105. Malpas J (Ed). Cancer in children. British medical Bulletin 1996;52:90-107.
106. Mamounas EP. Continuing evolution in breast cancer surgical management. JCO 2005;23:1603-6.
107. Marcus R, Cunningham D, Miles A (Eds). The effective management of non-Hodgkin's lymphoma. Aesculapius Medical Press, London; 2001.
108. Margolese RG. Local control, survival, and the Fisher Hypothesis; 2010.
109. Mauch PM, Armitage JO, Diehl V, Hoppe RT, Weiss LM (Eds). Hodgkin's disease. Lippincott Williams & Wilkins, Philadelphia, 1998.
110. McCarthy EP, Ngo LH, Roetzheim RG, Chirikos TN, LiD, Drews RE, Iezzoni LI. Disparities in breast cancer treatment and survival for women with disabilities. Ann Intern Med 2006;145:637-45.
111. McCleane G. The pharmacological management of neuropathic pain: A Review. Priory.com.Email: gary@mccleane.freeserve.co.uk
112. McCleane GJ. Anticonvulsants - epilepsy or pain. In: Press Ulster Medical Journal.
113. McCleane GJ. The cholecystokinin antagonist proglumide enhances the analgesic efficacy of

morphine in humans with chronic benign pain. Anesth Anal 1998;87:1117-20.

114. McCleane GJ. The cholecystokinin antagonist proglumide enhances the analgesic effect of morphine in chronic benign nociceptive and neuropathic pain. The Pain Clinic 1998;11:103- 7.

115. McCleane GJ. Topical application of doxepin hydrochloride, capsaicin and a combination of both produces analgesia in chronic benign neuropathic pain: A randomised, double-blind, placebo controlled study. In Press British Journal of Clinical Pharmacology.

116. McCleane GJ. Topical doxepin hydrochloride reduces neuropathic pain: A randomised, double-blind, placebo controlled study. The Pain Clinic 1999;12:47-50.

117. McMillan TJ, Peacock JH. Molecular determinants of radiosensitivity in mammalian cells. International Journal of Radiation. Biology 1994;65:49-55.

118. McQuay H, Carroll D, Jadad AR, Wiffen P, Moore A. Anticonvulsant drugs for management of pain: A systematic review. BMJ 1995;311:1047-52.

119. McQuay HJ, Moore RA. Antidepressants and chronic pain. BMJ 1997;314:763-4.

120. McQuay HJ, Tramer M, Nye BA, Carroll D, Wiffen PJ, Moore RA. A systematic review of antidepressants in neuropathic pain. Pain 1996;68:217-27.

121. Mohiuddin MM, Regine WF. Consenting the patient with early-stage breast cancer: Informed only after multi-discliplinary evaluation. JCO 2009;27:e158-9.

122. Moore A, Collins S, Carroll D, McQuay H. Paracetamol with and without codeine in acute pain: A quantitative systematic review. Pain 1997;70:193-201.

123. Mould RF. A century of X-rays and radioactivity in medicine. Institute of Publishing. Bristol and Philadelphia; 1993. PP. 126-47.

124. Nattinger AB. Variation in the choice of breast-conserving surgery or mastectomy: Patient or physician decision making?. JCO 2005;23:5429-31.

125. Newman LA, Kuerer HM. Advances in breast conservation therapy. JCO 2005;23:1685-97.

126. O'Neill P, Fielden FM. Primary free radical processes in DNA. Advances in Radiation Biology 1993;17:53-120.

127. Ohsumi S, Shimozuma K, Morita S, Hara F, Takabatake D, Takashima S, Taira N, Aogi K, Takashima S. Factors associated with health-related quality-of-life in breast cancer survivors: Influence of the type of surgery. Jpn J Clin Oncol 2009;39:491-6.

128. Osako T, Oguchi M, Kumada M, Nemoto K, Iwase T, Yamashita T. Acute radiation dermatitis and pneumonitis in japanese breast cancer patients with whole breast hypofractionated radiotherapy compared to conventional radiotherapy. Jpn J Clin Oncol 2008;38:334-8.

129. Owusu C, Buist DSM, Field TS, Lash TL, Thwin SS, Geiger AM, Quinn VP, Frost F, Prout M, Yood MU, Wei F, Silliman RA. Predictors of tamoxifen discontinuation among older women with estrogen receptor-positive breast cancer. JCO 2008;26:549-55.

130. Pancrazio JJ, Kamatachi GL, Roscoe AK, Lynch C. Inhibition of neuronal Na+ channels by antidepressant drugs. J Pharmacol Exp Ther 1998; 284:208-14.

131. Paterson RP. The treatment of malignant disease by radiotherapy. Edward Arnold, London; 1963.

132. Patt DA, Goodwin JS, Kuo YF, Freeman JL, Zhang DD, Buchholz TA, Hortobagyi GN, Giordano SH. cardiac morbidity of adjuvant radiotherapy for breast cancer. JCO 2005;23:7475-82.

133. Peckham M, Pinedo HM, Veronesi U (Eds). Oxford textbook of oncology. Oxford Medical Publications, Oxford; 1995.

134. Perez CA, Brady LW. Principles and Practice of Radiation Oncology, 3rd Edn. JB Lippincott, Philadelphia; 1997.

135. Pierce LJ, Levin AM, Rebbeck TR, Ben-David MA, Friedman E, Solin LJ, Harris EE, Gaffney DK, Haffty, BG, Dawson LA, Narod SA, Olivotto IA, Eisen A, Whelan TJ, Olopade OI, Isaacs C, Merajver SD, Wong JS, Garber JE, Weber BL. Ten-year multi-institutional results of breast-conserving surgery and radiotherapy in BRCA1/2-Associated Stage I/II Breast Cancer. JCO 2006;24:2437-43.

136. Pignol JP, Olivotto I, Rakovitch E, Gardner S, Sixel K, Beckham W, Vu TTT, Truong P, Ackerman I, Pas-zat L. A Multicenter Randomized Trial of Breast Intensity-Modulated Radiation Therapy to Reduce Acute Radiation Dermatitis. JCO 2008;26:2085-92.

137. Pinkerton CR, Plowman PN. Paediatric oncology-clinical practice and controversies, 2nd edn. Chapman & Hall, London; 1997.

138. Pizzo P A, poplack DG. Principles and practice of Pediatric Oncology, 3rd edn. Lippincott, Williams & Wilkins Philadelphia; 1996.

139. Plowman PN, McElwain T, Meadow A. Complications of cancer management. Butterworth-Heinemann, Oxford; 1992.

140. Pointon RCS. The radiotherapy of malignant disease, 2nd edn. Springer-Verlag, Berlin; 1991.

141. Portenoy RK, Lesage P. Management of cancer pain. Lancet 1999;353:1695-1700.

142. Post C, Gordh T, Minor BG, Archer T, Freedman J. Antinociceptive effects and spinal cord tissue concentrations after intrathecal injection of guanfacine or clonidine into rats. Anesth Analg 1987;66:317-24.

143. Potashner SJ. Baclofen effects on amino acid release and metabolism in slices of guinea pig cerebral cortex. J Neurochem 1979;32:103-9.

144. Potten CS, Merritt A, Hickman J, Hall P, Faranda A. The characterisation of radiation-induced apoptosis in the small intestine and its biological implications. International Journal of Radiotion Biology 1994;65:71-8.

145. Powell SN, Whitaker SJ, Edwards SM, Mcmillan TJ A. DNA repair defect in a radiation-sensitive clone of a human bladder carcinoma cell line. British Journal of Cancer 1992;65:798-802.

146. Price P, Sikora K (Eds). Treatment of Cancer, 3rd Edn. Chapman & Hall, London; 1995.

147. Pruthi S, Boughey JC, Brandt KR, Degnim AC, Dy GK, Goetz MP, Perez, EA, Reynolds CA, Schomberg PJ, Ingle JN. A multidisciplinary approach to the management of breast cancer, part 2:therapeutic Considerations. Mayo Clin Proc 2007;82:1131-40.

148. Punglia RS, Morrow M, Winer EP, Harris JR. Local therapy and survival in breast cancer. NEJM 2007;356:2399-405.

149. Rabinovitch R, Kavanagh B. Double helix of breast cancer therapy: Intertwining the halsted and fisher hypotheses. JCO 2009;27:2422-3.

150. Rabinovitch R, Kavanagh B. Reply to RG. Margolese. JCO 2010;28:e40.

151. Raine R, Wong W, Scholes S, Ashton C, Obichere, A, Ambler G. Social variations in access to hospital care for patients with colorectal, breast, and lung cancer between 1999 and 2006: Retrospective analysis of hospital episode statistics. BMJ 2010; 340:b5479.

152. Rouse RV, Warnke RA, Michie SA. Lymphomas presenting as histologically unclassified neoplasms: Characteristics and response to treatment. J Clin Oncol 1989;7:1281-7. processing

153. Royal College of Paediatrics and Child Health. Guidance for services for children and young people with brain and spinal tumours. Royal College of Paediatrics and Child Health, London; 1997.

154. Ryan PD, Kopans DB, Sgroi DC. Case 24-2005-A 58-year-old woman with early-stage estrogen-receptor-positive breast cancer. NEJM 2005;353: 617-22.

155. Sanders ME, Scroggins T, Ampil FL, Li BD. Accelerated partial breast irradiation in early-stage breast cancer. JCO 2007;25:996-1002.

156. Sanghani M, Truong PT, Raad RA, Niemierko A, Lesperance M, Olivotto IA, Wazer DE, Taghian AG. Validation of a web-based predictive nomogram for ipsilateral breast tumor recurrence after breast conserving therapy. JCO 2010;28:718-22.

157. Schaefer GO., Emanuel EJ, Wertheimer A. The obligation to Participate in Biomedical Research. JAMA 2009;302:67-72.

158. Shikama N, Mitsumori M, Yamauchi C, Takekawa H, Arakawa K, Sasaki S, Teshima T. Patterns of care study for postmastectomy radiotherapy in Japan: Its role in monitoring the patterns of changes in practice. Jpn J Clin Oncol 2006;36:499-503.

159. Smith AC, Brook IM. Inhibition of tissue prostaglandin synthesis during third molar surgery: use of preoperative fenbrufen. Br J Oral Max Surg 1990;44:251-3.

160. Solin LJ, Orel SG, Hwang WT, Harris EE, Schnall MD. Relationship of breast magnetic resonance imaging to outcome after breast-conservation treatment with radiation for women with early-stage invasive breast carcinoma or ductal carcinoma in situ. JCO 2008;26:386-91 Trent S, Yang C, Li C, Lynch M, Schmidt EV. Heat shock protein B8, a cyclin-dependent kinase independent cyclin D1 target gene, contributes to its effects on radiation Sensitivity. Cancer Res. 2007;67:10774-81.

161. Solin LJ. breast conservation treatment with radiation: An ongoing success story. JCO 2010;28:709-11.

162. Son BH, Kwak BS, Kim JK, Kim HJ, Hong SJ, Lee JS, Hwang UK, Yoon HS, Ahn SH. Changing patterns in the clinical characteristics of korean patients with breast cancer during the last 15 years. Arch Surg 2006;141:155-60.

163. Souhami R, Tobias J. Cancer and its management, 3rd edn. Blackwell Science, Oxford; 1998.

164. Spaulding TC, Fielding S, Venafro JJ, Lal H. Antinociceptive activity of clonidine and its potentiation of morphine analgesia. Eur J Pharmacol; 1979.

165. Stephen AE, Berger DL . Carcinoma in the porcelain gallbladder: A relationship revisited. Surgery 2001;129(6):699–703. doi:10.1067/msy.2001.113888. PMID 11391368.

166. Temple WJ, Russell ML, Parsons LL, Huber SM, Jones CA, Bankes J, Eliasziw M. Conservation surgery for breast cancer as the preferred choice: A prospective analysis. JCO 2006;24:3367-73.

167. Teoh H, Fowler LJ, Bowery NG. Effect of lamotrigine on the electrically-evoked release of endogenous amino acids from slices of dorsal horn of the rat spinal cord. Neuropharmacol 1995;34:1273-8.

168. Throckmorton A, Esserman L. Reply to MM. Mohiuddin, et al. JCO 2009;27: e160-1.

169. Toledano A, Azria D, Garaud P, Fourquet A, Serin D, Bosset JF, Miny-Buffet J, Favre A, Le Floch O, Calais G. Phase III trial of concurrent or sequential adjuvant chemoradiotherapy after conservative surgery for early-stage breast cancer: Final Results of the Arcosein Trial. JCO 2007;25:405-10.

170. Towfigh S, McFadden DW, Cortina GR, et al. Porcelain gallbladder is not associated with gallbladder carcinoma. The American surgeon 2001;67(1):7-10. PMID 11206901.

171. Treves N, Pack G. Carcinoma arising in the scar of thermal burns. Surg Gynecol Obstet 1952;95:579-88.

172. Treves N, Pack G. The development of cancer in burn scars. Surg Gynecol Obstet 1930;51:749-82.

173. Trousseau A. De la nevralgie Epileptiforme. Clin Med Hotel Dieu 1885;2:33-44.

174. Tucker SL, Chan KS. The selection of patients for radiotherapy on the basis of tumor growth kinetics and intrinsic radiosensitivity. Radiotherapy and Oncology 1990;18:197-211.

175. Underwood JCE (Ed). General and Systematic Pathology, 3rd Edn. Churchill Livingstone, Edinburgh, 2000.

176. Vlastos G, Verkooijen HM. Minimally invasive approaches for diagnosis and treatment of early-stage breast cancer. The Oncologist 2007;12:1-10.

177. Waljee JF, Hu ES, Ubel PA, Smith DM, Newman LA, Alderman AK. Effect of esthetic outcome after breast-conserving surgery on psychosocial functioning and quality of life. JCO 2008;26:3331-37.

178. Waljee JF, Rogers M AM, Alderman AK. Decision aids and breast cancer: Do they influence choice for surgery and knowledge of treatment options?. JCO 2007;25:1067-73.

179. Wapnir IL, Anderson SJ, Mamounas EP, Geyer CE. Jr Jeong JH, Tan-Chiu E, Fisher B, Wolmark N. Prognosis after ipsilateral breast tumor recurrence and locoregional recurrences in five national surgical adjuvant breast and bowel project node-positive adjuvant breast cancer trials. JCO 2006;24:2028-37 Lee RC, Ekaette E, Kelly KL, Craighead P, Newcomb C, Dunscombe P. Implications of cancer staging uncertainties in radiation therapy decisions. Med Decis Making 2006;26:226-38.

180. Ward JF. Mechanisms of DNA repair and their potential modification for radiotherapy. International Journal of Radiation Oncology, Biology, Physics 1986;12:1027-32.

181. Weichselbaum R, Fuke Z, Hallahan D, Haimovitz-Friedman A, Kufe D. Radiation-induced cytokines and growth factors: Cellular and molecular basis of modification of radiation damage. In: Yarnold J, Stratton M, McMillan T (Eds). Molecular biology for oncologists. Elsevier, Amsterdam; 1993. pp. 213-21.

182. Weissman DE, Burchman SL, Dinndorf PA, et al. Handbook of Cancer Pain Management. Madison, University of Wisconsin, J Med Educ 1985;60:552-7.

183. Werkoff G, Lambaudie E, Fondrinier E, Leveque J, Marchal F, Uzan M, Barranger E, Guillemin F, Darai E, Uzan, S, Houvenaeghel G, Rouzier R, Coutant C. Prospective multicenter comparison of models to predict four or more involved axillary lymph nodes in patients with breast cancer with one to three metastatic sentinel lymph nodes. JCO 2009;27:5707-12.

184. West CML, Davidson SE, Roberts SA, Hunter RD. Intrinsic radiosensitivity and prediction of patient response to radiotherapy for carcinoma of the cervix. British Journal of Cancer 1993;68:819-23.

185. Whelan TJ, Pignol JP, Levine MN, Julian JA, MacKenzie R, Parpia S, Shelley W, Grimard L, Bowen J, Lukka H, Perera F, Fyles A, Schneider K, Gulavita S, Freeman C. Long-term results of hypofractionated radiation therapy for breast cancer. NEJM 2010;362:513-520.

186. Whelan TJ. Use of Conventional Radiation Therapy As Part of Breast-Conserving Treatment. JCO 2005; 23:1718-25.

187. Whitaker SJ, Ung YC, McMillan TJ. DNA double–strand break induction and rejoining as determinants of human tumour cell radiosensitivity. A pulsed-field gel electrophoresis study. International Journal of Radiation Biology 1995;67(1):7-18.

188. Wiffen PJ, Collins S, McQuay HJ, Carroll D, Jadad A, Moore RA. Anticonvulsant drugs for acute and chronic

pain. Cochrane Database of Systematic Reviews 2005, Issue 3.

189. Withers H R, Taylor JMG, Maciejewski B. The Hazard of accelerated tumour clonogen repopulation during radiotherapy. Acta Oncologica 1988;27:131-7.

190. Woolf CJ, Wiesenfeld-Hallin Z. The systemic administration of local anesthetics produces a selective depression of C-afferent fibre evoked activity in the spinal cord. Pain 1985;23:361-74.

191. Xu X-J, Puke MJC, Verge VMK, Wiesenfeld-Hallin Z, Hughes J, Hokfelt T. Up-regulation of cholecystokinin in primary sensory neurones is associated with morphine insensitivity in experimental neuropathic pain in the rat. Neuroscience Lett 1993;152:129-32.

192. Zakhireh J, Fowble B, Esserman LJ. Application of screening principles to the reconstructed breast. JCO 2010;28:173.

193. Zellars RC, Stearns V, Frassica D, Asrari F, Tsangaris T, Myers L, DiPasquale S, Lange JR, Jacobs LK, Emens LA, Armstrong DK, Fetting JH, Garrett-Mayer E, Davidson NE, Wolff AC. Feasibility trial of partial breast irradiation with concurrent dose-dense doxorubicin and cyclophosphamide in early-stage breast cancer. JCO 2009;27:2816.

Index

D

E

F

Q

R

S